Becoming A Surgeon

Life In A Surgical Residency And Timeless Lessons Learned Therein

JOE I. GARRI, MD, DMD

Featuring: Elena Sheppard
Illustrations: Erin Wolfe

BECOMING A SURGEON:
Life in a Surgical Residency and Timeless Lessons Learned Therein
By Joe I. Garri, MD, DMD
1. MED024000 2. BIO017000 3. BIO026000
ISBN (paperback): 978-1-949642-61-2
ISBN (hardback): 978-1-949642-63-6
EBOOK: 978-1-949642-62-9

Cover design by LEWIS AGRELL

Printed in the United States of America

Address: Joe I. Garri, MD, DMD
6200 Sunset Drive
Suite #402
South Miami, FL 33143
Website: becomingasurgeonthebook.com
Website: JoeGarri.com
Email: drgarri@drgarri.com

Authority Publishing
11230 Gold Express Dr. #310-413
Gold River, CA 95670
800-877-1097
www.AuthorityPublishing.com

May you always live in the present,
inspired by optimism towards the future,
guided by the experience and confidence
gained from the past.

Joe Garri
1/1/2021

Dedication

Residency training is a difficult physical and mental process that physicians are asked to endure in order to achieve their career goals. The physician's family members undergo the process as well, most often through no decision of their own. They are at times forced to make immense sacrifices, not the least of which includes accepting the absence of their loved ones, who are frequently focused on their work at the hospital.

I dedicate this book to my father, whose life has always served as a great source of inspiration, to my mother, whose undying love and kindness always made me feel a deep sense of comfort, and finally to my sister and niece, in whom I see those wonderful qualities of my parents live on.

TABLE OF CONTENTS

The Third Year: Transition (Junior/Senior) Year

The Fourth Year: Senior Resident

The Fifth Year: Chief Resident

PROLOGUE

The thought of writing this book germinated during the two months between medical school and the start of my residency. I had just finished four years of medical school and was in awe of the changes that had taken place in my classmates and me. Taking the aforementioned into consideration, I envisioned the forthcoming changes during surgical training would be even more dramatic and profound. I decided to document the process. To that end, during my residency I took notes on every person or event that I thought would be pivotal in my transformation from a recent medical graduate into a practicing surgeon. The writing of this book was purposely delayed for years in order to allow for the true meaning of those documented pivotal people and events to become apparent. In other words, to allow for the impact of key people and lessons learned to be placed in better context for the reader. This book was never meant to be a diary of events, but rather a retrospective on the process of residency training in general surgery and to document how that process, as well as the people involved and the events experienced, can shape the heart, mind, and ethos of a surgeon.

Not all events I originally documented real-time made it to the pages of this book. The events chosen were the ones I thought would either be informative and entertaining to the reader or, most importantly, those that had a profound and lasting impact on my professional and personal life and from which I hope others might be able to learn. The events and people depicted in this book are all real and occurred as they are described. The names of the patients and most of the people described in this book—except for those who gave explicit permission—have been changed in order to protect their privacy. Some of the names and events described are a matter of public record and thus have not been altered in any way.

THE FIRST YEAR:

Intern

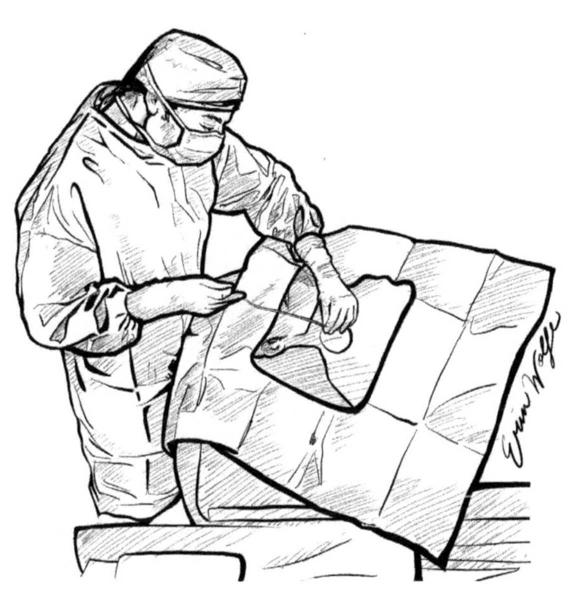

The First Day

I had moved to Miami two weeks before the start of my residency and found a place to live less than three miles from Jackson Memorial Hospital, the busy training hospital for the University of Miami Medical School. The week before starting, I had visited the residency director's office in order to do administrative paperwork, obtain my hospital ID card, and at that time was given the schedule of my rotations for the first year. The year was organized in monthly rotations through multiple surgical and non-surgical services. The idea was to give the intern—first-year resident—a working knowledge of multiple surgical and related specialties, and to allow him/her to learn the medical management of the surgical patient. I was to start in neurosurgery, specifically neurotrauma. The day before I was due to start my rotation, I called the page operator and obtained the pager number of the resident on call for the neurotrauma service. A tired-sounding intern answered several minutes later. He advised me that Dr. Andy Michaelsen, who was to be my immediate supervisor for my first rotation, had left instructions for me to meet him the following day at 5:30 a.m. on the eighth-floor neurosurgery ICU—intensive care unit. After I thanked the intern for the information, he promptly hung up but not before saying goodbye in the most unusual way: "Let me be the first to welcome you to the vegetable garden."

I found my way to the neurosurgical intensive care unit by 5:00 a.m. I made myself comfortable next to the nurses' station and waited for my workday to begin. While waiting, I observed the night nurses going about their duties quietly and efficiently. They would disappear into the individual glass cubicles where the patients were and would come out briefly only to walk in again. The entire unit was dimly lit at this time, and it gave one a sense of serenity and calmness. I have come to learn that this is the way most hospital wards look at night. At first light, as if by design, the lights on every floor get turned on around the same time. This act heralds the start of a brand-new day and is accompanied shortly thereafter by the arrival of the day shift nurses and a multitude of interns and residents who busily begin their daily routine. At night, however, the hospital wards usually appear serene and quiet, as if sickness and disease also take time to rest.

The night nurses barely glanced my way when they saw me sitting there. I got the sense that they were very much aware that a new residency year had begun. They seemed resigned to once again contend with a new crop of recently graduated physicians who would have to be shown—at times sternly—the way things were done at the hospital. I quietly smiled at them when they made eye contact, but in truth I felt somewhat intimidated and nervous.

Promptly at 5:30 a.m., Andy Michaelsen, MD walked in. He was a handsome, lean fellow in his late twenties. He was holding a cup of coffee in his right hand and a duffel bag in his left as he walked up to the nurses' station. After looking at me, he asked, "You are Joe, I take it?" When I replied in the affirmative, he smiled and extended his hand, which I shook with great enthusiasm.

After shaking hands, Andy led me to the resident's on-call room where he dropped off his bag. The small room was littered with X-rays and CT scan folders. They seemed to be everywhere, on the small desk, on the bunk bed, and on the chair next to the bed. At the end of the small room there was a door minimally ajar which led to a bathroom from which emanated the sound of a shower.

"Hey, Nick," Andy yelled into the room after he partially opened the door a bit more letting out some of the warm steam from inside. "Anything come in last night?"

"No," said the voice from within. "Everyone else is doing ok, but I had to re-intubate Rappaport." Nick, I soon came to learn, was the other second-year neurosurgery resident who had been on call the previous day and night and was cross-covering our patients. Henceforth and for the month, Nick, Andy, and I would take turns on call every third day covering the service overnight.

"This is our pile," Andy said while looking at me and pointing to a group of X-ray and CT film folders meticulously organized in the space between the desk and the wall. "Make sure you do not lose sight of them, and do not let the other services take them…we will never get them back." This was my introduction to one of the intern's most sacred responsibilities at that time, the hoarding and safekeeping of X-ray and CT scan films. Thankfully, this responsibility has become obsolete with the advent of digital technology, which allows for any doctor to view radiologic studies on any patient at any time simply by logging into the patient's chart from any computer terminal at the hospital. This, along with keeping a census of the names, chart numbers, and location of all patients on a particular service are the intern's primary responsibilities. Of course, that is besides doing all of the grunt work necessary to run the service. When films were not available and/or when patients could not be found (or were not seen during rounds because they were not listed on the service census), things would immediately take a turn for the worse for the intern. This would elicit the wrath of everyone on the team from the attendings to the most junior resident. Faltering at the custody of films and the failure to keep an accurate census were the two cardinal sins of being an intern.

I nodded in agreement and followed him out the door as he briskly started walking toward the chart rack, another remnant of the distant past as most, if not all, hospitals have instituted digital charts. Although the old-fashioned charts still exist in most hospitals, they only contain administrative paperwork and truly little, if any, medical information. He took out a printed list—the census—from his lab coat pocket that had the names of all the patients on the service. Simultaneously he grabbed a small chart trolley next to the main chart rack and started pulling the charts of the patients on our service and placing them on the trolley. We then pulled the trolley onto the end of the unit and started rounds.

Rounds were to be a ritual that I would perform every working day for the next five years and beyond to the present day. It is the systematic inspection of all the patients that a doctor or group of doctors carry on their service and for which they are responsible. The process entails visiting with the patient, asking pertinent questions, performing a physical examination, and evaluating all relevant data and information of events that occurred since the last rounds took place, usually the afternoon or evening of the previous day. Upon completion of all the aforementioned steps, a unique plan of action is formulated for each particular patient.

As we went through each patient, Andy would fill me in on that patient's particular story. Between patients he would give me a quick rundown of how the neurotrauma service functioned. "We are the trauma service within neurosurgery. We do not take care of anything else. All patients with aneurysms, brain tumors, strokes, etc. go to other services. We only take care of the ones with head-bunks."

He went on to explain how the patients with minor head trauma and without any surgical needs would go to the neurology service for observation. "We only take care of the real bad ones, the ones who have fractured skulls or brain bleeds, which is the reason why they are all 'gorked' (jargon for unresponsive). Unfortunately, the worst thing is, they usually stay that way." I half-smiled to myself now fully understanding the previous comment by the intern regarding the vegetable garden.

After we completed going over all the patients in the intensive care unit, we went to the regular floor to see the rest of the patients, all of whom were more stable and needed less acute care. In between rooms, Andy would give me a quick synopsis of the patient's history and condition, and he would then rattle off a long list of things that needed to be accomplished for that particular patient on that day: *Discharge Mr. Rawlings... Talk to social service about getting placement for Mr. Gonzalez... This patient needs medicine consult to come and control his diabetes...* etc.

It was now only 6:50 a.m. and we had seen about eighteen patients on the neurotrauma service. I had a list two pages long with all of the things that needed to be done for the patients that day. When Andy announced that we had seen our last patient for the morning, I was utterly exhausted from trying to keep up with him and everything he said. I was hoping now perhaps we would have some time for breakfast, but soon was disappointed when he promptly announced that if we did not hurry, we would be late for morning teaching rounds.

We took the elevator down to the first floor and dashed into the cafeteria where we each got a cup of coffee. Immediately after, we hurried up to the second-floor radiology department where the neurosurgery morning rounds were being held. The rounds were already in progress when we walked in, and the look the professor at the front of the room gave Andy was not lost on me. I made a mental note to make it a point to not be late for teaching rounds ever again.

The neurosurgery teaching rounds consisted of a format in which the senior or chief residents presented upcoming and interesting cases, and the professor leading the rounds would ask pertinent questions regarding surgical anatomy, surgical technique, neuroanatomy, and the management of complications. I was amazed at the degree of knowledge and specificity of facts that the residents were expected to know. The professor would pick residents at random and ask them questions that were appropriate for their level of training. If a resident did not know the answer, the attending surgeon would pick another resident from a more senior year. The residents were quite impressive in their knowledge base and in the manner in which they answered the questions. Even Andy, just starting his second year, seemed to have an extensive knowledge of neuroanatomy, pathophysiology, and surgical technique. Those teaching rounds on my first day impressed upon me how far I had to go, and how much reading I needed to do over the ensuing several years. I experienced a mixture of fear, insecurity, and awe upon pondering the future task at hand.

"How much reading do you do?" I asked Andy as we left the teaching rounds and began walking to the trauma building, where the neurotrauma service usually operated.

"Not as much as I need to," he said. "It is extremely difficult with the work hours we keep. You will see." He suddenly grabbed his belt and said, "Oh, I forgot this." Andy then proceeded to hand me my pager. This device, or one similar to it, would become my constant companion to be kept within arm's length at all times for the next five years of my residency and beyond. That particular moment as I took the pager from him and neatly hooked it to my belt, the pager became an instant symbol of the fact that I was now a doctor, someone who needed to be reached in order to make important decisions and help with patient care. Not too long after that, the pager became an instrument of torture, which upon going off meant more work and added tasks, most often when there was plenty of those to be had and new ones were not welcomed.

Andy walked me into the locker room of the trauma operating room so that I could change into my scrubs and leave my street clothes in his locker as I had not yet been assigned one. I hurriedly changed and walked into the operating room as our patient was being intubated. I think Andy could sense my nervousness at being in the operating room. He knowingly glanced my way while giving a chuckle. "Just follow my lead. Don't worry, our attending surgeon is one of the best surgeons and one of the nicest people you will ever meet. He will break you in easy." Just as he finished, Dr. Orret Gottenger walked into the operating room. A man of average height, with an easy-going and friendly disposition, Dr. Gottenger was the chief of the neurotrauma service. He was not only a much-respected surgeon, but I soon found out that Andy was right: He turned out to be a true gentleman, a caring doctor, and a great teacher. Over the course of the next several years, and after dealing with a multitude of attending surgeons, I interacted with less than a handful who measured up to him when it came to his personal and professional qualities.

Andy introduced me as the new intern on the team. Dr. Gottenger shook my hand and graciously welcomed me to the service. "I am expecting a transfer from the islands," he said to both of us and then turning towards me, "Andy will teach you the process of admission to our service and the ICU. Expect the transfer later in the afternoon." Then shifting his attention again, "Andy, after you see the patient, call me and tell me what you think."

We had three cases scheduled for that day. Our first case was a young woman who had been involved in a motor vehicle accident two months before and had sustained multiple skull fractures. Dr. Gottenger explained to me that some of the fractures were contaminated with debris during the accident, and subsequently the patient had lost a significant amount of the bone in the anterior aspect of her skull along the right forehead and hairline region. This left a substantial indentation in the front part of the patient's skull which was unsightly to her, but more importantly, it allowed for the brain to be exposed to injury without the usually protective bony shell which is the skull. I suctioned as Dr. Gottenger and Andy proceeded to make an incision along the top of the head from ear to ear and peeled the skin and deeper tissues down to bone from the forehead toward the eyes. The defect in the skull then became apparent. It was located on the front-right part of the head and was the size of the circumference of an apple, but with irregular borders. The dura, the layer of soft tissue that covers the brain, was visible at the bottom of the bony defect.

The purpose of the operation was to reconstruct the missing skull and protect the brain. To that end, Dr. Gottenger fashioned a metal mesh to cover the defect and secured it to the skull with screws. They allowed me to drill some of the holes and place some of the screws. After this was accomplished, we mixed an acrylic and covered the metal plate, creating a new skull contour at the same level as the intact bone. After irrigating the wound, we began closing the scalp skin.

"Done any sewing?" Dr. Gottenger asked.

"Enough," I said nervously, not sure if I had made a mistake in appearing too confident. He handed me the instruments in his hands and watched me for a few minutes while I nervously attempted to reproduce the suturing that I had seen him do moments before. I noticed that I had begun to sweat and that my hands were trembling slightly.

"You are trainable," Dr. Gottenger said as he removed his gloves and gown and left Andy and me to the task at hand.

"I think you should answer your beeper. I will finish here," Andy said after we both had been suturing for about ten minutes. It was then that I realized that the beeping noise I kept hearing throughout the operation was actually my pager going off. After looking at it, I noted that I had been paged six times during the two-hour operation. I called the numbers on my pager one by one and was confronted with a multitude of questions, none of which I had the answer to. My feelings of helplessness were ameliorated by the fact that Andy was there in the room with me. I was asked questions by the nurses, which I in turn relayed to Andy. He then told me what to tell them. Simultaneously to performing this task, I pondered what would happen the first time I found myself in a similar situation, except without Andy by my side. I would not have long to wait.

The fifth page was from the ICU. The nurse finally came to the phone. "Your transfer is here, and we need admission orders."

"I thought the transfer was due this afternoon?" I did not know what else to say.

"No, they are here. We need orders; the patient is intubated." I suddenly felt the grip of fear at the realization that I would have to face this issue by myself. Dr. Gottenger was already out of the room, and Andy was only halfway done with the scalp closure. He would have to continue operating for another thirty to forty-five minutes.

Stalling for time hoping Andy would soon finish and come save me, I took my time changing back into my regular clothes and leisurely walked from the trauma center to the main hospital building, the West Wing as it is called, where the neurosurgery ICU is located. Comforted only by Andy's promise that he would join me as soon as he finished with the first case, I felt the fear increase with every step I took. In the elevator headed to the eighth floor, I leaned against the back wall and closed my eyes and thought about my predicament. Even while wearing my pager, I felt a bit like an impostor, like I was still in medical school and it was all a game of playing doctor. Except now it was for real, and I would be expected to act and perform like a real doctor, which in fact I was, although a newly minted one. The pressure I felt was palpable. Then suddenly the elevator door opened, and I was startled back to reality.

"Are you Dr. Gottenger?" a nervous-looking woman in her late forties abruptly stood from her seat and asked me as I walked into the unit patient cubicle. I extended my hand to her, and then to the man beside her as I felt my voice quiver.

"No, I am Dr. Garri. I will be doing some of the preliminary admission paperwork. Dr. Gottenger will be here a little later."

For seconds I stood there in front of them not knowing what to do. I looked over at the bed and saw the patient. A young man in his late teens with his head shaved and staples on his scalp. He was intubated, and as I traced the tubing to the ventilator, I noticed the respiratory technician busily adjusting the knobs on the ventilator machine. He seemed to notice me at the same time and asked: "What vent settings do you want, Doc?"

I stared at him blankly. "I need a few minutes with the family," was the only thing I could muster.

He gave me a slight smile and to this day I am convinced he immediately understood my predicament. "I will just leave him on the settings he came with until you give me the new settings."

When intubated patients arrive at the ICU, they are ventilated by a handheld device called an Ambu bag but soon are placed on a ventilator machine, which breathes for them. This device needs to be programmed with certain settings such as respiratory rate, pressure settings, volume of each breath, etc., for that particular patient as determined by the physician. The respiratory tech had obviously realized that I was one of the new interns and had no idea what ventilator settings to put the patient on. In an act of kindness, he decided to cover for me and chose the settings to place the patient on himself, so as not to alert the patient's family to the fact that I was at a loss for what to do. I came to learn later that this particular respiratory technician was actually the supervisor of respiratory therapy for the entire hospital. I never did thank him, but over the course of the next few years, whenever I saw him about the hospital, I was always reminded of my first day as an intern and how he had come to my rescue.

"Tell me what happened." By this time, the two parents and I were sitting next to the bedside and I was holding a clipboard as I prepared to take notes in order to write the admission history. The mother proceeded to tell me that they were from the Midwest. Her son had recently graduated from high school and had decided to take a vacation cruise with friends to the Bahamas before his departure for college. He and his friends had rented bicycles and were riding them when a bus driver failed to stop at a red light and hit her son broadside at considerable speed. Harry, she added, had been taken to a local hospital where he was operated on to evacuate a blood clot from the brain and address other injuries he had sustained. As soon as the family became aware of what happened, they arranged a transfer to Jackson Memorial Hospital, the nearest US-based trauma center.

Over the course of the next half hour, I learned all about Harry from his parents. He was an excellent student who aspired to go to law school. He had been extremely excited about finishing high school and was eagerly anticipating his departure for college. His distraught parents were asking me questions that I could not answer. Was another surgery necessary? Was he going to recuperate fully? What was the next step? How long did I anticipate that he was going to be at the hospital? It occurred to me during the interview that from their vantage point, I was a doctor…a neurosurgeon at that. More importantly, they expected me to have answers to their many questions. There was no way for them to know that I had just graduated from medical school a couple of months before and that this was the first day of my residency. It did not seem appropriate for me to provide them with a long explanation of my situation. I stalled as best as I could. Over the course of the next few years, I would become quite accustomed to stalling when placed in situations where because of lack of knowledge and/or experience, I did not have answers to the questions that patients and their families would ask.

After completing a cursory physical exam, I excused myself, taking a large packet of films that had come with the patient, and went to sit at the nurses' station. I was pretending to write while collecting my thoughts. My mind tried to list all of Harry's injuries. He had brain trauma, a fractured collar bone, a lacerated liver, and a fractured tibia—leg bone—which had been treated non-operatively with a cast. Needless to say, I was overwhelmed. I did not know where to start. It was then that Andy walked into the unit and the sight of him made my heart leap with joy. His beeper went off as he approached me, and he seemed to be upset as he grabbed for it.

"I just left the OR two minutes ago and have been paged three times on my walk up here. I tell you, one of these days I am going to quit." Hearing him make this comment out of hand startled me a bit. How could he say this? Getting a neurosurgical spot was extremely difficult. He was getting to fulfill his dream of becoming a neurosurgeon and he was already thinking about quitting, after completing barely one year? How could this be? I was extremely enthusiastic about my surgical residency, so hearing a resident one year my senior speak this way was rather disheartening and disturbing. Could being a resident really be that bad?

Over the course of the next month, and then over the next several years, I would hear Andy make similar statements multiple times. Even in his last year of residency he would occasionally make these comments about quitting. It did not take me long to realize that this was merely how he let off steam. It was a sort of defense mechanism that he had developed for times when he felt particularly stressed or overwhelmed or just simply aggravated. It even became a joke among the residents in neurosurgery, as they all tried to guess when Andy was going to quit. It turned out that Andy did not quit; he became an excellent neurosurgeon. He decided to stay in academics and became an attending surgeon at Jackson Memorial Hospital. He now holds Dr. Gottenger's old position, chief of the neurotrauma service. Dr. Gottenger moved north to another state during my chief resident year after being recruited by another institution. I was sorry to see him leave.

After he finished answering his pages, Andy went over the information I had gathered. He then went into the patient's room, introduced himself to the parents, and proceeded to perform his own physical exam while asking the parents questions to reinforce and expand on the information I had gathered. As I watched him do this, I wondered if the parents could tell the difference in experience and confidence between Andy and me, causing them to lose confidence in my ability to participate in their son's care. It seemed to me that they should have been able to tell, as the contrast was obvious. However, they did not seem to take notice. In my future interactions with them, they never questioned my abilities or judgment and were always kind to me, particularly the mother.

"What do we do now?" I asked Andy after we were back at the nurses' station.

"Well..." he said. "We have to write orders, change all his lines, send labs, repeat the CT scan of the brain, get orthopedics to look at the films, and then call Dr. Gottenger." I attempted to write down everything he said, but the effort was futile as he was speaking very rapidly.

"Sit," he said. He proceeded to dictate in detail the list of orders that we needed while I dutifully transcribed them to paper. It became painfully obvious to me at this point that being a surgeon did not just involve performing surgery; it included the equally important and far more labor-intensive work of taking care of the patient, before and after surgery. It also became apparent that as a surgical intern, my job was not to perform surgery, or even to learn how to perform surgery. Rather, it was to learn the ins and outs of taking care of the surgical patient. I never imagined how much work this process entailed.

Andy got called for the second case and I was left alone again, this time with a long list of things to do. I made sure the labs got sent, I called the orthopedic service for a consultation, and eventually after getting the runaround, I got the resident who was responsible to do the consultations in the orthopedic trauma service. I had a tough time gathering all the supplies we needed to change the patient's lines as I was new to the ward and the hospital in general. This was a difficult task as I had no idea where the supplies were kept. Finally, I transported Harry down to the radiology floor and sat there while his head CT scan was repeated. In the middle of all that, my pager did not stop going off. I did the best I could answering the nurses' questions, and I deferred the ones I could not answer, making a list of them along with the associated extension so that I could call the nurses back after Andy had given me some direction as to what needed to be done. It was close to four o'clock by the time I was finished with Harry in radiology; I then proceeded to attempt to accomplish the many other "to do's" on my task list, which had grown progressively throughout the day.

At 5:15 p.m., Andy finally walked back into the ICU after finishing the last case for the day. He informed me that he and Dr. Gottenger had already seen the new CT scan on Harry. There was no obvious indication to operate, but we had to perform a ventriculostomy. I learned this was a small tube placed into one of the ventricles or fluid-filled spaces of the brain so that we could measure the pressure in the brain. If the pressure was elevated, we would need to institute certain therapeutic modalities, mostly consisting of certain medications and adjustments in ventilator settings, in order to lower that pressure. It is this increased pressure on the brain that leads to further brain damage after the initial traumatic event.

After donning surgical garb, I assisted Andy at bedside as he made an incision in Harry's scalp, used a hand drill to make a small hole in his skull, and inserted a tube until he reached the ventricle. He sutured the tube in place and placed a head dressing. We then connected the tube to a gauge to measure the pressure. The pressure was not elevated. We then changed the central line (venous catheter) inserted into Harry's chest, replaced all of his dressings, and finally assisted anesthesia as they came up to the unit and exchanged the ET tube (endotracheal breathing tube) through which Harry was being ventilated. Andy explained to me that when a patient is transferred into the unit from another facility, it is imperative that all tubes and lines be changed upon arrival, in an attempt to prevent infection. The idea seemed sound, but the amount of work to accomplish it was astounding.

We walked back to the on-call room where we had been that morning, located on one of the two hallways that ran through the ICU. When we walked in, there was a resident sitting at the small desk working on the computer. Andy introduced him to me as one of two chief residents in neurosurgery. He then went to the phone to page Dr. Gottenger.

"Your call schedule is up there on the wall," the chief resident said while still looking at the computer and pointing to the wall opposite the bunk bed. "You will be on call every third day starting tomorrow."

It was then that I realized how much I was sweating. The nearly two hours it had taken us to do all the line changes and ventriculostomy while wearing a surgical gown over my clothes had made me sweat profusely. I felt tired and sticky. I recalled walking into the hospital that morning wearing a shirt, tie, and clinic coat, noticing that most of the residents coming into work were wearing surgical scrubs. This was a practice that was technically not allowed, for infection control reasons: All medical personnel were supposed to come in wearing regular clothes and then change into scrubs if necessary. However, that process took altogether too much effort and time. From that day forth, I came to the hospital wearing scrubs whenever possible. Only during clinic and conference days would I come in wearing street clothes with shirt and tie.

Andy hung up the phone after talking to Dr. Gottenger. "I think this is it for the day. I will go look at the chest film on Harry to check the line and the tube and will let you know if anything else needs to be done pertaining to that." It suddenly occurred to me that I had not eaten all day. I was hungry. I wanted to leave.

"By the way," Andy added, "remember those two patients we discharged this morning? I suggest you go dictate their discharge. The charts should still be on the floor and if you delay the dictation for another day, it will be exceedingly difficult to track the charts down." When I looked at him inquisitively, he handed me a small, folded piece of paper from his pocket. "Follow the directions under the heading 'Discharge Summary.' I am so glad I don't have to do that crap anymore." He smiled and walked out of the room on his way to the radiology department on the second floor.

The thought of taking the stairs from the eighth to the twelfth floor occurred to me as I walked out of the ICU through the sliding doors, but I thought better of it as I was utterly exhausted by this point. The charts of the discharged patients were indeed in a small rack at the nurses' station. I took them to an adjoining small room which had a phone and looked at the paper Andy had given me. It contained instructions for the phone dictation system, and it had the list of items that needed to be included in the dictation of the discharge summary—dates of admission and discharge, a small narrative of hospital course, operations, complications, discharge medications and instructions, follow-up appointments, etc.

That first day, it took me the better part of one hour to dictate the two charts. Both charts were thick, and deciphering the doctors' handwriting in them was another challenge altogether. It was not long before I became an expert at these dictations. I could dissect a chart in minutes and pick out the pertinent information while at the same time dictating the narrative real-time as I went. By the end of my internship year, I was dictating discharge summaries in five to seven minutes. I learned to dictate while simultaneously looking through the chart searching for pertinent information.

As I dictated the discharge summaries, I attempted to remember the faces of the patients whose discharges I was dictating, but I could not. The entire day, including the patient's faces, were all a blur by this point. Upon finishing, I took a moment to catch my breath; my mind then wandered to Harry. Would I be dictating his discharge summary in a few days? A couple of weeks? Would he be going home with his parents to pursue his dreams of being a lawyer? It turned out that was not to be the case. Over the next few days, Harry's condition did not improve significantly. His mother was constantly by his side during the month that I rotated in neurosurgery.

"You are always here," she once told me one late evening when I went into his room to check his skull wound at the request of one of the nurses.

"You too," I said to her.

"He needs me," she answered sadly and then asked, "But how about you? Does your family not need you at home?"

"I don't have my own family...not yet anyway," I answered. I wondered about the stress on the family dynamics of the residents who did.

After several days, the walls in Harry's room were covered with pictures of friends and family. There were "get well" cards and pictures of him and his friends having fun, laughing, boating, and swimming at the local lake. The first couple of weeks he had multiple visitors. By the end of the month, it was just him and his mother. His father had to go back home and return to work. After a couple of weeks, Harry had not made much progress. He was responding to painful stimuli but not much else.

"Will he ever wake up?" I asked Dr. Gottenger one day during rounds.

"Unlikely," he said, "but there is always hope." The comment about the vegetable garden came to mind once again.

During the third week of my rotation, Dr. Gottenger and I performed a tracheostomy on Harry at bedside. This procedure inserts a breathing tube in the patient's neck that connects to the ventilator, which eliminates the need to have a breathing tube in the mouth. It is done for patients who are thought to require a ventilator for long periods—more than two weeks—or indefinitely. I was excited about this surgery as Dr. Gottenger and I did it alone without Andy, and he allowed me to actually perform it. Under his watchful eye and tutelage, he assisted me and carefully guided me through each and every step. "We need to start working on a chronic care facility for this patient," Dr. Gottenger said in passing as we finished.

Harry was transferred to a chronic care facility two weeks after the completion of my rotation. The intern who replaced me in neurotrauma shared that information with me while eating lunch together one day.

"Prognosis?" I asked.

"Poor," he answered.

It dawned on me then that most likely Harry would never wake up again and would never get to fulfill his dream of becoming a lawyer. I quietly thanked God profusely for allowing me the opportunity to embark on fulfilling my dream of becoming a surgeon.

It was after 9:30 p.m. when I finally walked out of the hospital that day and headed towards my car. I was tired and hungry but surprisingly very much excited about starting my residency. My walk was tall. I felt a sense of pride, excitement, and euphoria. I would experience these feelings time and again over the ensuing several years every time I took another step towards my goal. I felt deeply that I was where I was meant to be and doing what I was meant to do. As I walked, I mused at the thought that it might be fun to calculate how many more days I had until the completion of my residency, but I thought better of it. As I approached my car, my right hand reached into my pocket for my keys and along with them, I pulled a crumbled piece of paper. In my handwriting on that paper, there was a long list of the questions the nurses had asked me during the day. Next to each question was a name and phone extension where I could call them back with the answer. Most of the questions had been left unanswered. I prayed that none of the unanswered questions were of vital importance.

I did not eat that night, and while still wearing my clothes, promptly collapsed onto my bed right after walking through the front door. I woke up disoriented when my alarm went off at 4:00 a.m. I left for work an hour later—tired but fully inspired and feeling great excitement for the day ahead. I was not to see the inside of my apartment again for the next forty hours, after working nonstop the entire time with little to eat and without an ounce of sleep. I once again collapsed onto my bed and woke up startled when my alarm went off at 4:00 a.m. the following morning. Eventually my mind and body would get used to this pace but for the first couple of weeks, the experience seemed surreal. I walked around in a daze adjusting and learning to function under pressure, while in a state of extreme mental and physical exhaustion.

The Blood-Brain Barrier

"Aren't you happy to be on the safe side of the blood-brain barrier for once?" The anesthesia resident, Myla Griffis, had leaned towards me and whispered in my ear. I could barely hear her due to all the yelling. I had been rotating in anesthesia for several days now. This particular day we happened to be doing the anesthesia for a liver case. The attending surgeon had begun yelling at the chief resident from the moment that the case started. We were now well into the third hour and the yelling had not ceased. It was a constant, high-pitched whining that had given me a terrible headache. It seemed like the resident could not do anything right. I found the whole scene somewhat disturbing and a huge contrast to how the day started out. That morning started off pleasantly and jovially as Myla, the second-year anesthesia resident I had been assigned to, had jokingly asked me if I wanted to join her in "passing some gas." I laughed with her at this common anesthesia joke but now, in the middle of this case, I was wishing I had declined the offer (not that I had been given a choice).

I nodded without speaking as this day I was indeed happy to be on the safe side of the blood-brain barrier. This term refers to the physiologic barrier between the brain tissue and potentially deleterious substances carried in the blood. For example, certain antibiotics cannot be used for brain infections such as meningitis because this physiologic barrier does not allow the antibiotics circulating in the bloodstream to reach the brain tissue. The reference is often used by anesthesiologists sometimes in jest, sometimes not, to portray themselves as intellectuals and thinkers (the brain), while surgeons are mere messy technicians (the blood). The physical symbol of this phrase is the sterile drape in the configuration of a curtain that is placed by the surgeons while draping the patient to isolate the surgical—sterile—field from the nonsterile area, usually at the head of the table where the anesthesiologists dwell to monitor the patient. This sterile drape is usually taped or clipped to two IV metal poles that are placed on either side of the head of the operating table.

Anesthesiologists often compare themselves to airplane pilots. Their work involves cases (the flight) punctuated by two times of high concentration and potential danger, namely the induction/intubation (take-off) and emergence/extubation (landing), with a fairly peaceful time in the middle where the patient is closely monitored (midflight) while the surgeon does his/her work. At times, just like when flying through terrible weather, the anesthesiologists are kept busy throughout the surgery, working hard to stabilize an unstable patient, or to keep an unstable patient alive as the surgeon attempts a life-saving operation. However, most times during the case the patient is stable, which offers the anesthesia team a respite from intense activity. I was determined not to let this respite go to waste. I made it a point to observe surgeons at work.

My rotation in anesthesia had been an enjoyable one thus far, starting with the fact that the work hours were far fewer. After a twenty-four-hour call on the anesthesia service, the resident was allowed to go home after the shift was over rather than being asked to put in another twelve hours. It seemed that the anesthesiologists had surmised that performing anesthesia while tired and/or half asleep was neither safe for the patient nor a good learning experience for the resident. Surgeons, however, had not yet figured this out, as it was the norm to have residents work thirty-six-hour shifts every third day, while working twelve- to fourteen-hour days in between. Anesthesia also had the policy of lunch breaks, when another resident or nurse anesthetist would relieve the residents during a case so that they could go to lunch. A surgeon breaking for lunch during the middle of a long case was essentially unheard of, except for dire emergencies. Going to the bathroom did not qualify as a dire emergency. Surgery residents would grab a quick bite to eat between cases whenever possible. The old idiom of "eat when you can, sleep when you can" has always applied to the world of surgery. It is part of the surgeon's creed, particularly during training.

The "dead-time" in the middle of the case, where the anesthesiologist's job is to monitor the patient, is one of the greatest non-medical challenges in anesthesia, as boredom tends to creep in. If an attending anesthesiologist is in the room, they often use this time to teach the residents or medical students. When residents are by themselves, they usually use this time to read, look at their phones, or do board review questions while intermittently checking on the patient's vitals. These activities are frowned upon as it is expected that the anesthesia team will be fully concentrated on monitoring the patient. More than once during my residency, however, I saw anesthesiologists, residents, and nurse anesthetists doze off while in the middle of an operation. At one time I thought this was a stark distinction between anesthesia and surgery, as I could not conceive of a surgeon falling asleep in the middle of an operation. Then I learned better. More than once while working thirty-six-hour shifts during my residency, I found myself falling asleep while standing and holding retractors in the middle of an operation. Learning to sleep on my feet was never one of the skills I envisioned I would be learning during my surgical training.

This slow time during the middle of the case offered me an interesting opportunity. I began to study and observe the surgeons at work. Not necessarily to learn about the case, or even surgical technique, but rather to see how they acted during surgery—their protocol, habits, and demeanor. It was my attempt to pick out those desirable qualities that would make me a better surgeon in the future. I learned that, contrary to my previously held belief, surgery is not primarily and exclusively an endeavor of manual dexterity. Moreover, it is not necessarily the surgeons with the fastest hands and agility who are the most efficient in the operating room. There is a factor which is intellectual in nature, and a vital component that requires organizational skills and concentration. In fact, it is often not the surgeon with the best or fastest hands who operates the quickest. The quickest and most efficient surgeons are the ones who have formulated a well-thought-out plan of what they are going to do and are methodical in its execution. The surgeons who follow this protocol are the ones who keep the case moving at a steady pace and eliminate wasted motions and maneuvers. By doing this, they shorten the duration of the case, which in turn is beneficial to the patient in many ways, not the least of which is shortening the time the patient has to be under anesthesia.

Another great observation revolved around how different surgeons dealt with emergencies and stressful situations. The ones who panicked created panic around them. Not only would they and their surgical team panic, but this panic would soon extend to the anesthesia and nursing staff as well. This would often have a snowball effect that would diminish the ability—and thus the efficiency—of all personnel in the operating room to perform as they were expected and trained to do. I learned that panic was more contagious than the common cold and that one could catch it even while wearing a protective mask. On the other hand, some surgeons were cool under pressure. Even in the direst situations, they kept their composure and spoke in an even and steady tone. They seemed to exude confidence and were able to create an environment conducive to focus and concentration, which allowed for optimal performance under pressure. I aspired to be like one of these surgeons.

It was also interesting to observe the many different ways in which surgeons relieved stress during an operation. Some of them spoke through the entire case, some of them listened to music, some sang, and some incessantly yelled and screamed.

"COME ON GUYS...PAY ATTENTION! THE PATIENT IS NOT RELAXED, AND I CAN'T CLOSE THE ABDOMEN."

The screaming had become louder all of a sudden. From my seat next to the anesthesia machine, I looked up to see the masked face of Dr. Zach Wolfe who was peering over the curtain and yelling at the two of us on the other side. Myla was startled, and she immediately stopped reading, picked up a syringe containing a muscle relaxant, and with tremorous hands injected some of its contents into the patient's IV (intravenous) line. After several tense seconds, this allowed the abdominal wall muscles to relax, making it easier for the surgeon to close the abdomen. It turns out that the blood-brain barrier was not impermeable after all. For the rest of the case and until the attending and chief resident walked out of the room, Myla and I were on pins and needles the entire time.

Although the "blood-brain barrier" phrase when used colloquially applies best to the world of anesthesia and surgery, it also has broader meaning when it comes to the difference between the medical and surgical fields. The intern year is peculiar in that it involves several rotations on nonsurgical (medical) services. The purpose is to give the surgical trainee an understanding of how those other services work and how they approach patient care. Moreover, these rotations give the surgery intern a working knowledge of the other specialties and the ability to better relate, work, and coordinate with other services in the care of patients. The aim is to optimize the medical care being provided to the patient by enhancing the cooperation and communication between the surgeons and the members of other specialties of medicine. This excursion into other services does deliver the intended effect, but it also gives the young surgeon some interesting insights into how general surgeons are viewed by other physicians and specialties. The perceived, and sometimes real, differences are due to an inherent philosophical contrast between the surgical and medical specialties in how they approach patient care.

My initial rotation had been neurosurgery. During that rotation, I truly felt that all services worked well together and on behalf of the patient. Neurosurgeons, like many of the other surgical subspecialties, spend the first year of their training in the general surgery service. Dr. Gottenger, the attending surgeon and chief of neurotrauma, seemed to have great respect for and worked very well with his general surgery colleagues. He set the tone for his service, and there were few conflicts, if any. That was not the case with all other services, however, as I was to find out during my internship.

At times, there seemed to be a real love-hate relationship between general surgery and some of the other services in the hospital. A typical example was the relationship between the surgeons and the internal medicine doctors. Most of this was due to a combination of learned behavior, pride, and a certain lack of understanding as to the roles of different specialties and how they fit into the big picture.

The physicians who work in a hospital environment fall into two main groups: those that belong to the surgical areas (general surgeons, vascular surgeons, orthopedists, etc.), and those who belong to the medical specialties such as internal medicine, cardiology, and pediatrics. Certain other specialties such as radiology, for example, do not really fit into the two classic groups. Practitioners of this specialty perform many diagnostic and therapeutic procedures or interventions, but they are not surgeons in the true sense.

The medical specialties study disease processes in depth, and the treatment modalities they use are medications and procedures that are considered non-surgical—often referred to as noninvasive. To this end, internists (medicine specialists) are characteristically an intellectually oriented group of physicians who spend a great percentage of their day in discussions and study pertaining to their fields of expertise. Surgeons, on the other hand, are doers and tinkerers. They are trained to treat disease to a certain extent with their knowledge, but mostly through their hands by performing surgery. To that end, a great percentage of a surgeon's day, by necessity, is spent in the operating room, leaving less time for constant study and intellectual pursuits. Internists are mostly valued for what they know; surgeons are mostly valued for what they do.

This classical difference in the approach to patient care leads to different perspectives that can, in turn, lead to inherent conflicts between the different specialties, particularly in the resident ranks as they deal with one another. Some surgeons, even early in their training, develop an over-inflated sense of self-importance in thinking that only they can fix major health problems and truly cure, rather than just manage, disease. In contrast, some physicians in the medical specialties view surgeons as technicians with less intellectual capacity or medical knowledge. This mutual misperception sets the stage for some interesting and less-than-optimal dynamics.

Surgeons consult their medical colleagues for two main reasons. Consults are requested either when the patient has a medical condition that warrants a certain expertise, or for medical evaluation and clearance prior to a planned elective operation. Most medical consultants who are asked to perform preoperative evaluations are quite conscientious. They carefully evaluate pertinent data while making their assessment and recommendations in order to optimize the patient prior to surgery. They use sound judgment in deciding which of the patient's health issues need to be addressed in the short-term as they pertain to surgery, and which pose minimal risk and can be deferred until after the surgery. Nevertheless, some can be overzealous in requesting an excessive amount of lab data and preoperative tests, which in turn frustrates surgeons who are anxiously awaiting medical clearance in order to proceed with surgery.

This consultation trap was a recurrent theme during my internship. "Did you get the porcelain level?" I once heard a frustrated chief resident sarcastically pose this question to a senior resident in internal medicine whom he had asked for a preoperative clearance for a patient with diabetes who needed a hernia repair. There is no "porcelain level" in medicine. It was the resident's attempt at being facetious and making the point that the medical consultant was about to ask for a multitude of unnecessary tests that would only serve to delay the procedure and had little if any clinical relevance. As I read the consultant's note after rounds, it was obvious that the chief resident had a point. The medical consultant had asked for a long list of laboratory data and diagnostic tests, which not only meant more work for me but also did not seem pertinent to the medical clearance that we had requested. While explaining to the chief resident the next day that the surgery would have to be delayed until we got all of the results the medical consultant had requested, I heard him murmur under his breath in utter exasperation: "I am sure he didn't forget to recommend that we give the patient some potassium." Sure enough, towards the end of the consultant's note, there was the recommendation to add potassium to the intravenous line for a borderline but normal serum potassium level. I got the sense that the chief resident and this particular medicine resident had crossed paths before.

I was often conflicted with some of these interactions. On one hand, it seemed that if you request a consultant's input, you should follow or at least consider their recommendations. On the other hand, some consultants seemed to want to take care of all the patient's medical problems, no matter how minor and irrelevant, rather than concentrating on the issue at hand. Most often, the medical consultants won the day as they held the final say on whether to give the patient medical clearance for surgery. As interns, we were often caught in the middle and had to scramble to obtain all the laboratory data and preoperative tests recommended by the consultants, so that patients could be cleared prior to their scheduled surgery date. This process added countless workhours and unnecessary stress to an intern's already hectic life.

While struggling with how to deal with these inherent conflicts during my intern year, I soon came to realize that the main difference between the way the medical and surgical specialties dealt with patient care was more an issue of timing—meaning speed and aggressiveness. Surgeons, being used to dealing with conditions that could either get better or worse quickly, were used to a more aggressive and quicker pace when addressing patient care. Medical doctors by definition most often dealt with chronic conditions where patients improved or got worse at a more gradual pace, giving those physicians more time for thought and deliberation in their plan of action. One often got the impression that medicine doctors never seemed to be in a hurry for anything. This is not universal, however, as medicine doctors have come to learn the huge difference that rapid intervention can make in situations like heart attacks and strokes in saving patients' lives and brain function.

I learned this lesson early in my internship while on call one night at the VA hospital, which was located one block away from Jackson Memorial. The request had come from the medical service to evaluate an elderly man who had been admitted with diffuse abdominal pain and had now developed peritoneal signs. These signs, which typically include abdominal rigidity (sustained contraction of abdominal muscles) and rebound tenderness (pain upon vibration of the abdominal wall), are an indication that the internal lining of the abdominal wall is irritated due to an infectious or inflammatory process. It usually indicates a caustic or infectious process is occurring within the abdominal cavity and is one of the classical indications to perform an exploratory laparotomy (abdominal surgery).

On first inspection, it was obvious that the patient was truly sick. The gentleman was in his mid to late sixties, thin, and hardly moving in bed when I first approached him. He had been well until less than forty-eight hours prior when he had developed diffuse abdominal pain and diarrhea. When the pain worsened in the ensuing hours, he had decided to come to the emergency room. As the pain had been associated with some diarrhea, a presumptive diagnosis of gastroenteritis (stomach and intestinal infection) had been made in the emergency room and the patient had been admitted to the medical service for observation and supportive care. His pain progressively intensified, however, and "peritoneal signs" soon developed. A surgery consultation was called soon thereafter.

Even as an intern with little experience, it was obvious to me that the patient had peritonitis. His abdomen was distended, rigid, and although he had significant pain when I pressed on his belly, his pain was much worse when I quickly let go of the pressure and his abdominal wall returned to its normal position indicating rebound tenderness. The patient needed urgent exploratory surgery. After my exam, I grabbed the patient's chart and hurried to the nurses' station to call my senior resident.

After discussing the case with the fourth-year resident over the phone, I promptly expressed my humble opinion that the patient needed to go to the operating room immediately. After listening to all the pertinent information, the senior resident expressed his strong disagreement to my recommendations for immediate surgery.

"If we take him to the operating room now, we will kill him."

"What do you mean? If we don't take him, he will surely die." I firmly pressed my case as I knew peritoneal signs needed to be addressed urgently. The senior resident seemed slightly perturbed at having an intern question his judgment. I noted a hint of hostility in his voice not only towards me but towards the medicine team as well.

"I don't have to go up there to know that the patient is probably hypotensive (low blood pressure) and dehydrated as he has been under the care of the medicine team. He is probably very dehydrated and will need to be medically optimized and rehydrated before we take him to the operating room. Otherwise the stress of the anesthesia and surgery will kill him for sure. I will send Nadya to help you but start by doing this…" He gave me a fairly long list of things to order and do. "…And do it quickly," he added before hanging up.

Nadya Miocevic, the second-year resident on the service, walked into the room shortly thereafter. "Does he have an IV?" was the first thing she asked.

"Of course," I said while pointing to the IV line running to the patient's right hand. She examined the patient, picked up the flow sheet from the foot of the bed, and started studying it. The flow sheet is a piece of paper, usually on a clipboard, where the nurses record the patient's vital signs, intravenous fluid intake, urine output, and other significant data at regular intervals.

"Did you get the supplies?" she asked while still reading. I replied in the affirmative and pointed to the bedside table where I had placed all the supplies the senior resident had instructed me to get. She moved closer to the patient and after introducing herself, proceeded to perform a physical exam. Upon finishing, she washed her hands and picked up the flowsheet again.

"First of all, the IV is too small, the fluids are wrong, the patient needs a Foley catheter (catheter into the urinary bladder), and an NG tube (catheter inserted in the nose, which goes to the stomach)." Nadya pointed to the flow sheet she was holding in her hand. "Look, the blood pressure has been borderline low since he got here, the urine output has been decreasing steadily and there is none recorded in the last eight hours, and he has vomited twice since this morning."

As she spoke, she pointed with her finger at the pertinent numbers, as if to prove her point. I had looked at the flow sheet while doing my consultation, but I had concentrated on the temperature and vital signs and had missed some of these other data points. In the next ten minutes, we placed two larger (wider lumen) IV catheters in the patient, one in each arm, each connected to a liter bag of normal saline—the appropriate IV fluid. A Foley catheter had gone into the bladder only to reveal a small amount of dark urine, and we inserted a long nasogastric (NG) tube through the nose into the stomach. Once this tube was put to suction, large quantities of yellow-green fluid quickly collected in the canister.

"Please page the doctor taking care of this patient," Nadya instructed a nurse who was now close by. A few minutes later the medical intern walked into the room.

I could tell he was an intern by looking at the pockets of his lab coat; they looked like mine. It is not long after starting to work at a hospital that you begin to accumulate small booklets, papers, and other items that you stuff in your lab coat pockets. You carry drug-dosing books, cards with normal lab values, pamphlets with codes for dictations, booklets with hospital phone extensions, patient censuses, etc. These are added to items such as the ever-present stethoscope, small flashlight, and reflex hammer that all interns usually carry. After a few weeks, the lab coat pockets become extremely full, but somehow you refuse to part with these things, as they might come in handy when you least expect them to. It is not until sometime during the third year that residents begin to shed some of these items. The result is that you can usually tell the seniority of the resident by how full or empty his/her lab coat pockets are. The interns and medical students have lab coat pockets that look like they are about to burst. The chief residents usually have their pockets empty except for possibly a stethoscope. Some of them only carry a pen, if that, because they know that when the need arises, they can always borrow a pen or a stethoscope from a nearby medical student, intern, or junior resident. Chief residents rarely see patients alone, as they almost always travel with an entourage.

Nadya questioned the medicine intern as to why the patient had not been properly worked up and medically optimized. When the intern quietly replied that they had ordered abdominal films, Nadya lost her composure a bit and started to list the things she thought the medicine team had done wrong or at least had failed to implement in a timely manner. As she rambled on, the list touched on more frequent physical exams, not allowing the patient to eat in case he needed surgery, more fluids, the right IV fluids, the NG tube, the Foley, and stepped-up intervention when they noticed that the patient was not making any urine. The points came out rapid-fire, leaving the medicine intern and me with little to say. It was a good lesson for both of us, but I got the sense that some of it was lost on him because she was berating him and questioning the competence of his team rather than teaching him how to properly manage the situation in the future. It was clear that the medicine team had not appreciated the rapid deterioration of the patient and had not acted in a timely manner in order to address it. However, I thought the best course of action in this instance, rather than berate, was to teach all involved how to do better so that the mistake would not be repeated. Although Nadya's intentions were in the right place, her execution left a bit to be desired and added to the general friction sometimes seen between the two specialties.

Nadya told the medicine intern that we were taking the patient to the operating room and inquired as to how to contact the patient's family. It was obvious that the patient was very sick and was in no shape to participate in a long discussion as to his medical condition, let alone be able to understand the situation well enough to give informed consent for the operation that he needed.

"Should I cancel the abdominal films we ordered?" the intern inquired after he gave us the family contact information.

"Forget that! This man has a surgical abdomen, and we should concentrate on getting an EKG (electrocardiogram), chest X-ray, and things anesthesia is going to want." Nadya did not leave any opening for discussion. She told me that she was going to book the case and instructed me to contact the next of kin to get consent.

I was surprised after a short while how much the patient seemed to improve by our intervention. We had pushed four liters of fluid through the IV lines in a rather short period of time. The urine had become much lighter, and the patient seemed far more awake and responsive. Now that the abdomen was not as distended, he seemed more comfortable as well. The change was utterly amazing.

"Now he is ready," the senior resident seemed to emphasize the point as he helped me wheel the stretcher into the operating room approximately three hours later.

I was allowed to participate and assist in the case. It turned out that the patient had a perforated colon from an obstructing cancerous lesion in the horizontal section of the colon called the transverse colon. We washed his abdomen, resected the segment with the cancerous lesion, and performed a colostomy where we brought out both segments of the colon through the abdominal skin so that he could evacuate his feces as he healed. The plan was to take him back in three months when he was better, to reconnect his colon.

Our patient had a rocky stay in the intensive care unit after the surgery, but eventually made it out of the hospital alive. It was a good save, and it impressed upon me the need to be aggressive and expeditious in the diagnostic work-up and pre-operative preparation of the critically ill surgical patient. Similar experiences during the course of my residency served to reinforce these principles as I gained a deeper understanding of how quick, aggressive assessment and intervention can be crucial and lifesaving in treating surgical disease. The leisurely pace often afforded to the medical diagnostician is rarely allowed for the surgeon.

Despite differences in the perspective and philosophy of various specialties, I came to learn that the great majority of doctors are highly intelligent individuals who are motivated to do the right thing for their patients. The conflicts brought about by some of the differences in philosophy when it comes to patient care are sometimes more apparent in the resident ranks, as most residents are overworked, stressed, and prone to overreact to minor differences of opinion. As doctors progress in their training and gain some experience and perspective, and particularly after completing their training, most medical and surgical practitioners come to understand that they are part of a bigger team with the goal in common of treating patients and making them better. This goal is better achieved by bridging the gaps and overcoming the figurative blood-brain barrier in all of its manifestations.

Trauma 101

The trauma service at Jackson Memorial Hospital is housed in a separate building from the main hospital. It is called Ryder Trauma Center. This four-story, modern building is a self-contained trauma unit with its own resuscitation area (resus), operating rooms, and radiology department including a state-of-the-art CT scanner. The entire second floor is intensive care unit (ICU) beds and administrative offices, the third floor is the main ward housing patient rooms, and the fourth floor contains the rehabilitation and burn units. This building and the people who work in it constitute one of the busiest and best trauma centers in the entire country.

While I was there as an intern, the trauma service was separated into two different teams, red and blue. Each team consisted of six to eight medical students, an intern who manned the ward, a second-year resident who oversaw the resuscitation area, and two senior residents. The two senior residents on the red service were a fourth-year surgery resident from the US Air Force and a chief resident from Jackson Memorial. The blue service seniors were a fourth-year resident from Jackson and a trauma fellow. A fellow is a trainee who has already completed a general surgery training program and has undertaken further training in one of the subspecialties of surgery, such as trauma, pediatric surgery, plastic surgery, etc. These fellowships were usually one (surgical oncology, colorectal) or two years (cardiothoracic, trauma) in duration, although some were as long as three years.

I had been assigned to the red team, and for the first time in my training I was going to get to work with one of the general surgery chief residents from Jackson. I started my rotation with great excitement and anticipation. Not only was I interested in the trauma field; I was looking forward to working with one of the chief residents in general surgery. After all, I would be a chief resident in five years, and I wanted to see the quality of surgeon that my program could produce. Up until now I had mostly rotated with chief residents from other services, and I had only worked with the general surgery chief residents when I cross-covered their services while on call. This rotation was going to be different; I would get to work with the chief resident on a daily basis.

During orientation on the first day of the rotation, I was instructed on my duties. There was the floor of course, which was the exclusive responsibility of the intern, and then there was the "every other day" on call. We were expected to come in at 6:00 a.m. every day for rounds, be at morning report at 7:30 a.m. sharp where all cases from the previous day were presented, and all pending patient issues were discussed with the incoming team. Upon finishing with this conference, we would promptly begin the workday. When on call, sleep was not an option. We had approximately thirty patients on the floor on any given day, and once the intern on the other team went home, his/her patients became the responsibility of the intern on call. There were many new admissions and discharges every day, and a seemingly insurmountable amount of floor work. Post call, one made rounds after the morning report and tried to tidy things up before going home—hopefully by noon, only to have to come back the next day at 6:00 a.m. for another thirty-hour shift.

As if that were not enough work, we were expected to come down to the resuscitation area to help with the new trauma patients as they were being evaluated and treated. Patients who met trauma criteria usually arrived by ambulance or helicopter.

"The intern's job on resus is always the same," the charge nurse had told us during orientation. "It is to stick, stick, and stick—otherwise known as the intern's three sticks. You are to stick your finger in the anus and do a rectal exam to check for blood, stick a Foley (a catheter inserted through the urethra into the bladder) to assess the patient's fluid volume status (patients who had lost a lot of blood would not make much urine due to low blood volume), and stick a needle in the femoral (groin) artery in order to get a blood sample." If the medical students were around, we were to instruct and teach them how to do these three things when appropriate, which usually meant in patients who were stable and not "crashing." Even if there were medical students around who were proficient with the three sticks, it was made clear to us that we needed to be there to supervise them and make sure the job was done right. This job usually took less than ten minutes, except that it always took you away from the many things you needed to do on the floor. These interruptions occurred up to twenty-five times on a busy trauma call day, which meant that no matter where the intern was at the time of the trauma alert, he/she had to drop everything, go down to the resus area, gown and glove, wait for the patient to arrive, do the three sticks, and then hopefully leave before being assigned any other tasks, in order to get back to the many pending duties up on the floor.

It was on the morning of my third call that I looked down at my pager and read: "25YOM (year old male) with GSW (gunshot wound) to chest. ETA three minutes." I figured this would be a quick trip to resus. By now, I had learned that when patients came into the resuscitation area awake (after minor trauma, for example), and especially if they were intoxicated, it was always a struggle to accomplish the three intern sticks. However, when the patients came in comatose or in extremis (near death) and therefore unresponsive, the job was much easier as the patients could not put up a fight to these rather painful maneuvers that the intern had to perform on them.

When patients have significant trauma, which meets the criteria for care in a trauma center, time is of the essence. Thus, all the diagnostic maneuvers and initial therapeutic modalities must be done simultaneously in a short amount of time, in order to quickly diagnose and assess any potential life-threatening issues and initiate treatment as soon as possible. From the patient's perspective, arriving at trauma-resus is an extremely traumatic experience, no pun intended. As the patient is brought into the trauma bay, he or she is immediately accosted by a team of up to seven or eight medical personnel. While being asked a multitude of questions about medical history, events, and certain facts (date and time) in order to assess cognitive status, there is usually an anesthesiologist assessing the airway, two nurses attempting to gain vital signs and start two IV (intravenous) lines, a trauma surgeon assessing for injuries, and two or three others cutting off all the clothes in order to fully expose the body to check for injuries. This all takes place while the patient is lying on a hard wooden or plastic board to prevent further damage in case of spine injury or fracture. Then along comes the intern and the three sticks. When the patient is unresponsive, these things are accomplished quickly and efficiently. When the patient is awake and cognizant, however, the trauma bay protocol can be a struggle as the patients naturally rebel against all these uncomfortable maneuvers performed on them simultaneously. When patients arrive awake but disoriented or confused due to injury, intoxication, or other factors, this battle can be epic and more akin to a "pile-on" wrestling match.

It was early in the morning that day and I had a long list of things to accomplish for the patients on my service. I had slept well the night before and was full of energy. It took seconds to come down the stairs from the third to the first floor. As I started to put on the protective gear that we always wear for resus patients (gown, hat, mask, booties, and two sets of gloves), I happened to glance up at the members of the trauma team who were already dressed and waiting for the patient. My eyes rested on the chief resident who was looking straight at me with an obvious grin under his mask. For a moment I surmised that I might be the source of his amusement after having done something wrong while donning my protective equipment.

"Put on extra gear, Joe," he then said. "They lost vital signs en route. We are about to do the big whack."

Dr. Jack Rio was the type of guy who lived, ate, and slept surgery. We all called him Jack but when referring to him in the third person, we called him Rio. His scholastic achievements in medical school not being stellar—a fact he freely admitted—he had relied on an unshakable perseverance and determination to gain admission to the general surgery program. After being admitted, his work ethic earned him a reputation around the hospital as an excellent resident and he garnered a great amount of respect during his residency years. He had great hands and was an extremely aggressive surgeon, a quality that perfectly complemented his self-assured, confident personality. He was reputed to have been a great football player in high school and he had the demeanor and body of a jock. His six-foot-one frame had at one time been extremely powerful and muscular. Over the course of the residency, however, he had developed a bit of a belly as his time for exercise had been squeezed by the surgical residency and his family responsibilities—Rio had four daughters. He always looked unkempt, and I never saw him wear anything but scrubs during his entire chief residency year, even for conferences, for which professional attire was mandatory. As he was larger than life, no one seemed to want to mess with him, and you got the sense that he was one of those people who exist outside the normal rules and get to break them with impunity.

As the chief resident on our team, Rio was my immediate supervisor and did rounds with me on the trauma service every morning. He was never interested in minutia, and only wanted to be told the big picture. "Just take care of it," he would say when I brought up information that he was not interested in, such as an abnormal lab value, or issues pertaining to a patient's discharge. When dealing with a problem that was over my head, however, he did take the time to come and help every time I asked. Over the course of the rotation, a part of me began to like the way that Rio dealt with the service. I hoped that someday, like him, I would be able to leave the details to others and just enjoy doing surgery. I got the sense that for him surgery was more like a sport than anything resembling work. It was obvious to all that he was having great fun being a surgeon.

"He needs a whack," Rio was fond of saying when he decided a patient needed to go to surgery. On occasion, particularly when a patient needed the type of surgery that he was fond of doing, like a major abdominal or thoracic procedure, he would say that the patient needed the "big whack."

Not all of Rio's habits or actions were well received. In fact, he had a habit of using the interns as his personal assistants. He would often call me to the operating room at the end of a trauma case so that I could transport the patient to the ICU—a job usually reserved for the resident-surgeon of record on the case—while he went with the attending to eat at an all-night sandwich shop that was just outside the trauma center. One time he demanded to borrow the set of regular clothes that he knew I kept in my locker so that he could go to a dinner being hosted by a pharmaceutical representative. I relented and told him he could keep them. He was such a nice guy that it was hard to refuse his requests. Nevertheless, I will admit that transporting patients for him when I had a million other things to do wore thin after a while. Despite all his idiosyncrasies, however, it was hard not to like him.

"What do you mean?" I asked Rio.

He was still brimming as he answered me. "We are going to really whack him right here; you know...open his chest. And you, my friend, are going to help me." He motioned me into the resus room so that we could take our positions to be ready for what was about to happen. It was then that a voice came over the loudspeaker. It was the voice of the ambulance driver bringing the patient to the trauma center.

"Repeat, the patient has lost vital signs. ETA one minute." It then dawned on me what we were about to do. It brought with it a mixture of excitement, exhilaration, and guilt—for it meant that our patient had just expired in the ambulance on the way to the hospital.

Trauma surgery is different from any other surgical practice in that often you don't have time to develop a doctor-patient relationship before operating. Even when covering the emergency room, there is a consultation process that allows the surgeon to visit, speak to, and examine the patient prior to deciding whether the patient requires surgery. Although some of these consultations are short, there is still time for the patient and surgeon to get to know each other to a certain degree, and for a patient-doctor bond to develop, albeit a weak one. In trauma, however, all too often the patients arrive on the brink of death. In these cases, the trauma surgeon must decide whether to operate without talking to or having any input from the patient. As such, there is a danger that the surgeon may think of the patient less as a human being and more as a type of injury or as an impending operation. During my trauma rotations, I had to constantly remind myself not to fall into that trap—i.e., to remember that all patients who come through the resuscitation bays are human beings just like me, who unfortunately had sustained serious or life-threatening injuries, most often through no fault of their own.

An "ER (emergency room) thoracotomy" is a last-ditch effort to essentially bring a patient back from the dead. It is done under dire circumstances when the patient has just expired or is about to expire, usually after deep trauma such as stab or gunshot wounds. Opening the chest on the spot allows for direct access to the heart, in order to assess and repair any injuries, or perform direct heart compressions in order to circulate the blood to vital organs, particularly the brain, while measures are taken to treat whatever issues need to be addressed. This procedure also allows access to the aorta—the main large artery carrying blood from the heart to the rest of the body—which can be clamped in order to prevent further blood loss. Moreover, clamping the aorta also helps to direct whatever blood is left in the patient's circulatory system to perfuse (flow into) the brain, a matter of vital importance.

The emergency thoracotomy has a probability of being effective in saving a life of less than one in a thousand (0.1 percent). The chance of success must be weighed against the real risk of exposing the entire surgical team to communicable diseases in the patient's bodily fluid, because this procedure is usually done in dire situations when speed is of the essence, most often in a setting other than the operating room. Taking these concerns into consideration, this operation has understandably been restricted to patients with sharp chest trauma (gunshot wounds, stab wounds, etc.) who lose vital signs just before arrival at the trauma center, or while in the presence of the trauma team, instances that are fairly rare but offer the best hope of survival. Our patient met the criteria, and Dr. Jack Rio was ready and excited about the opportunity. Saving a patient's life through this procedure is one of the biggest rushes known to surgeons; for those who accomplish it successfully, it is an experience they will never forget.

I peeked out the trauma bay door as the double-doors to the trauma center opened and three paramedics came in running while pulling and pushing the stretcher. One was ventilating the intubated patient with an AMBU bag as they sped towards us. I went back to join Rio on the left side of the patient's bed as he finished opening the large instrument tray that had been placed on the side table for our use.

"You are here with me; let the medical students do the other stuff." He pressed a large suction into my hand. Instinctively I checked to make sure it was functioning. The patient was brought into the room followed by the rest of the trauma team who began their work immediately.

The patient was shirtless, and as he was being transferred from the stretcher to the bed, I saw a jet of dark brown fluid come from my right and hit the patient's chest, causing the fluid to splash messily onto the gowns of all of us who were close by. My face turned to witness Jack Rio holding a plastic container of betadine disinfectant, which he was squeezing tightly, causing a jet of fluid to escape the bottle. In his right hand, he held the biggest surgical handle and blade that I had ever seen.

"Vitals?"

"None." The exchange between Rio and one of the nurses was lightning fast. Almost simultaneously, I saw Rio cut deep with the knife from the patient's sternum (breastbone), along the left chest just under the nipple, and all the way down until the sharp blade touched the bed. He made the same cut again, except much deeper this time. He dropped the knife on the side table, inserted the fingers of both hands in the wound, and forcefully spread the ribs apart while letting out a quiet groan, thereby revealing the amount of force needed for this maneuver.

The gush of blood emanating from the patient's chest was unexpected. My suction was useless as two to three liters of blood spilled from the chest onto Rio and myself. Suddenly blood was everywhere, all over my gown, the bed, my booties, and the floor. "Turn this." Rio had produced a large retractor from the tray, inserted it into the wound, and was pointing at the handle. I turned the handle as fast as I could, and the ribs began to spread apart. Halfway I heard the unmistakable sound of one of the ribs breaking. "Keep going," I heard Rio say. "We need access."

Rio, using the large scissors he was holding in his right hand, began cutting something I could not see deep in the chest. His hands were moving extremely fast, but his voice was unhurried and steady. "The first thing you have to do is cut the pulmonary ligament to gain access to the aorta." His left hand was now buried in the chest almost to his elbow as he seemed to be almost blindly feeling for something. "There, you feel for the aorta and with a finger you break the parietal pleura..." I was not listening anymore. I was enthralled at what I was seeing. The ER thoracotomy is the type of operation that surgical residents dream of doing. It is an experience that physicians tell stories about for years afterward.

Rio then inserted a large clamp into the chest, aiming the tip towards what he seemed to be holding in his left hand. After closing the clamp, he triumphantly announced that he had clamped the aorta. “Now, let’s look at the damage.” Rio used scissors to cut the pericardium (lining of the heart), at which time another rush of blood spilled onto the table. He grabbed the suction from my hand and continued to suction around the heart.

“Heart looks good.” He was pulling on and turning the heart with his left hand while suctioning with his right and inspecting it for injuries all the while. I struggled to see but could not. My vision was blocked by Rio’s hand and, to make matters worse, my protective face shield had blood and betadine splattered all over it and was getting foggy. “Back here,” he announced. “It’s the pulmonary artery. Give him fluids and hang blood.” Rio raised his head to emphasize his wishes to the nurses. He then placed my hand to hold the heart out of the way and told me to squeeze it every couple of seconds. He proceeded to work deep in the chest where I could not see.

“What’s going on?” The voice was that of Dr. Oz Dragan, the surgical attending on call. He had been operating with the fourth-year resident and had left the operation to come help us. He walked into the room in full battle gear ready to work.

“Got a couple of holes back here in the pulmonary artery,” Rio replied as he continued to struggle to get a better view. They both began to work through what seemed like a small opening between the ribs for two sets of hands. When they attempted to suture, I saw the sharp needle come extremely close to my hand several times.

“Don’t worry, I won’t stick you.” Despite Rio’s promise, I instinctively pressed my hand onto the heart and away from the needle every time I saw the needle come towards the chest.

“It’s like freaking Kool-Aid,” Rio said referring to the blood, which had taken on a light-pink hue. Blood was already hanging, but it was being mixed with the other intravenous fluids that had been given earlier. They had been working in the chest for several minutes and I could sense that things were not going well. Rio and the attending were both sweating now, and their frustration was obvious as they struggled to repair the damaged vessel. Light-colored blood kept emanating from behind the heart, but in gradually decreasing amounts.

"It's been twenty minutes, guys," came from one of the nurses in the room.

"How long?" The attending stood erect to stretch his back. The resuscitation table was low and all three of us surgeons were bending over to be able to work and have a view of what we were doing.

"Twenty minutes since he got here," the head nurse repeated.

"That's it, Jack, let's stop." I saw the attending put his hand on Rio's forearm, gently insistent. I sensed that Rio was not ready to give up, but he said nothing and stopped his efforts.

Rio was obviously frustrated as he threw the instruments on the tray. "Joe, close the chest. I am off to have breakfast." As my eyes followed him to the door, I noted that a small crowd of medical students, other residents, and some of the ancillary staff had gathered outside the glass walls and were looking into the room. It must have been a striking scene. Blood was everywhere. On the stretcher lay a man with his chest wide open, exposing his heart and lungs floating in a pool of blood.

"Here Joe," it was Dr. Dragan's voice this time. "Let's go over the operation." He also invited some of the medical students on our team to come to the room for a teaching session. He asked them to put on protective gear and stand by the partition away from all the blood. We then went over the anatomy and surgical maneuvers in detail. The attending pointed out to me where to make the initial incision, how to expose the aorta, how to open the lining of the heart vertically in order not to injure the nerves traveling to the diaphragm, which run in close proximity. We further dissected where they had been working including several large openings in the vessels that ran from the heart to the lungs. There were multiple tears in the left lung as well. He told me how these operations were not as common as they had once been before the advent of AIDS, due to the potential risk of exposure to medical personnel while doing a procedure that had a very low probability of a successful outcome. As the procedure was rarely done nowadays, he felt it was important to get the most educational benefit from it as possible, even if the outcome was bad. "… as almost always is the case," he said. "Now we can close the chest."

I began to close the chest in single layer with a large nylon suture provided by the nurse. The closure was not pretty. As the resuscitation table was low, I occasionally straightened out to stretch my back and, in the process, lifted my head to where I could survey the room. The curtains had been drawn and I was alone now, except for a nurse who would come in and out once in a while to make sure I had whatever I needed. There was something surreal and macabre about the scene. The body on the stretcher, all the blood, the chest incision half-closed in a haphazard and gross fashion. Once finished, as I walked out of the room, I removed all the bloody garments and threw them into the red container by the door. My scrubs stuck to me uncomfortably, thankfully from sweat and not blood.

The resus resident walked towards me carrying "the bricks," as we called the two large radios that the second-year resident had to carry at all times. These radios were for communication with all the county and city ambulances. All ambulance traffic in the city of Miami had to call in their runs to the trauma center. It was the second-year resident's responsibility to triage and direct all ambulance traffic in the city.

"Sorry I could not help," he said, "but I had three other rooms going." He pulled me gently by the arm. "Let's go talk to the family. You gotta get used to doing this."

On the first floor of the trauma center, between the resus area and the lobby, there are two or three small rooms used for family conferences. When family arrives to the trauma center seeking information about their loved ones, they are brought into one of these rooms. Usually the second-year resident, along with a social worker, goes into the room after the patient is assessed and discusses the findings and management with the family. This particular family was rather large, and they had been brought into another, larger room near the lobby. The social worker stood by the doorway as the second-year resident and I walked into the room. There were perhaps ten people in the room, several of whom were standing and some of whom started approaching us as we entered the room.

"He did not make it," was the first thing out of the second-year resident's mouth as we were still walking towards the family on the opposite side of the room. The comment was made almost in passing and before we had identified ourselves or learned which ones were the close family members. As soon as he made the comment, two elderly ladies who were standing by the wall to my right promptly collapsed to the floor. The scene turned chaotic as the family began to loudly wail in despair. We immediately had to mobilize help and call for other residents and nurses to attend to the two family members who had now become patients themselves.

That night around 2:00 a.m., I received a page from Rio inviting me to grab some food. I was not hungry and had lots to do but I got the sense he wanted to talk. After walking to the sandwich shop across the street from the trauma center, I found Rio sitting in a back booth eating. I picked up a soft drink and sat across the table from him.

"I heard things were crazy with the family," he inquired as he stuffed a sandwich in his mouth. I described how we had to deal with the ladies who had collapsed along with the rest of the grieving family. Thankfully, both relatives recovered quickly and did not require further treatment or admission to the hospital.

"If we had gotten to this guy a little earlier, I think we could have saved him," Rio offered while shaking his head from side to side as he chewed. I nodded my head in the affirmative but said nothing. We sat there quietly in deep thought for several minutes while he ate. Then as an afterthought after a few seconds, Jack added: "By the way, when you are giving a family bad news, make sure everyone is sitting down. Oh yeah…and make sure you sit or stand by the door, sometimes you need to make a quick exit."

I took notice and followed his advice religiously when I became a second-year resident and had to talk to family members of patients arriving at the trauma center, particularly if the news was bad. This is one part of the job I have always found extremely distasteful and nerve-wracking about trauma surgery, as most of the time the family is not aware of the patient's condition and are not really prepared for bad news, particularly if it's news of a loved one's death.

Rio's pager went off. He looked at it, stood up, and grabbed his drink. "Stay and finish. They are ready for me in OR with an abdominal washout." I was left alone and decided to reward myself with a few minutes of quiet contemplation. My body was tired, but I was beginning to get that second wind that comes at around 3:00 – 4:00 in the morning as you realize you have made it through most of your call and your shift will eventually come to an end in several hours. I craved a shower.

I took a little time to reflect on what had taken place that morning. The case would make for an interesting discussion during morning report. I wondered if I would ever get the chance to do it again. How would I react if I were ever in Rio's shoes? Would I be able to perform well enough to save a life?

I did get my chance to perform this procedure again, when I was a chief resident rotating in the trauma service during the last two months of my residency. The incident was one of the most heartbreaking and disturbing experiences of my many years of surgical training. As for Dr. Jack Rio, he went on to become a cardiothoracic surgeon. He was developing a great reputation and a promising future, when one night while driving to dinner after a case with one of his partners, his life was tragically cut short in a motor vehicle accident.

THE NIGHTINGALES

"After the experience that I had with my surgery, I've decided to become a nurse." Terri Neely seemed excited about her decision. She had been my patient at one point and our initial meeting had been under the worst of circumstances. It was obvious at that time that she had no idea what she was going to do with her life. Now she seemed to have found her calling and had determination and purpose. I was happy for her. This conversation took place during my fifth year of residency, mere months before I was to finish the program.

Terri had been a most unusual patient, from whom I learned quite a bit about surgery, and about life. As Terri discussed her future plans, I pondered whether all nurses went into their field with the same idealism and enthusiasm. I am certain most do, but the interactions I had with a few of them during my training, especially during my internship year, made me wonder.

As an intern, one learns early on how to be efficient and organized. Being efficient is part of becoming a good resident, as it can mean a few more minutes of sleep or perhaps going home a little earlier at the end of a long day. In addition, interns develop organizational skills to optimize their efficiency by learning how to get from the ancillary staff the help they need to get their work done. Some do it with charm, while others attempt a more forceful approach. A few even go so far as to use bribery if necessary. For interns, all is fair in love, war, and getting the work done.

Nurses fall into that category of ancillary staff whom residents interact with on a daily basis. They work hand in hand with residents in the care of patients and are a valuable resource of knowledge and guidance for residents who are smart enough to realize their value. In a large teaching hospital like Jackson Memorial, nurses are overworked just like the residents and the rest of the staff. They struggle to stay empathetic and helpful under an ever-increasing patient load and a raft of responsibilities. Nurses work in all areas of the hospital and are an integral part of any service. Most nurses are nurturing and caring and have a congenial relationship with the residents; some are feared by interns and residents alike.

As an intern, one's first interaction with the nursing staff is on the floors. Nurses are the hospital's first line of human interaction with patients. They are responsible for the day-to-day care of patients. At the beginning of the three daily shifts, nurses check on all the patients on the floor. They record their vital signs and other information such as fluid intake and urine output. They query the patients as to any changes in the way they feel, and they report any complaints promptly to the first line of physicians, the interns. In addition, they have a long list of responsibilities that include documentation of events on the floor, admission and discharge of patients, executing doctor's orders, et al. My interactions with nurses as an intern and throughout my residency were overwhelmingly positive. I admired their dedication and respected their commitment to a difficult job.

I always considered floor nurses a great help in my daily responsibilities and in taking care of patients. At times, however, they seemed to be my personal tormentors, responsible for ninety percent of my daily pages. I tried to learn every way possible to minimize the number of calls by nurses. There were some obvious ways, like writing legibly; making sure to include orders for diet, activity, vital signs, etc. in my admission orders; and making sure medication orders were accurate for dose, interval, and route of administration. These measures helped significantly in reducing the number of pages from nurses to clarify ambiguous orders or orders that the nurses could not decipher due to "doctor's handwriting."

Some interns went a step further to minimize pages by writing detailed "contingency orders." These were designed to anticipate likely events that could happen with the patient and instructing nurses on what to do for each anticipated event. "If the temperature is above 101, then do this... If the patient does not void in six hours, insert a catheter," etc. Although contingency orders helped, sometimes writing them was more trouble than it was worth as one was forever trying to figure out potential "ifs."

After a while, I learned to accept that I would most likely not get to sleep during on-call nights. Once this became my overall attitude, it was much easier to not get aggravated every time I got a call for a Tylenol order or sleeping medication in the middle of the night. Nevertheless, several floor nurses still managed to get under my skin. There was one in particular on the general surgery floor on the eleven to seven night shift who made it part of her nightly routine to check all medication orders for each and every patient to make sure none was expired. So that patients would not remain on certain medications indefinitely, most medication orders had a one-week expiration date. In theory, this prompted interns and residents to review the orders for every patient weekly, and not renew medications that the patient did not need, or that they had already taken for the required amount of time, such as antibiotics that are usually prescribed in one-week regimens.

This particular nurse made it her mission to call me every night I was on call to give me a list of patients who needed their orders renewed. At that time, when I was on call, I would often be covering the patients on my service as well as the patients of two to three other services. Although I was happy to renew the orders on any patients on my service (those whom I knew), I tried in vain to explain to her that patients on other services should have their orders renewed by the doctors on the primary team when they showed up for work the next day, as they knew the patients well and were in the best position to decide which medications the patients needed. She always insisted that she would not give the medications to patients whose orders had already expired, thereby giving me no choice but to do as she asked and review medication orders on patients who were not under my care and thus were unknown to me. Failure on my part to do so could have resulted in certain patients not getting needed medication doses, because the nurse in question would simply refuse to give it.

There was nothing I could do with this line of reasoning. Even appealing to the charge nurse on the floor was of no use. I can't count the number of hours that I spent on call reviewing the charts of patients on other services so that I could figure out which of the long list of medications should be renewed. My pleading to the interns on the other services to renew all expired medications prior to going home usually fell on deaf ears, as the exhausted interns did not want anything to keep them from going home after a long day at the hospital.

This particular nurse also seemed to enjoy paging interns in the middle of the night to ask for orders when such orders were already written on the chart. Contingency orders did not seem to work with her; she called for every patient complaint even if the treatment for that complaint was already ordered in the chart. "Mr. Smith has insomnia," or "Mrs. Johnson wants Tylenol for a headache." Telling her that these orders were already in the chart did not faze her; several minutes later she would call with a similar request on another patient. I was convinced that she thought it was easier to call for a new order than to check the medication sheet to see if that situation was already addressed in the existing standing orders.

One particular call night when I had several emergencies to deal with and several consults pending from the emergency room, I finally had the dreaded but anticipated confrontation with this particular nurse. While writing admission orders at three in the morning on a very sick patient and anticipating going to the emergency room where I had two consults pending, the nurse approached me with two charts in her hand to get me to write Benadryl orders on patients that had insomnia. These two patients happened to be on my service, and I was very much aware that they both had Benadryl orders already, as I had been the one who had written them one or two days before.

"Please, I am really busy now," I said. "If you look at the orders you will note that the medications were already ordered by me in the last couple of days. If you just looked before calling, it would eliminate a lot of the pages you make and perhaps I could get a little sleep when I am done." The nurse could sense my aggravation but did not seem in any way sympathetic.

"I have a lot of work too and don't have time to look through all the orders or the med sheet." As if that answer was not bad enough, what followed was even worse: "...besides, if I don't get to sleep, you should not get to sleep either."

My attempt at trying to explain to her that while she worked an eight-hour shift, I was working thirty-six hours on a regular basis, did not elicit a favorable response.

When seven a.m. rolls around, you get to go home, whereas I have to continue to work a full day." I had reached my boiling point by this time.

"Not my problem, doctor. Remember, I did not choose your profession for you; you did that all on your own."

Her answer, as exasperating as it was, I have never forgotten. For although it was arguably cruel, it was also true. That particular interaction made me aware of the "superhuman" expectation that others sometimes demand from physicians and particularly surgeons. I no longer remember that particular nurse's face or name, but from that one interaction—as frustrating as it was, and as mad as it made me—I learned the solemn responsibility and sacrifice expected when one chooses to become a member of the healing professions.

Perhaps the most difficult nurse I worked with during my internship by far, was the charge nurse of the surgical floor at the VA hospital across from Jackson Memorial. Thankfully, I only worked there for two months during my intern year, but the struggles I endured in that service were momentous and disheartening. Part of the problem was that because of hospital and union rules, the VA floor nurses were not allowed to perform many procedures that were standard for nurses at Jackson Memorial Hospital. Things such as blood draws, EKGs, or blood cultures were not done by nurses at the VA hospital, but were the sole responsibility of the intern on call. I was introduced to these policies during my first night on call at the VA hospital, concerning a patient who had a fever.

It was the first night in a long time when I thought it might be possible for me to get a couple of hours of sleep while on call. The pager went off sometime close to midnight. "This is Ms. Colon on 9 North; Mr. Randolf in 947 has a temperature of 101.7." I knew Mr. Randolph; he had been admitted with acute cholecystitis several days before and had his gallbladder removed (cholecystectomy) two days prior.

"Ok, please give him Tylenol, send a CBC—" But she did not let me finish.

"We do not draw blood here, doctor. You have to do it."

I could not believe what I was hearing. Nurses that don't draw blood? I was about to inquire what it was they *did* do, but thought better of starting a confrontation. "Ok," I replied, "please have the supplies at bedside and I will come up to draw the blood momentarily."

In the same monotonous and uncaring tone of voice, she responded, "We don't get supplies for you here, doctor. You have to get them yourself."

Burning mad, I walked the few flights of stairs from my call room to 9 North. I found Ms. Colon and two other nurses sitting in a small room by the nurses' station drinking coffee and chatting.

"Why is it that you guys don't draw blood again?" I could not contain my anger.

"We are not allowed. Hospital rules." After answering, the three nurses continued to sip their coffee. It was obvious that I had interrupted an interesting conversation, as they did not seem so happy to see me.

"Where is the supply room?"

One of the other nurses pointed and told me it was around the corner. I left them and went to the door of the supply room only to find out that it was locked. "Where is the key?" I was back in the nurses' station, fuming by now. Ms. Colon took a key from around her neck as if to make a point and handed it to me without saying a word or even looking at me. I then went on a scavenger hunt to try to find all the supplies I needed. After several minutes and several trips back to Ms. Colon to retrieve a few other things, the blood draw and blood cultures were done.

When I inquired as to what paperwork I needed to send the labs, one of the nurses simply pointed to a drawer in the nurses' station. The drawer was full of many different forms from which, after some effort, I extracted the ones I needed. After labeling all the blood tubes and filling out the paperwork almost as if designed to add insult to injury, I once again heard the voice of Ms. Colon from inside the room where the three nurses were sitting and chatting.

"If you don't take it to the lab yourself, it will not get there until late tomorrow morning." I thought I heard them laugh as I walked towards the elevator carrying the blood bottles to the lab.

Multiple similar episodes dealing with the same overnight nursing crew left a bad taste. To this day, I shudder when I think of Ms. Colon's voice over the telephone. The sound of her voice alone used to raise my pulse considerably. Unfortunately, during the two months I covered the VA at night and dealt with this particular nursing crew, similar scenarios were more common than not.

I remember another episode when I was called because a patient had chest pain. As this could potentially be a serious issue (e.g., a heart attack), I anticipated that I might get a little more cooperation. That was not to be the case. Besides the blood draws, getting the respiratory technician to start oxygen, etc., I had to do an EKG myself. Finding the EKG machine was the first challenge. I had to inquire where it was, get the key to the room, take the machine to the patient's bedside, read the instructions on how to use it—as it was an antiquated machine somewhat different from the ones I was used to. Finally, I placed all the leads on the patient, and started to do the EKG only to find out that there was no paper in the machine, which would normally provide a printout of the patient's EKG tracing. Obtaining the paper was another ordeal, which took over half an hour. After unsuccessful attempts at finding it where the nurses said it would be, I ended up having to go to the ICU on the second floor to get it.

Exasperating is the most appropriate word I can use to describe my interaction with some of the nurses at the VA hospital during that particular rotation as an intern. I loved working with veterans and caring for them, for I have always believed they are the best our society has to offer. However, my early experiences with some of the nursing staff at the VA made it so that I did not like working there. In fairness, I found the VA ICU nurses to be top notch as well as most of the floor nurses, although there were certainly some bad apples. At the time, I could not help but think that some of these nurses should not have been allowed anywhere near patients. If the passion for it was never there or had been lost for some reason, health care practitioners should not be put in a position where their indifference can actually cause harm.

With time, the floor nursing situation improved at the VA, and services were added such as night phlebotomists who could do blood draws or perform other related tasks to relieve the workload on the busy residents. Unfortunately, I did not have the luxury of those services during my intern and second year of training. By the time I returned to the VA hospital for my senior rotations, Ms. Colon was no longer working there. She was not missed by most, especially me.

Besides the ups and downs with the floor nurses, there were certain units in the hospital known for having nursing staffs that were tough on residents, and especially interns. Two such places were the trauma resuscitation unit, and the ICUs, particularly the trauma ICU. The trauma resuscitation area is located on the first floor of the trauma center. It is here that trauma patients are brought in via ambulance and helicopter by paramedics. As most of these patients are critically ill and injured, they require expert care to be delivered in a timely fashion. More than the doctors, it is the nurses on that unit who are responsible for making it run smoothly.

The nurses who run and work in the trauma resuscitation unit are usually experienced emergency room nurses who have taken further training in trauma care. They are extremely sharp and able, and they have two main objectives: To make sure that trauma patients get diagnosed and treated in a timely manner, and to make sure they are triaged and moved from the unit as soon as possible to make room for other patients. To this end, these nurses push the residents to do their job in an efficient and timely manner. At times, these nurses can get quite aggressive and forceful in accomplishing this task.

From the first time I started going down to resus to help during my trauma rotation, it seemed that I could not do anything right. Either I was in the way or could not fulfill my intern responsibilities in a timely manner. If I took too long to draw the blood, the nurses would immediately call for the senior resident to do it. It became obvious from the beginning that they ran the show. At times I even saw them arguing with the second-year residents as to the proper plan of care and simply refuse or even contradict the second-year resident's orders when they felt they were not appropriate. More than once I saw second-year residents utterly frustrated, and even reduced to tears from having to deal with the trauma resus nurses.

Although these nurses did not have the extensive medical school training that the residents did, they had the advantage of having worked on the resus area for many years. Through repetition and study, they had learned how to manage the trauma patients, and they knew much more than interns and junior residents who had limited experience with the trauma service or were in their first trauma rotation. These nurses could be intimidating but were also a great resource and could offer helpful suggestions when one was lost as to what to do next in a particular situation.

Another area with a notoriously difficult nursing staff is the intensive care unit. These nurses are extremely good and have extensive training in the care of critically ill patients. Nurses are also strong patient advocates, and in certain wards like the ICU, nurses are fierce in the way they take to heart this solemn responsibility. They keep a close eye on the residents and interns to make sure they do not do anything that could lead to a negative outcome. These nurses can be blunt and upfront about questioning orders and will flatly refuse to follow a resident's order if they think the order is not appropriate—even to the point of insisting that the attending give approval of the order before they follow it. This can make it awkward for the residents and their interactions with patients. Although it is usually the senior residents and fellows who make the decisions in the ICU, it is the interns and junior residents who do the daily activity, implement most of the procedures, and have the most interactions with nurses. After rounds, it is usually the interns who write the orders and execute the treatment plan that was agreed upon.

I once experienced the uncomfortable sequelae of such an interaction while in the trauma ICU, trying to obtain consent from one of the patients in order to place a central intravenous line. These lines, as opposed to the regular peripheral IVs that one places in the arms, are placed in the larger veins of the neck and/or chest. They are used when the patient does not have good veins in the arms, or when certain medications need to be given that cannot be given via the other lines. These lines are a little more complicated to place and have the possibility of more significant complications such as bleeding or pneumothorax (air within the space between the lungs and the chest wall) when the lung tissue is damaged inadvertently by the needle.

One morning, while I was obtaining consent for a central line, the nurse approached the bedside to adjust some of the monitors. She overheard me talking to the patient and promptly interjected, "You are not going to do that without your senior." It was the policy of the ICU that when procedures such as central lines were to be done by the interns, that the senior residents had to be present to supervise. I was very much aware of this and had been instructed by my senior to get everything ready and then call him. Somehow the nurse, not seeing the senior present, surmised that it was my intention to do the procedure alone. Making such a statement in front of an already-concerned patient proved to be counterproductive.

"Are you doing this for the first time?" the patient inquired with fearful eyes.

"No," I answered.

Although technically correct, I knew the patient had some grounds for concern. This was to be my second central line, the first one being a failed effort in that I was not able to enter the vein after three attempts, requiring the senior resident to take over and finish the job. I tried to keep my composure while informing the nurse that the senior would come as soon as we were ready. I told the patient that the procedure was better done by two people and that my senior had extensive experience in doing these lines.

"Why is he not doing it then?" The question was expected, but I did not have a ready answer for it. The only response that came to mind was to say that it was the policy of the ICU to have the interns do the lines. This of course was not entirely true. By their second year, most surgery residents have done plenty of central lines and it was the unspoken, accepted protocol among residents that this was the opportunity for interns to learn to perform this procedure while being supervised and guided by more senior residents.

The placement of the central line went smoothly, as I got the line on the first stick. In the back of my mind, there was the added satisfaction of showing the nurse that I could perform the procedure without a hitch. She was not impressed. It was a painful realization several minutes later while reviewing the post-procedure chest X-ray to note that the lung on the side of the line had been punctured and the patient had a pneumothorax. One of the more difficult things that I had to do as an intern was to go up to the ICU and tell the patient, in front of the nurse, that his lung had been punctured during the procedure. I further had to explain that to remedy the situation we would have to insert a small tube through his chest wall into the pleural space so that we could suck out the air. The tube would have to remain in place for several days until the puncture in the lung had a chance to heal.

The patient was visibly upset, and I did not have the guts to look the nurse in the eyes. The patient made his wishes known that he wanted someone else to do the procedure. I told him the fourth-year senior resident would be the one doing it. Several minutes later, after collecting all the needed supplies for the procedure, I sheepishly went to collect the senior resident. He came over to the bedside and with an air of confidence of which I was envious, he proceeded to explain to the patient what had happened and what needed to be done.

"Dr. Garri will be placing a small tube in your chest," the senior resident was saying. I thought I should intervene.

"The patient requested that you do the chest tube."

The senior resident was not aware of what had transpired before his arrival. He took a seat next to the bedside, looked at the patient, and empathetically explained the situation. "The complication that you had is fairly common and could just as easily have happened if I had placed the line. Dr. Garri is a very capable doctor and will be able to do the chest tube without a problem. I will be here to make sure everything goes ok."

The patient immediately calmed down and agreed to let me do it. I was not so sure this was a great idea as this was to be my first chest tube placement. I surely did not want to make matters worse.

Although I had never done a chest tube before, I had watched many of them being done. Under the senior's direction and the watchful eyes of the nurse, the procedure went smoothly. A few minutes later sitting side by side in radiology, the senior and I were looking at the post-procedure chest film to check the position of the tube. While checking the film, I was explaining to him the reason for my previous comment about him doing the procedure by explaining what had taken place earlier with the nurse and how I had felt that her comment while I was getting the consent had made the patient lose confidence in me.

"You will have many complications during your residency," he said, speaking from dearly-earned personal experience. "It is better to deal with them honestly and expeditiously." He turned on his chair to face me as if to give emphasis to what he was about to say next. "Nurses, just like patients, will trust you when you come across as someone who appears confident and knows what he is doing."

Although I could not fully appreciate the extent of my inexperience at the time, later, as a senior resident and looking back, I became fully aware of how interns lack the knowledge and experience to deal with many situations they face in their first year. Nurses serve the important role of protecting patients from well-meaning interns and residents who can easily get in over their heads. As the years went by and my knowledge and experience increased, I noted that I was not getting in the way as much, and when taking care of patients, nurses were less and less likely to object or interfere with what I was doing. It was not lost on me that this change in how I was treated by the nurses occurred at the same time that my experience and self-confidence grew.

From my years as an intern, resident, and now attending surgeon in private practice, and after having worked with a multitude of nurses in all types of different situations, I've come to develop the utmost respect for their work ethic and their dedication to helping others. I've become the surgeon I am today in no small part by modeling great mentors, some of which have been nurses. I've learned from them the meaning of dedication, selfless service, and empathy. Some of the lessons learned from nurses were taught by example and gentle cajoling, while others were learned through "tough love"—for which I paid a dear price in extra effort, loss of sleep, and considerable mental aggravation. However, no matter how the lessons were taught and learned, looking back at them now, I am most grateful to all the nurses I've come in contact with throughout the years for those lessons, and for their selfless efforts in helping me take care of patients in need.

The First Hernia

The primary reason medical students go into surgery is that they love to operate. Why else would one endure the psychological and physical hardships that a surgical residency entails? Most interns, especially those in large university training programs, are initially disappointed with how little operating time they get during the first year. The internship year is mostly focused on giving the surgical trainee a broad education in the surgical specialties, and an understanding of how to care for the surgical patient before and after the operation. In large programs, there is an endless amount of work to be done on numerous patients. This workload falls on the interns primarily, which leaves little time for the operating room.

Most interns look at operating room time as their reward for putting in long, hard hours of work. Similarly, it is a long-held belief among surgical educators that the primary motivator and morale booster for surgical trainees is the ability to operate. Residents tend to complain about the long working hours and the difficult working conditions, but they are ultimately happy to endure those hardships as long as they are getting plenty of operating room time.

An intern's introduction to the operating room occurs in a subtle way. You might be asked to come and help with retraction during certain operations. Then again, you might be involved in suturing lacerations in the operating room. If you are particularly fortunate you might even be in a situation where you are the primary surgeon in small operations such as a biopsy or drainage of an abscess. These are high points in any intern's day, but the ultimate prize sought by one and all is the opportunity to do a "real" operation.

There are two operations in general surgery that have classically been considered the purview of interns and junior residents—the appendectomy (the removal of an infected appendix) and the inguinal (groin) hernia repair. These operations, which capture the imagination of experienced surgeons and all surgical trainees, can be extremely difficult technically and have been known to humble the most confident of interns and even senior residents. Nonetheless, most interns covet the opportunity to perform one of these "real" surgeries, and the first time an intern gets to do one of these is a seminal event, an occasion for celebration indeed.

Sometime during the latter part of my intern year, I was due to rotate in the surgical oncology (Elective 1 or E1) service. I was excited about this rotation because of the promise of a significant amount of operating room time. Not only does the intern in this service do a lot of breast biopsies, but in my case, I got to operate with the chief of the service, which meant the opportunity to do some inguinal (groin) hernia repairs—an elective procedure for which this chief was known and did on a regular basis. My opportunity to do appendectomies had come and gone unfulfilled during my trauma rotation. All of the emergency surgery at Jackson Memorial Hospital was done by the trauma service, which covered trauma as well as emergency room consults. During that rotation, a few patients had come in with acute appendicitis, but the operations were all claimed by the more senior residents, as my trauma rotation took place in the middle of the year and most of the second-year and senior residents had not yet gotten their fill of these procedures. Thus, the opportunity for me to do a hernia repair was something I very much looked forward to, as this would most likely be my last chance to perform one of these landmark operations during my internship year.

I had spent a great deal of time reading about this operation. My studies had informed me that hernia repairs, or herniorrhaphy as the procedure is technically called, had captured the imagination of many of America's and indeed the world's best surgeons. Many surgeons who historically were considered the fathers of the specialty of general surgery in the United States and the rest of the world had tackled the problem of groin hernias. Some of them had come up with their own techniques to surgically treat groin hernias. Many of these techniques are in use to this day and bear the name of the surgeons who developed them. It had been fascinating to read about some of these operations: the Bassini, the McVay, the Shouldice, the Lichtenstein technique, et al. Having an operation or a technique named after you is a great honor indeed.

My day finally came. I was to operate with Dr. Henry Willoughby, the chief of the service on a patient with a groin hernia. I arrived early in the preoperative area to meet and evaluate the patient. Mr. Zachs was a man in his forties, a professor at the University of Miami, who was otherwise healthy except for a left groin hernia. He told me how the hernia had been present for several years but had recently gotten slightly bigger and it was beginning to bother him. He had finally taken some time off to get it repaired. Eventually, Dr. Willoughby walked in and said hello to the patient in the preoperative holding area. As he was leaving to head to the locker room to change, he quickly asked me if everything was ready, to which I replied in the affirmative.

When interns and junior residents begin to operate, they of course have a certain amount of anxiety. You try to study the anatomy and read as much as you can about the disease process and the surgical techniques to treat it, because you are sure to be asked a multitude of questions during the procedure—not only about the disease process, but about the technical aspects of the operation and particularly the anatomy involved. You try to go in as prepared as possible, and you hope you remember all the information that you've read. Moreover, you hope that your hands will perform as you want them to, as there is plenty of pressure involved the first few times interns and residents do operations with which they are inexperienced.

The mixture of anxiety, nerves, and anticipation can wreak havoc on a young surgeon's confidence, and the first few minutes of an operation can set the stage for the rest of the case. A surgeon's confidence is always extremely important, but never more so than when the young surgeon is first learning to operate. At this point, the trainee has no previous reference on which to rely when things go wrong, and it is rather easy for the young surgeon to have his confidence shaken from the slightest mistake or unanticipated mishap in a case. When those instances occur, it is extremely easy for the young surgeon to panic, allowing things to spiral out of control.

From the beginning of this operation things did not go well for me. "I hope you did not shave the groin!" was the first thing Dr. Willoughby said when he walked into the room after the patient had been put to sleep. I was already scrubbed and gowned, standing at the patient's side after he had been prepped and draped, exposing his groin area which was half-shaved. Shaving the surgical site is a standard protocol to follow for all operations as a way to theoretically reduce the possibility of infection, although some surgeons prefer to drape the hair out of the way rather than shave it. Unbeknownst to me, given that I was operating with him for the first time, Dr. Willoughby was a member of this camp.

"Yes, I did," I said nervously, though I quickly added, "but only the one side." Dr. Willoughby was one of the most respected senior surgeons in the program and soon thereafter became the department chairman. He was known, though, for occasional off-color comments. He walked toward me and stood on the opposite side of the table. He took a few seconds to look at the patient's groin, and then looked up at me.

"After we finish, I am going to send you to talk to his wife and explain to her why her husband is going home with only half of his pubic hair." For a few seconds, I could not tell whether he was joking or serious. I then heard him laugh under his mask. "Now, let's go."

Dr. Willoughby asked the scrub nurse for a marking pen. He held it out for me and asked me to mark my incision. For a few seconds, my mind went blank. I was still thinking about the shaving mishap, and I found my mind completely devoid of all information on the anatomical landmarks and where to make my incision. My hand was shaking as I took the pen from his hand. My motions were slow and deliberate in an attempt to stall for enough time to remember the information.

"Well?" Dr. Willoughby was beginning to get impatient.

I mumbled something that even I could not understand. He could surely tell by now that I was nervous, and he attempted to make it easier for me. He asked me several direct questions and gave me some clues: "Where is the iliac spine?" "The pubis?" "The inguinal ligament?"

Things were now beginning to click, and I decided to take it from there. I told him where the incision should go and drew it on the patient. He took the pen from my hand and drew some cross marks where he wanted me to stop, since apparently, I had marked the incision a little too long for his taste. He then grabbed some local anesthesia and injected it along the planned incision and then some into the deeper tissue planes.

My mouth was about to open and request the surgical knife when I turned towards the nurse and saw the knife in her hand already extended towards me. It seemed that even she was getting a little impatient. I extended my left hand and she put the knife in it.

"God help us, a lefty!" Dr. Willoughby's voice had a jovial quality to it. I was beginning to feel more comfortable.

"Bilingual," I said as I put the knife to the skin and started to make my incision.

"You mean ambidextrous?"

"That too!" I laughed as my anxiety lessened slightly. He did not seem amused. I made my cut.

"Maybe next time you can cut the skin rather than scratch it," he suggested.

Once again, the sarcastic/jovial nature of Dr. Willoughby was coming through. I made a second cut all the way through the skin this time. Dr. Willoughby then placed retractors in the wound as he invited me to start my dissection. All the while, he began asking me about the layers that we were encountering in the dissection, and he would occasionally point to an anatomical structure and ask me to name it. I found it difficult to answer questions and work at the same time, so I had to stop to answer his questions.

It was then that I learned an important lesson: You are likely to overestimate your ability as a surgeon when you watch others do surgery, compared to when you are the one actually doing it. As an intern, I had spent a significant amount of time holding retractors and assisting other surgeons. Many times, I had been utterly frustrated as I saw residents struggling to perform specific tasks called for during certain operations. From my perspective, it seemed that these tasks they were struggling with were easy to do. I was sure that I could do them much faster and without any struggle. I was about to learn differently. What in my mind was conceptually easy, I simply could not get my hands to do. I felt slow, clumsy, and utterly useless at times during this first hernia operation.

"Ok, one of the things you are going to have to learn to do is to work and talk at the same time. At this rate, I will not make my meeting." Dr. Willoughby began to get more impatient.

I would eventually learn that Dr. Willoughby was a remarkably busy man and his schedule was always full of meetings. He began to do more and more of the operation. I did not mind; I was beginning to get completely lost in the anatomy. One of the things that residents learn early when they begin operating is that anatomical structures are much more difficult to identify in the live body than they are in books and in cadavers. In a textbook they are color-coded and depicted free of all adjacent soft tissue and structures. In true human dissection, these structures are encased in soft tissue, which makes their identification much more difficult. This is particularly true in inguinal hernias, where the bulging hernia tends to obliterate all the soft tissue planes and makes finding anatomical landmarks that much more difficult.

Before long, I was facing a lump of tissue which I knew contained the hernia sac as well as the spermatic cord, but it was impossible for me to tell which was which. Dr. Willoughby picked up the mass of tissue and slipped under it a large piece of rubber tubing (Penrose drain), which he used to pull the mass and separate it from the rest of the wound.

"Dissect the sac," he commanded, more to make a point than to actually allow me to do it. I did not know where to begin. It all looked the same to me and it was difficult to differentiate hernia sac from normal structures. "Where would the sac be located?"

I did know this answer. "The antero-medial aspect."

He held the tissue out to me. "Well, find it then."

My hands were holding dissecting scissors that I intended to use for the dissection.

"Let's make sure this man can still have babies after we are done." He took the scissors from my hands and instructed the nurse to hand me a hemostat, a much blunter dissecting instrument which minimized the amount of damage I could do. The baby reference was meant to remind me about the vas deferens, the anatomical tube-like structure that carries the sperm from the testicle to the penis and is one of the structures contained within the spermatic cord.

I began a clumsy, feeble attempt at dissecting the sac and soon it became obvious that he could not take it anymore.

"Here," he said, while using a moist gauze to separate the hernia sac from the rest of the cord within a few seconds. I marveled at what I was seeing, and I hoped that someday my skills would be comparable. He separated the sac entirely down to the base and shoved it back through the defect in the abdominal wall, the entire time pointing out to me the pertinent anatomy.

Although some of the newer hernia techniques advocate the use of a synthetic (Prolene) mesh in the repair so as to generate scar tissue, which in turn would lower the incidence of recurrence, Dr. Willoughby is one surgeon who falls into the more classical view that, when appropriate, standard techniques not utilizing foreign bodies (mesh) should be used. He informed me that we would not be using mesh. He helped identify and dissect the two tissue planes that we were to suture together in order to repair the defect in the abdominal wall, thus preventing the hernia from recurring.

The nurse then handed me the needle holders and forceps. The next step of the operation was even more of a struggle for me. Under the watchful eye of the professor, I attempted to place the sutures that would bring the two ligaments together. He would comment after each stitch and made me repeat most of them if he thought I was doing them wrong. When it was time to tie, things went from bad to worse. I had spent a great deal of time during medical school and throughout my internship year practicing my hand ties. Many nights, weekends, and at slow times while on call I had practiced my suturing and tying. I practiced the single and two-handed ties over and over again. By now my confidence was pretty high in my ability to perform these ties well at a fairly rapid rate.

Performing these ties deep in the wound, with bloody gloves and under pressure, was a completely different ballgame.

"Granny knot.""Air knot."

"Loose knot."

Dr. Willoughby called out after each of my ties that he did not like. He made me redo them until he was satisfied. I was much relieved when the last knot was tied. Next came closure of the wound, which presented its own challenges. Then, finally, it was all over. We put Steri-Strips (small adhesive strips) to cover the incision, removed the drapes, and just like that, my first hernia repair was done.

It had not been totally smooth, but I had completed my first groin hernia repair—albeit with some help and a great deal of difficulty. No matter, a great feeling of accomplishment, pride, and satisfaction came over me, and I could not wait to get home to call and tell my family, and just about anyone I knew. That feeling made worthwhile all the on-call nights, the long hours of work and study, and the many hardships I had overcome during my short time in residency. I knew there would be more tough times, but they could be endured with pleasure if I remembered to look forward to once again having the feeling of pride and satisfaction that I felt that day.

Over the course of the next five years, I was to perform close to fifty hernia repairs. I learned the many different techniques for performing this particular operation and learned to treat the many complications that can occur if this condition is left untreated. Toward the end of my training, I felt some sense that I had mastered groin herniorrhaphies while retaining respect for its nuances and potential, unexpected difficulties, which make this particular operation challenging at times even for the most experienced and talented of surgeons.

Although I soon forgot my second, twentieth, and even my last groin hernia repair, it will be almost impossible for me to ever forget my first "real operation" and my experience with Dr. Willoughby that particular day. It was the realization of a dream that brought with it a great deal of personal validation, satisfaction, and pride. The possibility that someday I would indeed become a surgeon was now within my mind's ability to grasp and accept as a future reality.

THE SECOND YEAR:

JUNIOR RESIDENT

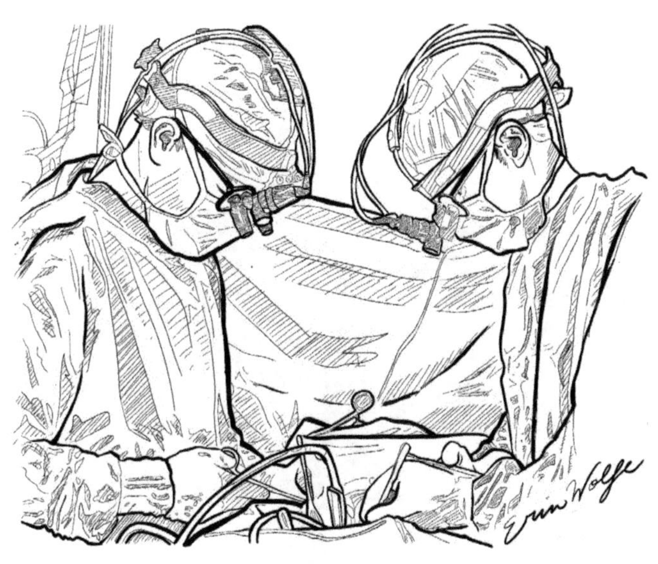

STAR POWER

While the internship year was divided into twelve month-long rotations, the second and all subsequent residency years were structured in two-month rotations, which allowed for residents to spend more time devoted to each discipline. I had started my second year in the trauma service and after being there for two weeks, I had already acclimated a bit and had gotten used to the rhythm of the service. The radio call began like any other that morning: "Miami Beach Rescue to JMH (Jackson Memorial Hospital)."

I was carrying the two large radios—affectionately called "the bricks"—which the second-year trauma resident always carries, through which all ambulance traffic to the trauma center and to the city of Miami is triaged and routed. It is the job of the second-year trauma resus resident to take these calls from the ambulances, triage them appropriately, and make sure they go to the correct facility in the city. When it came to trauma victims, there were criteria as to which patients needed to come to a level 1 trauma center like Jackson Memorial Hospital. Any penetrating injury—such as gunshot or stab wounds—to a vital cavity—head, chest, or abdomen—met those criteria.

"JMH K" was my answer, thereby informing the crew on the rescue truck that I was listening and ready for their information.

"JMH, we have a male with gunshot wounds to the head. Vitals are pulse 120, systolic blood pressure of sixty. ETA is five minutes."

"Rescue, proceed to the JMH trauma center and advise of any changes en route." I had been in the process of completing a consult in the emergency room. I immediately stopped what I was doing and started walking towards the trauma center resus area, a mere forty to fifty yards away.

I was tired, as this was technically not my call day; I was supposed to have gone home by eight or nine a.m. immediately after change-over rounds. In those days, however, the trauma teams alternated calls every other day. One team would come in, work twenty-four hours, and sign out to the other team, only to return the next day for another twenty-four-hour shift. As the second-year resident on the service in charge of the trauma resuscitation area, my schedule was no different. I was alternating with one of my best friends that year, Dr. Tarik Borges, who was an oral and maxillofacial surgery resident doing a year of general surgery. A native of Tennessee, he spoke with a heavy Southern accent and was known among his friends as "Elvis."

Tarik had a wife and two young kids, and he had expenses that he could not cover on a resident's salary. As such, he had taken a job with one of the air-ambulance companies. Moonlighting during residency was strictly prohibited, so he kept this endeavor secret except from a few of us who might find themselves in a position to have to cover for him, as I was doing that particular morning.

The night before had been extremely busy, and sometime around three a.m. I had received a page to a cell phone. When I called the number, the Southern accent and familiar voice were unmistakable.

"Hey Joe, this is Tarik." At three a.m. this call could only mean one thing. Tarik was stuck somewhere and needed me to cover for him. It turned out that the day before, Tarik had flown with the air-ambulance company to Cartagena, Colombia, to pick up a patient and transport him to Iowa. He was calling me from somewhere in Iowa with an interesting story.

"As we were taking off to fly back home," he said, "one of the engines blew."

"Are you ok?" My immediate concern was for his safety.

"Yeah, I'm alright." Tarik sounded stressed. "I tried to get the pilot to continue on one engine so that I would not be late for call, but he refused. He said it was too dangerous and that the plane might crash." I was not sure that this part of the story was true but such behavior was within the realm of possibility when it came to Tarik.

"Sorry bud," he continued, "they are flying me commercial, but I won't be able to make it to the hospital until after one p.m. I need you to cover for me."

I told him it would be no problem. Tarik and I were great friends and I liked working with him. No matter how tired I was, it would be a pleasure to do him this favor. At morning report, I was trying to come up with a way to tell the trauma surgery attending that I would be covering the radios for a few more hours, without getting Tarik in trouble. However, Tarik had already taken care of that.

"Joe," the attending began, "I just received a call from Tarik. He is having a bit of a family emergency and will not be in to work until after one o'clock this afternoon."

"No problem. I will take care of the bricks until then," I said, relieved that I did not have to come up with my own lie, or worse—a story line that differed from the one Tarik had already given. The attending gave me a somewhat puzzled look as if he had not anticipated that I would have agreed so readily.

"Please call neurosurgery." I was addressing Jen-Jen, the secretary on the trauma desk, while beginning to put on the protective gown, booties, gloves, and face shield for the trauma case as was the norm. From the rescue crew communications, I knew the injuries were limited to the patient's head, so I anticipated that I was going to need neurosurgery's help. Thankfully, the neurotrauma service operated routinely at the trauma center and I knew at this time of day they would not be that far away.

What I heard next over the radio was truly unexpected: "JMH, this is Miami Beach Rescue, we have a name for you... Gianni Versace."

Calling a victim's name over the radio was never routine; it was the first time I had experienced it. The name did not register with me, so I was somewhat perplexed as to why it had been given.

"Ask for the name again." Jen-Jen had suddenly stopped entering the text page which went to all the doctors on the trauma team so they would convene at resus. She was now looking at me.

"This is JMH to Miami Beach Rescue; please repeat your last transmission."

The radio communications through the bricks were simultaneously played through speakers throughout the resuscitation area and other locations on the first floor of the Ryder Trauma Center. This was done so that the entire trauma personnel would be alerted simultaneously about trauma patients due to arrive, to allow time for everyone who was to participate in the action to come and assume their place and start getting ready. Simultaneously the trauma desk secretary, upon also hearing the transmission, would send a text page to all members of the trauma team in case they were elsewhere and could not hear the communication through the speakers. Thus, many people heard the transmission real-time as my communications with the rescue squad was taking place. One of them as per protocol was Jen-Jen, the trauma desk secretary.

The voice came over the radio a few seconds later. "JMH, the name is Gianni Versace." The name still did not register, and I could not figure out why the ambulance crew felt it necessary to give the name of the victim over the radio. However, Jen-Jen knew. "That's the fashion designer who owns a house in Miami Beach."

I had been in Miami for just over one year by then and also lived in Miami Beach. This information was news to me, but I was not known for my sartorial prowess, as my usual garb at the time was limited to surgical scrubs in different shades of green.

"Why would they be telling us the name?" I inquired from Jen-Jen.

Now some of the nurses were beginning to gather around the trauma desk listening to the transmission. Jen-Jen again knew the answer as she had been through similar episodes before. "It is because they want us to be ready for all the media people who are going to be descending on us in the next few minutes. They are alerting us to be ready for some crowd control."

I was aware that the media monitored the transmissions to the trauma center. While on the roof of the Ryder Trauma Center to pick up patients brought in by helicopter, I often saw media trucks parked on the top floor of the adjacent parking garage. TV crews filmed us as we went out with a stretcher to the helicopter in order to pick up particular patients. On more than one occasion my family and friends let me know that they had seen me on the local news as TV stations used that footage when running stories about trauma victims who were brought to Ryder. Once the media realized who our next patient was going to be, the amount of attention and interest focused on the trauma center was going to be intense.

Unfortunately, it turned out that it was not just the media we would have to contend with. Within the next couple of minutes, as the members of the trauma team were beginning to come down and congregate in the resus area, there were many others who began to show up as well. The call had come mid-morning, a busy time in the hospital when there were many people around. They had obviously heard my conversation with the rescue personnel and were attracted like bees to honey. Nurses, medical students, other ancillary staff, and others began to migrate toward the trauma resuscitation area. Before the paramedic truck got there, a fairly large group of people had already gathered. I did not have time to worry about that. I had to get ready. Then the voice came over the radio one more time: "JMH, this is Miami Beach Rescue. We have lost vital signs. Repeat, we have lost vital signs. ETA two minutes."

When the double-door to the trauma center opened to let in the ambulance crew and the patient, I could see that many more people were gathering outside as well. The rescue team came running in with the patient on a stretcher and one of the paramedics performing CPR while another was ventilating the intubated patient with an Ambu bag. As soon as the patient was transferred to the trauma stretcher, I positioned myself on his right. My left hand went to his neck to palpate for the tracheal rings to make sure they were midline. With my stethoscope in my right hand, I auscultated (listened to) the right and left lung for breathing sounds. I could hear breathing, which confirmed that the breathing tube was well-positioned and the patient was being ventilated in both lungs. Simultaneously my left hand was palpating for a pulse in the neck; there was none. By this time, the EKG leads were already positioned. I looked at the monitor for a heart rhythm; there was none as a flat line was clearly evident on the monitor. I directed members of the trauma team to restart chest compressions.

As the intern started chest compressions, I opened the patient's eyes and looked at the pupils. The eyes were both swollen with the left showing signs of contusion or bruising. Both pupils were dilated and did not respond to light. The anesthesiologist concurred with my findings that the breathing tube was well-positioned in the trachea; he took over the job of ventilating the patient. I came around at the top of the bed and palpated the patient's head. My fingers immediately fell into two holes in the back of the head about the size of quarters. Ragged bony edges could be palpated in the periphery, but I could tell the holes were deep indeed, consistent with findings of gunshot wounds.

I caught the eyes of one of the paramedics who was now standing by the resus bay door. "Any other injuries?"

He shook his head no. "Just the head, two shots. We did not see any exit wounds."

By this time, the nurses had IVs on each of the patient's arms and fluids were being pushed. Blood had been collected and sent to the lab. The intern and one of the medical students were alternating doing chest compressions. We quickly turned the patient—as per protocol—to make sure there were no back injuries. There were none. There was nothing else to do except wait for neurosurgery and continue with what is called the ACLS (Advanced Cardiac Life Support) protocol. I was told by the nurse that neurotrauma was aware and were coming over.

While still giving chest compressions, two quick head X-rays were taken at ninety degrees to one another to locate the projectiles in the skull. As far as I could tell, there were two entrance wounds in the back of the skull and there were no exits. One of the bullets was most likely located close to the front of the skull and causing all the bruising and swelling around the left eye. The patient had a neck collar partially obstructing the neck from view so I could not confirm whether or not there might be an exit wound there, although the rescue crew had already stated that they had not seen any.

One to two minutes later, Dr. Gottenger walked in. He was the chief of neurotrauma with whom I had worked on that service a year prior during my first rotation. I was happy to see him. "What's going on?"

He was wearing scrubs most likely after coming straight from the operating room, and as he put on his second set of gloves, I gave him a quick description of the situation. "He has two gunshot wounds to the back of the head, no heart rhythm, and his pupils are dilated."

Dr. Gottenger quickly maneuvered himself next to me at the head of the table. He palpated the head as I had previously done and quickly found the two holes. "Stop compressions!" His eyes went over to the monitor behind us as the intern stopped compressions and everyone stepped back from the table. A flat line was now again showing on the EKG monitor. Dr. Gottenger then opened the patient's eyes and inspected the pupils each in turn.

"There is nothing we can do here; we are going to call this." Everyone stopped their activities, stepped back from the stretcher, and slowly began to walk out of the room. Dr. Gottenger was taking off his gloves when he turned a little towards me.

"We are going to have to talk to the media. You want to come?" I was a little behind on some consults and now had to do all the paperwork for this event.

"Not if you don't need me." I did not relish the thought of having to take time from my busy workload. I wanted to make sure to finish everything pending so I could bolt out of the hospital the moment that Tarik Borges walked into the hospital to relieve me of the bricks.

The curtains to the trauma room had been drawn, but the moment I walked out of the room I realized that the news had traveled fast. There were many people in the trauma resuscitation area now. While typing the resuscitation encounter note in the computer adjacent to the trauma desk, the numerous conversations going on around me regarding the event made it difficult to concentrate. Many were speculating as to the cause of the shooting. Some thought it was a robbery attempt, which seemed unlikely to me as the shooting had taken place in the middle of the morning in a very populated area of South Beach. Soon after, the public relations people from the hospital had to be called to deal with all the reporters who were converging on the trauma center. They were also instrumental in dealing with the chaos taking place in the trauma resus area. After a few minutes, people finally began to slowly file out, and I was left to finish my work.

The media session went off without me as my attention was focused on my paperwork and on the consults pending in the emergency room. The trauma was light for the rest of that morning, and I was thankful for the quiet time. Upon finishing another consult in the emergency room, I had stopped by the radiology room to check some radiographs. At that time, all radiographs taken in the emergency room and in the trauma center were placed on one of three viewing boards located in a small room on the first floor. The radiologists sat in this room and read the radiographs as they were brought in. It was also the job of the second-year resident in charge of resus to personally review all films taken on all patients brought to resus so as to document pertinent findings in the resus encounter note.

I had looked at the films on the emergency room board and was now sitting in front of the trauma board looking at several films from patients who were still in the trauma bay. There were two buttons on the machine that would allow me to scroll through a series of films until I found the one needed. I was scrolling when two head radiographs came into the viewer. They were radiographs of a skull on lateral and frontal view. Two large projectiles were clearly evident within the skull. One of them had traveled from the back of the skull and was lodged in the front of the skull by the eyes. Small metal fragments were evident throughout the trajectory. The other projectile had stopped somewhere in the middle of the brain.

"Is it true that they brought Versace there?" While looking at the radiographs, I had answered a phone call from one of my fishing friends who was not a doctor and was not in any way associated with the hospital. He had obviously heard about the incident from news reports. By now the news about the shooting was on the radio and TV. My friend knew that I was rotating in trauma that month and called to inquire about what I knew.

"Yes, but he did not make it. As a matter of fact, I was just looking at the skull X-rays. There are two bullets in the brain."

"Take the films," he immediately replied.

At first his suggestion seemed like a joke, but when he insisted, it became obvious that he was serious. "Take them," he repeated, "they will be valuable, I am sure we can sell them." It was difficult for me to understand how someone could think of such a thing at such a time. Even worse, it was quite disturbing that my friend thought so little of me as to seriously believe that I would give any consideration to his request.

Putting aside the insensitivity of his suggestion, just the thought of stealing films to try to sell them was disturbing and macabre. For a few seconds, I pondered what would make someone think of such an idea in the middle of a tragic event. Then I thought about all the people who had come down to the resuscitation unit upon learning of the patient's identity. In our modern, celebrity culture, there was no denying the strong pull of the curiosity many people feel about the lives of those who inhabit that world.

It was not until about an hour later that I had occasion to visit the radiology room one more time to review films on some of the new patients. While scrolling through the board, I noticed that the skull radiographs with the bullets were missing. I thought perhaps the radiologists had taken them down from the board for safekeeping, but they denied doing that. After talking to the radiologists, technicians, and clerks, I became convinced that the radiographs had been stolen. It seemed that my friend was not the only person to think of taking the films. The thought of it made me sad.

Several days later, Andrew Cunanan, the man believed to have shot Mr. Versace, was surrounded by the police in a boat house in Miami Beach. The old boat houses, which have since been replaced by boat slips, were located on the west side of Millionaire's Row. This is a broad, six-lane section of Collins Avenue north of 41st Street in Miami Beach, which is lined on both sides by luxury condominium buildings. When the news came over the TV that he had attempted suicide, the trauma center was asked to prepare for a similar situation to the one that had taken place days before. Unfortunately for Mr. Cunanan, he was declared dead at the scene and was never brought to the trauma center.

Dr. Tarik Borges eventually made it to the hospital a bit after two p.m. He was apologetic when he saw how utterly exhausted I looked. "No problem, Tarik," I said with a smile, as I gave him the radios, which seemed to be getting heavier by the minute. I signed out to him and walked to my call room to pick up my bag. As I exited the trauma center building and walked to the parking lot across the street, I could see that there was still much excitement around the trauma center. There were police all around and many press people in the main lobby and just outside the door. There were multiple TV station vans and trucks all around the trauma center and in the parking lot across the street. As for me, I was extremely happy to finally be going home.

Over the course of the next several days, the hospital censured a significant number of employees who, without medical indication, had logged onto the hospital computer to seek information regarding the death of Mr. Versace. My trauma chart entry, his lab results, etc., suddenly had become a great source of interest. Many hospital employees could not resist the curiosity to seek information regarding the event. In an environment where patient privacy is highly valued, it is a challenge for hospitals to control access to information needed for patient care while at the same time ensuring patient privacy. This particular event taught me about the strong lure that popular culture has for most of us, including medical professionals who know the importance of patient confidentiality and who are theoretically trained not to let such issues cloud their emotions or change anything about how they carry out their job.

About two weeks after the incident, I ran into an acquaintance who was a lab tech in the blood bank lab on the second floor of the main hospital. Trauma resus patients routinely had their blood drawn as part of the resuscitation protocol and sent to the blood bank lab for type and crossing in case blood transfusions were required. The trauma resus resident working that day was considered the doctor of record of any patient for the purpose of ordering those lab studies, and the name of that resident was thus included on all lab paperwork.

"I saw that the request on the blood slip on Versace had your name on it. Did you take care of him?"

After I answered in the affirmative, he drew me closer. "You know, we took some of the blood and ran an HIV test on it. Do you need to know the results?"

"Nooooo!" As I said it, I motioned to put my hands over my ears, turned, and walked away.

The way the question was framed was most likely a well-intentioned attempt to give me pertinent information in the case that I had somehow been contaminated with the patient's blood through direct contact, needle-stick injury, etc. At that time during the middle to late part of the 1990s, an AIDS diagnosis was still considered fatal. For those of us in the medical profession and particularly in surgery, that was a reality we all lived with and was ever-present in the back of our minds. Needle-stick injuries and other forms of contamination with patients' bodily fluids were always a concern. If that ever happened, we would make it a point to ask the patient or next of kin to allow us to perform an HIV test on them, to figure out if the medical personnel were at risk. In the trauma resus area, however, if the patient in question expired and no next of kin was ever found, the test would be performed by administrative decree, again in order to know how to advise the health care provider involved. I never knew nor did I inquire as to whether this HIV test was done due to someone being contaminated or simply by some of the lab techs involved who were curious as to the results.

As I walked away down the hall after my interaction with the lab tech, I felt the strong pull of curiosity to know the information that he offered to share. Running in my mind through the entire scene of what took place in the trauma bay one more time, I searched for the slightest possibility that I might have come into contact with the patient's blood, which would justify me knowing the answer. I remembered the sharp bony edges as I palpated the skull, but thankfully I had not been pricked or contaminated in any way. As I resigned myself to never knowing that answer, I became acutely aware how the strong gravitational pull of all stars, both celestial and of this world, affects us, including those who like to think of themselves as being immune.

Mr. Cunanan had assaulted several homosexual men shortly before his fatal attack on Mr. Versace. This led to some speculation at the time that Mr. Cunanan might have been targeting men who possibly could have infected him with HIV. These rumors were short-lived, however, when press reports revealed the HIV lab test results taken during Mr. Cunanan's autopsy were negative. Mr. Versace's family has always insisted that so was he.

Becoming A Doctor

Residents interact with medical students throughout the course of their residency. It is in the second year, however, that the resident begins to assume more of a supervisor/teacher role. During the internship year, the surgical trainee is mostly concerned with taking care of him or herself and are totally focused on getting their work done. Most interns, not being far removed from medical school themselves, lack the self-assuredness and confidence to assume the role of teachers.

It is not until the second year that the surgical trainee truly internalizes the profound difference that the first year makes in their ability to perform as physicians. Interns enter a residency with a solid medical education, but they lack the experience that comes from taking care of patients, and the self-confidence that comes from performing as a physician with a certain degree of autonomy. During the clinical rotations, medical students are closely supervised, and everything they do, including their notes and orders, needs to be cosigned by the residents. The moment that medical students become interns, they are exposed to situations where they become the responsible parties and have to make decisions without immediate back-up or supervision. When this responsibility is first encountered, it is usually accompanied by a significant amount of anxiety. This feeling can last for some time, but eventually dissipates as the interns gain experience on the job.

It is not until the resident commences his/her second year, has had time for introspection as well as the chance to work with medical students and interns, that he/she begins to realize the remarkable change that has taken place over the previous year. The internship year is a key element in the process of the medical student transitioning to a full-fledged physician. This change does not take place at the graduation ceremony from medical school as that ceremony is meant to signify, but rather through the hard work and clinical interaction of the internship year of any medical or surgical training program. Rather than an immediate transformation, it is more of an imperceptible, gradual evolution.

Medical school is broadly divided into two years of didactic instruction and two years of clinical work. During the third and fourth year, the medical students rotate through the different medical and surgical specialties. There are rotations that take place during the third year in fields considered core such as internal medicine, general surgery, obstetrics, et al. During the fourth year, there are typically two more extensive rotations called sub-internships in medicine and surgery. The remaining rotations are essentially electives where students choose fields of medicine in which they would like further exposure and experience.

Medical students by and large greatly enjoy their surgery rotations. It gives them the opportunity to experience the awesome power of surgery and what a significant difference it can make in a patient's life. They also learn firsthand the great sense of satisfaction that comes from the ability to quickly and dramatically change the progression or outcome of diseases, some of which can even lead to a fatal outcome, if not for the intervention of the surgeon. The workload involved in the surgical rotations during medical school is extensive, but most students endure it with a great sense of enthusiasm and vigor.

Surgical residents deal with students at different levels of their clinical education. During most rotations, the resident works with third-year students. These students are inexperienced as they are just beginning their clinical rotations and are working with patients for the first time. Fourth-year medical students who are doing either externships or electives are much more experienced and can be a source of great help to interns and residents alike. What is almost universally common to all students is their enthusiasm and desire. The clinical rotations are the first time in their long educational journey that medical students get a taste of what it is like to be a physician. For the overwhelming majority of them, this is the realization of a dream. Their optimism can be infectious, and at times reminds tired and wary residents what it was like for them to first discover what being a doctor really meant.

I always enjoyed working with medical students. Not only were they a great source of help in getting the work done, but their presence always created a much more educational and academic environment. Even as an intern, it was always my philosophy to teach them what I could and fan the fire for medicine which I knew they harbored. However, medical students can also be a source of anxiety for residents, particularly interns. Medical students tend to ask many questions that interns and even residents are not always able to answer. Some interns dealt with this situation by staying away from medical students to a great degree. I decided early on to embrace my ignorance and was quick to let them know when I did not know the answer to their questions. I did make it a point, however, to try to find the answer when I had the time so that I could share it with them later.

As I began my second year, however, the amount of knowledge and experience gained from my internship year was becoming evident and my confidence in dealing with medical students grew commensurately. Now I was able to answer most of their questions and felt that I could contribute to their education in a significant way. It was a great pleasure for me to share with them the passion I felt for surgery; they responded in kind by exhibiting a great desire to learn. It was my experience that students love their surgery rotation, and most of them, even if just for a fleeting moment, entertain a career in surgery at one point or another during the rotation.

For those who seriously considered a surgical career and asked for my advice as to whether or not I thought it was worth it, I always found it hard to advise them one way or the other despite my strong personal commitment to the specialty. In order to explain to them what surgery residency was like, I used to convey a conversation I once had as a medical student, when I asked a chief resident the same question. He had a way to elucidate the issue that I have not yet heard surpassed by anyone else to this day.

"What kind of activities do you really enjoy?" he asked in response to my question. I commented that I liked to SCUBA dive and play golf.

"Let's take golf," he said. "Now, suppose that you are given a job which is to play golf all the time, every day for at least twelve hours per day. Then every third day you have to stay up all night and play golf. Then at any time when you are at home, you can be called in the middle of the night so that you can wake up and go play golf, and so on..."

From his explanation, I was beginning to get the picture.

He added, "Surgery training is like doing something you really like to do, except doing it to the point that it makes you sick of it, as it is all you do. Not just for the five years during your training, but then for a majority of the time for countless years after that while in practice. If you can live with that and think you would still like surgery, then by all means, you should do it."

That explanation more than any other encapsulated for me what it had been like to be a surgical resident and a practicing surgeon after that. Thankfully after these many years, I am still as passionate as ever about being a surgeon.

Despite their level of interest in surgery, I always found it special to work with third-year students and be a part of their introduction to surgery. During my trauma rotation as a first- and second-year resident, it was my job to spend a significant amount of time teaching students how to do basic procedures like intravenous lines, blood draws, and the repair of simple lacerations. It was interesting to see how different students reacted to such tasks. Some were extremely motivated to do more and more. Others, especially those who were less hands-on and had already ruled out surgery as a future career, tended to be a little more timid about taking on extra responsibilities, especially if it meant performing procedures or spending time in the operating room.

Besides the hard work involved, another aspect of medicine that medical students and young doctors rarely think about—but which becomes very real as medical students start their rotations and interact with patients, for some students painfully so—are the health risks that all physicians face in one way or another as part of carrying out their chosen profession. Medical students from their first year of medical school learn about communicable diseases and the mode of transmission for each. At that time though, these risks are abstract and esoteric. During the surgery rotation, these risks become a clear and present danger as rotating medical students, just like all residents and attending surgeons, are routinely exposed to patients' blood and other bodily fluids as part of their day-to-day activities.

Lea and Junco were husband and wife, both of whom were third-year medical students when I was rotating through the trauma service. They had decided to do their rotations together as having the same schedule would allow them more time with each other. I was fond of them, as they were excellent students who did their work efficiently and well. Although neither of them desired to pursue a career in surgery, they were both extremely enthusiastic about doing the ward work and spending time in the operating room.

I was called to help on a case one day and while scrubbing, I saw Lea walk out of the adjacent operating room with a distressed look on her face. As I was expected in the operating room promptly, I did not have time to inquire as to her distress. After finishing the case, I walked up to the floor to assess what was going on with the service. The call team usually had four to six medical students on at one time, and Lea and Junco were two of the medical students on call that day. After failing to find them on the floor, I assumed that they were either eating or taking a break. I was later informed by one of the other residents that they had gone to physician's services because Lea had sustained a needle-stick injury in the operating room. It was not difficult to imagine how bad she felt. Unfortunately, I had already experienced needle-stick injuries myself, and I was very much aware of the fear and trepidation each of those incidents brought to mind, particularly anyone's first time.

It was about two hours later when I got to see Lea and Junco again. They had come from the infirmary and Lea was still visibly upset. "I heard what happened," I offered as they approached. Lea did not talk, but it was obvious that she had been crying. Junco handed me a piece of paper.

"We are going to need consent from the patient for HIV and hepatitis testing." I told them I would take care of it as soon as the patient was awake enough after the surgery to give consent.

Junco seemed upset as well. He shook his head, and it was obvious that he felt bad for his wife, but he also seemed mad. "I can't believe it. He sticks my wife in the operating room and does not even apologize or seem to care." He was referring to the attending surgeon involved on the case.

I tried my best to diffuse the situation. "These things happen, and they are never intentional." It took me several minutes to explain to them that the attending probably felt terribly about the whole thing, but his first priority was to take care of the patient under his immediate care in the operating room. I further told them that unfortunately, no matter what precautions you take, accidents do happen when you are in a setting like the operating room, with surgical blades, needles, and other sharp instruments around. I shared with them my own personal experiences with needle-stick injuries. I said that the data available suggest that the chances of contracting a disease like HIV or hepatitis are exceedingly small. This information may be comforting, but it never eliminates the angst felt by those who experience such an injury, as I had already learned firsthand.

They had gone to the employee health office and Lea had gotten blood drawn for baseline labs and had received a tetanus injection. The next step was to talk to the patient and find out if she was infected with any diseases that could be transmitted via contamination with bodily fluids. It just so happened that the patient was an elderly woman who had presented with a gallstone related infection. Her profile suggested that she was a low risk for having any of the concerning infections. To be sure, however, we would need to test her blood and I promised them that I would talk to the patient as soon as possible.

Their last question centered on whether Lea should take AIDS-related medications until the results were back. The recommendations at the time were to take a particular medication called AZT, starting as soon as possible after the injury. Data suggested that if the patient was positive for HIV, taking this medication after needle-stick injuries would decrease the chances that the person injured would contract the disease. As the side effects of these medication were minor in the short-term as far as was known at the time, I told Lea and Junco that it would be my recommendation to strongly consider taking the medications as I had done when I was stuck the first time.

It was not my prerogative to send them home; this was the decision of the chief resident. But I did tell them to go take a break for a while. "Come back to the floor when you guys feel better. We will cover for you here." They seemed thankful and went off toward the cafeteria. As they walked off, I thought about how scared I had been as a medical student when I sustained my first needle stick while drawing blood. Of course, you take all precautions to avoid such injuries, and during medical school you are taught the proper use of needles and other items you need for blood draws, starting intravenous lines, etc. However, no matter how hard you try to prevent it from happening, it is inevitable that injuries occur. For physicians and nurses, especially those involved in the surgical specialties, occupational injuries are a reality. You try to take every precaution to prevent them, but when they do occur, one is never prepared. Although HIV is perhaps the most feared risk, other diseases such as hepatitis C are a more significant concern due to a much higher probability of transmission during these types of injuries. By the time surgical residents finish their residencies, most of them have sustained several needle sticks and other sharp injuries. It is something you never get used to, and every time it happens, it is a cause for worry and concern. The first time it happens can be psychologically devastating. I felt terrible for Lea. After I called and recommended it to the chief resident, he agreed to let Lea and Junco go home for the night and settle their emotions before returning to work the next day.

That next day, with a nurse standing by my side, I found myself at the patient's bedside explaining to her why we needed her blood to test it for HIV and hepatitis. Thankfully, the patient was extremely nice, understanding, and quickly agreed to the test. She further expressed concern for Lea and told me to tell her that she hoped everything would work out okay. And so it did. All the tests came back negative on the patient and on Lea several days later. Upon receiving the patient's negative results, Lea immediately stopped taking the AZT. She and her husband graciously expressed their gratitude for my help. For the rest of their rotation, neither of them was very keen to go to the operating room and scrub.

Both Lea and Junco did very well during their surgery rotation, and both graduated from medical school with honors. Not surprisingly, they both went into nonsurgical fields and currently are in private practice together in the same office. They occasionally refer me patients. Their trust in me is as gratifying as it was to have them as my medical students during their surgery rotation many years ago. I've genuinely enjoyed seeing their transformation from medical students to excellent, empathetic, and caring physicians. We are all grateful that their needle-stick story, as well as their lives together, had a happy ending.

As for me, I've unfortunately sustained several other needle-stick injuries since that time, thankfully none for the last several years and none that resulted in permanent consequences. Every time one of those incidents occurs, the echoes of prior episodes of psychological distress related to such incidents come to mind, and I'm reminded of Lea and her introduction to the potential health risks that physicians assume for the privilege of practicing their chosen profession. I've come to think of these occupational injuries as a preventable but often unavoidable rite of passage on our way to becoming surgeons and an ever-present risk of practicing our chosen profession.

The Heart Of The Matter

Most of us began the second year excited. Finishing our internship was a great accomplishment, and it was a relief to no longer be the person at the bottom of the totem pole. The second year promised more responsibility and operating room time. Moreover, there were particular rotations in the second year that all general surgery residents looked forward to, such as trauma and cardiothoracic surgery.

Heart surgery is a two-year fellowship after the completion of general surgery. This specialty is considered by many to be the quintessence of surgery. There is something about operating on the heart that appeals to the imagination of all surgeons. As it is a difficult specialty to get into, it attracts the best and brightest of the general surgery graduating class. Furthermore, the training fellowship is one of the most demanding of all the subspecialties.

During my second year, general surgery residents spent two months on the cardiothoracic service. One month was spent at Jackson Memorial Hospital, and the other month was spent at the VA hospital, located one block away. Both services were extremely busy, and these two months were among the most demanding of the year. Although all residents had the hope of operating on the heart, as a second-year resident one rarely had the opportunity to do that. In the operating room, the resident's responsibility was to harvest the leg vein that is often used for the "bypass" grafts, and to hold the heart while the attending surgeon and the fellow connected the grafts to the coronary arteries of the heart and the aorta. One also would get to help the fellows open and close the chest. At the VA hospital, however, the involvement of the second-year resident was more significant. Often, he/she and the fellow did most of the case, while the attending surgeon had limited involvement. Some residents even had the opportunity to perform the suturing of the grafts to the heart native vessels; this was considered to be a great privilege among the lucky second-year residents who got to do it. I happen to have been one of the lucky ones.

The second-year residents would also round on all the patients on the service both in the ICU and on the floor, and they would do daily rounds with the fellows. In addition, there were multiple patients all over the hospital who had chest tubes that required daily follow-up. These patients were almost exclusively the responsibility of the second-year resident, who after getting all the floor work done was expected to go down to the operating room and assist in the surgeries. The fellows in cardiothoracic surgery had a reputation for being difficult to work with, as they were always on edge due to the immense amount of stress they were under.

It was not long after the start of our second residency year that my fellow residents started talking about the first-year cardiothoracic surgery fellow covering Jackson Memorial Hospital. Although most residents liked him personally, they found it extremely difficult and frustrating working with him. I was a little apprehensive myself as the start of my rotation approached. Comforted by the thought that there were still two weeks to go before the start of my rotation, I had decided to not think about it anymore. I was determined to drive that bridge from my mind until it came time for me to cross it. This mental respite did not last long, because the week prior to the start of the rotation I was paged by the first-year cardiothoracic fellow saying that he wanted to set up a meeting with me and the other two residents who were scheduled to start the rotation. He then called a second time several hours later with a date and time for the meeting. This was highly unusual as I had never heard of or experienced a pre-rotation meeting of this sort.

Dr. Gregorio Esposito was all of five foot six and spoke with a heavy Italian accent. He was a little older than the rest of the fellows, as he had already finished a cardiothoracic fellowship in Sicily when he decided to come to the United States and start his residency all over again. The reason for the nickname that some of the residents had for him (Mussolito) became obvious during that first meeting when he spelled out what he expected. He outlined in great detail how he wanted the service to function. We were to show up for rounds at 5:00 a.m., and we were to get everything ready for him before he showed for rounds at 6:00 a.m. He even spelled out how he wanted the patients presented to him during rounds, how the chart notes were to be written, how the consults were to be done, and he made us take note of everything he said. I knew on that day that it would be a tough month working with him. At the end of the meeting he demanded we give him all of our contact information including our home phone number, cell phone number, etc. One of the residents refused to do so, at which point Gregorio did not seem too pleased and asked the resident to wait a bit after our meeting so that they could talk privately. I gave him all my contact numbers, as I was dying to get out of there.

It took only one day in the cardiothoracic surgery service for me to comprehend the immense amount of work that had to be done. The fellows were of little help, as they spent their entire day in the operating room. It was left to the three of us residents and the rotating medical students to get the work done. I also found out rather quickly that after all the cases were finished, utterly exhausted as they were, the fellows would go home. This left us to care for the sick patients in the ICU and the patients on the floor, an awesome responsibility indeed. Only when there were truly critical patients in the ICU would the fellows stay in an on-call room close by. Needless to say, they were available for consultations and questions, but they did not share in the ICU or floor work. I understood their behavior. By the end of the day these guys were utterly exhausted and thus somewhat limited as to how much help they could or would be willing to offer. Having them close by, however, was a great psychological comfort, especially when dealing with complicated postoperative patients.

Dr. Gregorio Esposito had an exasperating habit of calling the residents multiple times per day before and in between cases to inquire as to what we were doing. He seemed to be the classic control freak. It was not long before I began to resent these calls as they took valuable minutes away from the work I had to do. During rounds, he was regimented and would make us rewrite our notes or re-start patient presentations again and again if we did not do things exactly the way he wanted them done.

For a fellow, Gregorio dressed very well to rounds. While most of us found it more expeditious to show up to work in scrubs, he always came in wearing shirt, tie, and blazers for morning rounds, even on weekends. This gave him a certain professorial look and demeanor. As superficial as it might seem, his attire conveyed the unspoken message to one and all who interacted with him, especially patients, that Gregorio Esposito was very professional, focused, and took his career very seriously. Looking back at it now, it is because of him that I developed the same philosophy of dressing the part when dealing with patients anywhere outside of the operating room. Even including all the attendings I dealt with as a resident and since then, very few have matched Gregorio's ability to dress the part of the gentleman surgeon.

As rounds began, he would pull out a small notebook from his breast pocket in which he wrote down pertinent information on the patients so he could share it with the attendings later. His handwriting was minuscule. To my eyes, surgical loops would be required in order to read it. He generated enormous lists on each patient of things he wanted done. Quite often during rounds he embarked on long teaching diatribes, which often were a mixture of medicine and philosophy. Moreover, his delivery was extremely peculiar.

He was fond of saying highly unusual phrases and retorts, which always made me wonder where he had picked them up. Once during rounds, while looking at a chest X-ray on a patient with fluid on his pleural space, he pointed to an area of blunting on one side of the chest; he explained to us that this meant there was residual fluid in the chest and that the patient would need another chest tube, as the original chest tube had not been perfectly placed. So as to drive the point home, he shook his head and exclaimed: "The resident who placed this chest tube should have known that with so much fluid present, the patient needed the tube placed more inferiorly in the chest." He then added a phrase that I will never forget: "Good medicine comes from good judgment which is the result of good experiences which in turn come from the correction of bad experiences that are the result of bad judgment."

After such a profound statement said in his peculiar accent, there was nothing much left to be said. He promptly dismissed us after that, leaving us to marinate on that bit of Mussolito wisdom.

Once one dug a little deeper, it was hard not to like Gregorio. Toward the end of my rotation with him, I had made peace with his idiosyncrasies, having learned to coexist and work with him. I think the feeling was reciprocal; he even told me that he appreciated my work ethic. Days before the end of my rotation, he asked me and the medical student rotating through the service, Rachel, to meet him for a beer after work. The story he told us was inspiring and explained to a certain degree some of his unusual behavior.

It seemed that Dr. Gregorio Esposito had finished cardiothoracic surgery in Italy only to realize that he wanted more, which for him meant coming to America. He dreamed of coming to the United States and learning some of the newer techniques that he had read about in journals but had not been exposed to during his training. After giving it serious consideration, he decided to take a chance and come to the States to learn some of those techniques. Being single, he did not have family responsibilities to worry about, but he did tell us that parting with his parents had been difficult. After arriving in the United States, and barely able to say but a few words in English, he started taking language classes. Soon thereafter he began studying for his medical exams, while he simultaneously took odd jobs to make ends meet.

A few years later he took his board exams in order to apply for a residency. He had learned that to do cardiothoracic training in the United States he would have to redo his general surgery training. He had managed to get a preliminary position in a hospital in New York City, and had been told that he had little chance of continuing in the program after the second year. As he told Rachel and me that afternoon at a local pub, "When I started, no one believed that I would make it." He had studied hard and worked even harder. "I was determined to show them all that I could do it."

He quickly became known for being the most diligent resident in the program, and on residency standardized (inservice) exams he scored the best among his peers. "I made it impossible for them to deny me a categorical spot." He was obviously proud of what he had accomplished. He was fulfilling a dream and he was determined to become the best cardiothoracic surgeon that he could. I remember that both Rachel and I had been moved by his story, and when left alone for a few minutes while Gregorio stepped into the restroom, she shared with me how the story had inspired her, as she had similar dreams. She was from Spain and was going to medical school in Ireland. It turned out that she also wanted to be a cardiothoracic surgeon in the States. The look in her eyes as she spoke gave one the impression that she was letting herself consider the possibility that if Gregorio could do it, she could do it too. In turn, I instinctively was swept by the same feeling and began to ponder the possibility, and maybe even hope, that she could.

With time, my respect for Gregorio grew. It must have been difficult to deal with the hardships that he faced. To his credit, he had overcome them and was now on his way. We became friends that year but did not talk much once he started the second year of his fellowship. He went on to do a subspecialty in pediatric cardiothoracic surgery, and eventually he set up practice somewhere on the West Coast. I have not kept in touch with Gregorio, but he did teach me a great deal during that short month we rotated together, not only about medicine and surgery, but about how hard work and overwhelming dedication can sometimes overcome difficult obstacles. There are still times I think of him when facing a difficult professional impasse in my own career.

In contrast to Dr. Gregorio Esposito, Dr. Seth Oscar, the second-year fellow at the VA hospital, was the complete opposite. A tall good, ole-boy from Louisiana, his laid-back attitude and Southern drawl complemented his relaxed demeanor. He came to work in scrubs, old tennis shoes, and a lab coat, which more often than not, was wrinkled and dirty. The VA hospital's cardiothoracic service was not as busy as at Jackson Memorial Hospital, and only one second-year resident rotated on the service at a time. I did not have any interns or medical students working with me, and very much missed working with Rachel during the second month of my rotation as she had already gone back to Europe.

Rounds with Seth were rather slow-paced, a welcome change compared to rounds at Jackson Memorial. We did rounds together and got most of the work done as we saw each patient, as he often pitched in and helped write notes, orders, etc. We would then go for a quick breakfast, and from there directly to the operating room. There were not many teaching sessions during rounds with Seth, as he much preferred telling jokes and flirting with the nurses. He had an extremely jovial nature and I liked him immediately upon meeting him.

In the operating room, Seth was all business. To my eyes, he had excellent hands and an impressive ability to focus.

While working with him in the operating room, he did teach quite a bit and let me do a great deal during the operations. He explained in detail and taught me how to open the chest through the sternum in order to approach the heart. He taught me how to dissect around the sternum, how to hold the saw, how to make the cut in the middle of the sternum, and how to enter the pericardium (the fibrous membrane that encases the heart). At the end of the case, he would teach me how to close the chest wall with wires. He showed patience as he allowed me to struggle and do the closure while he assisted me. By the end of the rotation, I was capable of performing the chest opening and closure in an expeditious manner. These techniques later came in handy while a senior resident in my trauma rotations.

Seth was also cool under pressure. Whether it was the attending surgeon yelling at him, or the patient deteriorating rapidly, he was always composed and his hands steady and sure. "My hands only have one speed…fast," he once told me just after completing an exceedingly difficult case. His example became pivotal for my career, teaching me much about how a surgeon should ideally perform during dire situations. It was Seth more than anyone else whom I emulated later in my training when facing situations of extreme pressure in the operating room.

The operation we most often performed during that VA rotation was the coronary artery bypass graft known by the acronym of CABG and pronounced "cabbage." The operation consists of opening the patient's chest in order to have access to the heart, then inserting conduit tubes in the right atrium (compartment) of the heart and in a femoral vein in order to place the patient on the heart bypass machine. This machine continues to circulate the blood through the patient's circulatory system while the heart rhythm is brought to a standstill through a combination of cold temperature and certain medications—in essence causing the heart to stop beating. As the vessels of the heart wall are exceedingly small, it is much easier to perform the bypass grafts while the heart is not moving. The grafts usually go from the chest wall, or the aorta, to the small (coronary) arteries that run on the outside surface of the heart and provide blood to the heart muscle itself. These are the vessels that tend to get occluded during atherosclerotic arterial disease. Once the grafts are completed, the heart is warmed, normal heart rhythm is again established, the hoses—conduit tubes—that run from the patient's vessels to the bypass machine are removed, and the patient's chest is closed.

I remember one particular morning when we had just begun a bypass operation on an unstable patient from the medical ICU. This patient had severe atherosclerotic disease of his coronary vessels and was suffering from heart failure. Taking him to the operating room was a risk and he knew it, but it was most likely the only way we had to save his life. As per our routine, I was opening the chest while being assisted by Seth. I had just finished splitting the sternum with the saw blade, placing the sternal retractor, and was in the middle of separating both halves of the sternum thereby exposing the heart, when the anesthesiologist's voice interrupted Seth's teaching: "We have V-fib."

Seth put his hand on mine to prevent me from moving. "Check the leads," he said as his gaze fixed on the heart monitor that traced the patient's heart rhythm (EKG). The anesthesiologist adjusted the leads under the drapes while we all looked at the monitor. "Leads are okay; he is in V-fib."

Contrary to what I was expecting, Seth made a highly risky, split-second decision. I was anticipating that he was going to stop the operation while we performed three electric shocks to the chest wall and the rest of the protocol as per the ACLS (Advanced Cardiac Life Support) protocol to get the patient out of this fatal arrhythmia (heart rhythm). Ventricular fibrillation is the name given to a cardiac rhythm when the heart beats in an irregular and inefficient fashion. If not treated within a matter of seconds to a few minutes, it invariably leads to death. It is universally accepted that upon diagnosing ventricular fibrillation, the indicated intervention for such a rhythm should be initiated immediately per the protocol of the ACLS algorithm. This involves three consecutive electric shocks to the chest wall (with progressive increases in energy) followed by chest compressions if the rhythm is not converted back to normal by the successive shocks.

Instead of asking for the small, electric paddles which we would now need to use as the heart was exposed, Seth alerted the nurse that he was going to put the patient on bypass. Seth had decided that he would place the patient on cardiac pump and freeze the heart rather than attempt to reverse the arrhythmia. When the anesthesiologist realized what we were about to do, he firmly objected and asked why we were not going to shock the patient. Seth, working all the while, explained to him that the patient's heart was receiving almost no blood supply due to the coronary occlusion, and that even if we were able to temporarily reverse the rhythm, it would be for naught, as the patient's heart could not take the stress of the anesthesia and the surgery.

Seth had decided that the only way to salvage the situation was to put the patient on the heart bypass machine as soon as possible, and in essence, put the patient's death on hold. He would then re-establish a normal heart rhythm once the heart had been revascularized with the new vessel grafts that would bring adequate blood flow to the heart muscle. Needless to say, this course of action was highly risky and extremely unorthodox; however, neither the anesthesiologist nor I were in any position to stop him.

What happened over the next few minutes has always stayed with me as the prime example of a surgeon working at his/her peak in the midst of a dire emergency. Every movement he made was extremely precise and accomplished the desired effect. He placed the retractor on the sternum to fully expose the heart and proceeded to insert the hose in the right atrium that would allow us to put the patient on the heart bypass machine. All this was accomplished with utmost efficiency in what seemed a matter of seconds, although I knew it had probably taken several minutes.

Even my inexperienced hands seemed to respond to the challenge as I suctioned, retracted, and cut sutures as I helped him complete the task. I knew that if we did not get this patient on pump soon, he would not wake up from the surgery, and even if he did, he might end up with some brain damage from the temporary lack of oxygen. My concentration was so intense that I was not aware of anything else going on in the room. I experienced tunnel vision as if I were watching a movie, in slow motion, of our hands performing a well-choreographed dance. We worked in complete silence until the task was completed and the patient's blood began to circulate with the help of the perfusion machine (heart bypass machine).

Later, during the critical part of the operation when the attending surgeon and Seth connected the grafts, I held the heart in a steady position, wondering the entire time whether the patient was going to wake up after the operation. Technically, he had been dead as we put him on pump. It had been a gutsy call for Seth to make. I pondered how much confidence in one's surgical ability it took to make a decision like that. Would I ever reach that level of confidence? Did I even want to? Especially if it meant having to make these kinds of decisions and putting someone's life in my hands to such a degree.

Dr. Ted Stone was the attending assigned to us for that day. He walked into the room five minutes after the patient had been placed on pump. He had already scrubbed the first time he walked in, and I moved out of the way as he reached the table and stood in my previous spot across the patient from Seth.

"Everything okay?" he addressed Seth while adjusting some of the drapes around the patient's open chest. When he heard the events that had just transpired, his eyes went from what he was doing and looked straight into Seth's face. He held them there without saying a word. The eyes of the two surgeons held each other's gaze over their surgical loops for a few seconds, and then almost simultaneously they lowered their heads to look at the surgical field and resumed working. They did not exchange a word during those uncomfortable first few minutes, each of them consumed by their own thoughts. I assumed Seth was second-guessing his decision while Dr. Stone was pondering the repercussions should Seth's high-stakes gambit not work out. At this point, there was nothing else to do but continue with the surgery, all the while desperately hoping that all would turn out for the best.

Once the critical part of the case was finished, the attending stepped back from the operating room table and sat by the computer writing his notes; he seemed to be lingering, I thought. Seth and I went through the routine to warm and restart the heart. Neither he nor I said anything as we were exhausted, each of us letting the events of that morning sink in while anxiously awaiting the endgame. The tension in the room was palpable as the heart did not start in the normal amount of time. After a little while, however, the heart began fibrillating as Seth continued to pour warm saline solution on it. The irregular contractions continued for a bit, and then all of a sudden, the heart began beating rhythmically. I felt like letting out a scream, but instead raised my head and looked across the table at Seth. I was staring right into his thick surgical loops as he had already raised his head and was looking at me. I could easily convince myself that I saw him let out a great sigh of relief behind his mask. He was standing tall and triumphant as he extended his gloved hand my way. I did the same and we shook hands over the patient, both extremely relieved that things had worked out, at least temporarily. "Congratulations, great job," he let out as we shook hands. I congratulated him in turn.

It was then that Dr. Stone approached the table again and looked at the heart beating rhythmically within the patient's chest. He was standing somewhat behind me looking over my shoulder at the heart, and then at Seth. My peripheral vision caught his movements, although I dared not look his way. I heard his voice close to my ear. "You guys were lucky; you almost had an MDK." He then turned and walked out of the room.

"MDK?" I gave Seth a puzzled look.

"MD Kill," Seth said with some gravity. "He is saying that we almost killed this guy."

I was never able to tell if Dr. Stone had taken this episode in stride or if he was really mad at Seth and me. He was the kind of guy who was hard to read, but both Seth and I liked him and looked up to him. Dr. Stone was in his early forties and seemed to be living a great life. He had joined one of the best cardiothoracic groups in town, was young, relaxed, and drove a beautiful, modern sports car. He had taken a part-time position at the VA hospital helping with the overflow of heart cases. He always seemed to show up for the cases just in time to help the fellow with the grafts and never was around for all the preliminary work that had to be done to get the case up to that point. For weekend rounds, he would show up around 9:00 AM, always looking dapper, relaxed, and holding a cup of black coffee. To the residents and fellows, he seemed the epitome of what could be achieved professionally and what life was to be like after we finished. I remembered one day after rounds Seth telling me that he wanted to be like Dr. Stone when he grew up. It was Dr. Stone's group that Dr. Jack Rio joined upon completion of his cardiothoracic fellowship. After a long case one night, they both left the hospital in Dr. Stone's sports car to get something to eat. Shortly after leaving the hospital, they were involved in a car accident that tragically took both of their lives.

Thankfully, our patient did not sustain any hypoxic (low oxygen) brain damage from the surgery and sailed through his stay in the ICU and then the floor. Two weeks later the patient was ready to go home and Seth, who was running late that day, asked me to delay the discharge until he got to the hospital. Seth walked in as I was finishing giving discharge instructions. He shook hands with the patient and wished him well. He told the patient that his heart was revascularized and fixed, adding, "You have the heart of a twenty-year-old. Please take care of it. Make sure you don't go back to the smoking and your other bad habits."

The patient looked at him with a broad smile on his face. "Why would I want to do that? If my heart is all fixed, then why not continue the drinking, smoking, and bad habits? I figure that I have another twenty years before I mess it up again. I am sure you will be right here still fixing hearts…and breaking them."

We all laughed. It seemed even the patients were aware of Seth's reputation as a ladies' man. We walked the patient to the room door where the transport service was waiting for him with a wheelchair to take him to the first floor. Accompanied by his wife and a nurse, he cheerfully waved to all the floor nurses while being wheeled down the hall towards the elevators.

"We did right by him." Seth had a satisfied and proud look on his face. We were both happy and relieved that things had worked out the way they did. Credit for an "MDK" was not something Seth or I wanted on our record. It had been a great save.

Toward the end of my rotation I walked into the fellow's room one day and saw Seth as I had never seen him before. He seemed obviously preoccupied, nervous, and did not respond at my obvious attempts at humor. "What is wrong, Seth?" I asked.

"I am about to call my chairman and quit the program," he answered while sitting at the desk and staring at the phone.

"What in the world are you talking about? You have less than half a year to go."

This conversation that had started off very strangely ended with Seth sharing a profound, deep secret: "I have a phobia of flying," he confessed.

I still did not see what this had to do with his training program. He explained that part of the second-year fellow's responsibility was the procurement of hearts that were to be transplanted at Jackson Memorial Hospital. To this end, fellows were sent to hospitals near and far to harvest the hearts and bring them back to Miami. He had kept this phobia to himself during the interview process, as he was afraid that they would not take him into the program if it became known. He had eventually confided in the other second-year fellow, who had mercifully agreed to go on all the harvests that required flying if Seth covered his duties at the hospitals while he was gone, and went on all harvests that required traveling by ambulance. Apparently, the arrangement had worked perfectly until now, as the other fellow was on vacation, out of the country for two weeks, and Seth had received a call to get ready for a harvest that night. I thought back to my cardiothoracic rotation at University Hospital and the multiple transplants that we had done that month, each of which required one of the fellows to travel to the hospital where the donor was, in order to harvest the heart.

"You don't understand, Joe. I went to a harvest on a small plane during the beginning of the year and almost died." He was obviously very distressed at the thought of having to do it again. "I nearly passed out and almost ruined the organ (heart) from my hands shaking so bad. I get panic attacks just from thinking about having to get on a plane."

I suggested that he ask one of the first-year fellows to go, but apparently, they were not allowed as they were not yet proficient at doing the organ-harvesting procedure. "Then talk to the attendings," I suggested, "I am sure they will understand, maybe one of them will go."

Seth was sure that they would not understand and would fire him on the spot for refusing to go. Technically, that was one of the requirements for the fellowship and he had lied to the program director by not divulging the information that he would not be able to fulfill this particular responsibility.

"How about trying a sedative?" I suggested, but I quickly realized how irresponsible the suggestion was. If a resident or fellow were ever caught working under the influence of any drug or alcohol, he/she would be fired on the spot for sure. Moreover, this would be an obvious ethical breach as any physician partaking of this behavior could put a patient's health and/or life in jeopardy.

It took me hours to convince Seth to agree to go on the trip. I tried every conceivable reason I could come up with. It was not acceptable for him to consider quitting his fellowship just four months before finishing it. I had heard rumors of residents and fellows who had quit their training due to nervous breakdowns and the like, but the thought of Seth thinking about quitting this close to finishing his training was ludicrous. He was such a great surgeon and such a nice guy. Moreover, he had invested almost seven years in making his dream of becoming a heart surgeon a reality.

When the time arrived for him to leave for the airport, I was not sure that he was going to go. He had not made a decision as the time to leave approached and seemed to be getting more anxious by the minute. I offered to call the program chairman and explain to him the situation myself, but Seth would not have it. I was out of options and did not know what else to do. For a time, it seemed like he was not going to be able to pull himself together. We had been talking for what seemed like many hours, and I was feeling exhausted from playing psychiatrist.

Finally, the confirmation call came in letting him know that the plane would be waiting for him in one hour. It was go-time for him to start heading toward the airport so as not to be late. "Take it one step at a time, Seth. You will be back here and done with this nightmare in no time." I grabbed his arm and insisted we walk to his car. He did not seem happy but did not resist. In the elevator and while walking through the parking lot I continued to encourage him as best I could. As his car drove off, I wondered whether he would make the plane. If he did not show after all the plans for the transplant had been set in motion, it would definitely be a disaster, not only for him, but also for the patient who at the time would have been getting ready to receive the new heart.

Seth rose to the challenge. He went on to harvest the heart that day and two others before the year was done. I saw him on the last day of his fellowship. He was making plans to move to Kentucky to start a new job. He had a big smile on his face as he was extremely happy to be finally done with his training.

Residency and fellowship training are an extremely difficult and time-consuming process. Pulling one's weight and fulfilling one's responsibilities is ingrained in the surgical trainee from the first day of residency. This becomes the overwhelming concern of the resident, sometimes to the detriment of the resident's family, health, and other personal concerns. When a particular resident deals with all those demands while at the same time dealing with physical or personal handicaps, the challenge becomes mammoth. What under any normal circumstances is an exceedingly difficult ordeal at best, in the presence of personal handicaps can become an insurmountable challenge, leading to unfinished careers and broken dreams.

Seth's predicament was unusual in that it concerned a fear of flying. However, the underlying apprehension that some residents have regarding failing to perform their assigned duties, for one reason or another, can be very real. This is in part due to the longstanding culture among surgeons that they are to perform at all costs and under extreme pressure no matter the personal sacrifice. Admitting personal difficulties, weaknesses, or the need for help is not part of the surgeon's belief system, sometimes to their detriment and that of their patients. Some of these issues would become a great source of debate and discussion later on during my second year when the resident's union (CIR) was being discussed and established at Jackson Memorial Hospital.

Two years later, while on vacation during my fourth year of residency, Rachel (who was then my girlfriend) and I decided to drive to Kentucky to visit Seth. He had taken a job as a cardiothoracic surgeon in a small town near Louisville. The drive to his home was extremely pleasant and visually inspiring, as the rolling hills along with the many farms and the beautiful homes that are typical of that part of the country were on full display throughout the latter part of the drive. Being from a small town in Louisiana, Seth had always been drawn to the quiet, country life. I envisioned him being happy there in this part of the country and in his new job.

Seth was a perfect host and welcomed us into his new home, which was surrounded by the small horse farm that was part of the property. One morning he insisted that I take a bath in the huge guest bathtub that was located on the first floor of his house. Sitting there, looking out of the large panoramic window as his horses leisurely fed in the pasture, I felt incredibly happy for him. He had put in many years of training and had overcome many personal demons to get here. That night after dinner, Rachel left us alone for a while and I could not help but ask him if he was happy.

"I really am," he said. "And you know what makes me the happiest?"

He placed his hand on my shoulder to emphasize what he was about to say next. "I will never have to get on another airplane again in my life."

The Final Six

Although the University of Miami graduates six general surgeons per year, the internship class contains more than thirty residents. These residents are categorized differently depending on their educational track. Six residents out of the intern class are considered categorical surgery residents. These six have been accepted to the general surgery program and are programmed for graduation in five years as general surgeons or a bit longer if they decide to invest one or two years in research as part of their training.

The remaining residents are considered preliminary, of which there are two groups. The designated preliminary residents are those who are already accepted to other surgical specialties or anesthesia. As part of their training, these residents are required to do either one or two years of training in general surgery. Specialties such as ENT, orthopedics, and urology for example, have this requirement. The other group is called undesignated preliminary residents. These residents seek a position in general surgery, but for a host of different reasons, have not secured one. They accept preliminary positions in the hope that during the following years they might be able to secure a categorical spot. This can occur in different ways. Sometimes categorical residents decide to undertake one or two years of research thereby leaving a senior residency spot available for those preliminary residents who have completed the prerequisite junior years. Another possibility is that one of the categorical residents will quit the training program. After working with my fellow five residents for close to two years, I was convinced that this opportunity would not be an option in our year as I never envisioned the possibility that one of us would quit.

The beginning of the third year is a critical transition for undesignated preliminary residents. Although there are spots in the second year to accommodate the categorical residents and several preliminary residents, the third year contains rotations only for the number of residents who will eventually become chief residents and graduate. Thus, after the second year all undesignated preliminary residents who have not secured a categorical spot are not allowed to continue with their training. They must either transition to other specialties or scramble to find a categorical spot elsewhere. This time of the year was always particularly sad for me, as it was difficult to say good-bye to great preliminary residents, some of whom would never realize their dream of becoming surgeons. By this point in the second year, some of the undesignated preliminary residents had chosen to pursue other nonsurgical specialties. There were some, however, who would not give up on their dream and were determined to struggle on.

Although my class started out with several preliminary residents who intended to pursue general surgery, by the end of the second year there were only two who remained dedicated to the idea. Both were foreign medical graduates who worked extremely hard for two years and were seeking to secure a categorical spot. I had every reason to believe that a spot would not open up in our program, as the six categorical residents in my class all seemed committed to continue. I was saddened at the expectation that in a few months, the two preliminary residents who had chosen to continue the struggle would have to leave our institution to seek opportunities elsewhere.

Rick Lopez was born and had attended high school in the States but had eventually gone to live with his family in Colombia where he graduated from medical school. He was smart, driven, and worked quite hard...sometimes perhaps too hard as if he had something to prove, perhaps because he did.

I had the pleasure of working with him during my internship year in a service that required three interns. He spent significant time reading and was always prepared for rounds and conferences. I very much enjoyed working with him. It was a natural thing for me to like him, as we mutually shared a passion for surgery, as well as a firm commitment to invest the time necessary to learn the didactic and technical aspects of surgery.

Ray Castro was the other preliminary surgeon. Born in Guatemala and the son of a surgeon, Ray came into the program much more knowledgeable about surgery than most of the categorical residents senior to him. It was obvious that he had learned a great deal from his father. I never had the opportunity to work with him directly, but I had plenty of interactions with him during conferences and rounds. He soon developed a reputation as a conscientious and responsible resident. He got his work done and never complained. He had an air of confidence about him that was unusual for residents in the first or second year. He was amicable, fun to be around, and seemed to be liked by attendings, residents, and patients alike. I always had positive interactions in my dealings with him and liked him very much as well.

As the middle to latter part of the second residency year approached, I became acutely aware that this might be the last few months that all of us would be working alongside Rick and Ray. I very much empathized with both of them as I saw the strain they were under as they juggled their considerable workload as residents while scrambling to secure their professional future. As sad as I felt for them, I was at the same time relieved that none of the categorical residents in our class were going to quit, as it would have been extremely difficult and nerve-wracking for anyone to have to choose between the two of them. Unbeknownst to me, that difficult decision would ultimately have to be made, although thankfully not by me.

Apart from the excellent preliminary residents, I was fortunate in that my fellow categorical residents were truly first class. Most of them had graduated with honors from medical school, and some had done significant amounts of clinical research. They were all intelligent and hardworking. Truly devoted to surgery, their motivation was clearly evident in the way they approached their responsibilities. We believed we were the strongest group of residents in the program at the time. This might not have been the consensus among others, but we believed it to be true.

Besides me, there were three other male residents and two female residents. Among the male residents was Dr. Chad Yarborough. He was from the Midwest, a genuinely nice and devoted family man whose father had graduated from the surgery program at the University of Miami. He turned out to be the one resident I spent the most time with, as early during my first year we started studying together on a weekly basis. Over time, we developed a close friendship. Dr. Tony Cicilio, also the son of a surgeon, was born in Los Angeles but had gone back with his family to Italy after his father finished his transplant fellowship in California. He was without a doubt the hardest working resident in our class and up to this day is one of the hardest working surgeons I know. The last male resident in our group was Dr. Rahimi Husain. Our program took one resident per year from Kuwait. They always sent their best students, as it was extremely competitive to be honored with the scholarship that would enable medical students from Kuwait to come to the University of Miami to train in surgery. Rahimi followed the tradition of his predecessors, as he was extremely bright and hardworking.

Women who go into surgery are special, as surgery even to this day is a male-dominated profession, in which extraordinarily little thought is given to female sensibilities. The two women in my class were indeed special, and it was my pleasure to know and work with them during my training. I first noticed Dr. Tracy Trott during my general surgery interviews in medical school. While waiting for our interview appointment in the lobby of a busy New York City hospital, my classmate and friend Scott and I noticed a striking young woman dressed in a business suit walking through the lobby. Later that morning we realized she was one of the other candidates interviewing along with us.

It was surprising to see her about two weeks later when Scott and I traveled to Miami together for our general surgery interview there. While being given a tour of the hospital in Miami, I had exchanged some polite words with her and had found out that she was from Philadelphia but was living in South Florida at the time. While on the elevator, she confided in me that Miami was her number one spot, not divulging the reason why.

"You know, I am being highly recruited by this program, I will make sure to insist that they take you, if they really want me to come here." I rationalized the statement as flirting rather than the blatant lie it was. She gave me a quizzical look and polite smile which I took as a positive, as there was always the possibility that she would have opted for a more negative response.

During the first week of residency, Tracy was the first person I saw when I walked into the room for our scheduled orientation meeting. "See…" I said, "I kept my promise." She did not seem amused then but eventually I did overcome her warranted mistrust.

Tracy and I became rather good friends during the residency. It turned out that one of the reasons she wanted to come to Miami was that she was engaged to a surgeon in the community; he later took on a faculty position with our program. She often made it a point to tell me how crazy she thought I was when we first met during our residency interview.

Dr. Stacy Stiles was the last of my fellow categorical residents. She was an honor student in medical school, had significant research experience, and was excellent with her hands. She was pretty, with long blonde hair, and was thin and tall, but not frail. Although I liked her very much, I was not close to her during residency despite my efforts to the contrary, not necessarily for purely altruistic reasons. The way the residency is set up, one hardly ever works with the residents in the same class.

My interactions with Stacy were primarily limited to conferences, rounds, and occasional meetings at the cafeteria or wards.

From what I knew of my fellow residents, we were all happy and motivated with our career choice. Of course, there were times when we all complained about working too hard, or having problems dealing with a particular senior resident or attending. This was par for the course. I would venture to say that most surgery residents during the course of their residency have some doubts about their choice. General surgery residency is quite a challenge both physically and mentally. It is normal for people involved in such an arduous process to question how they ended up there to begin with. Of course, for most this is only temporary, and soon they connect once again with the reason why they chose surgery in the first place. Nevertheless, when one begins to question the decision on a regular basis, and begins to think realistically about quitting, the situation becomes much more serious.

It was March or April of the second year, and I was on call during a slow night. I had finished my work on the floor by about 9:00 p.m. and had decided to go down to the cafeteria for something to eat. As I paid for my food, I glanced at the nearly empty dining room and saw Stacy sitting by herself in one of the back tables. She seemed deep in thought. It was always a pleasure to find one of my co-residents in the cafeteria when I came down to eat. It gave me a chance to visit and talk about mutual areas of interest—a nice break from the daily responsibilities.

"Stace, may I join you?" I asked as I walked towards her table.

"Please," she responded with a forced smile. I could tell she was not happy.

"How are you doing?" I tested the waters carefully as Stacy seemed to be in the midst of some sort of crisis.

"Living the dream!" This was usually said sarcastically by residents when they found themselves particularly overworked or stressed.

Deciding not to press her, I started talking about my day and issues on the floor. I figured she would eventually open up if she wanted to share her troubles with me. Up to that time, we had never had a long, deep discussion on any serious topic. Most of our conversations had been short, lighthearted, and related to residency issues and events. This time I sensed that she was dealing with something significant. Her customary sarcastic sense of humor was gone.

Eventually she got around to what was on her mind, albeit in a roundabout way. “Are you happy? Here, I mean….in residency?” Her question and change of subject took me a bit by surprise.

“I have some bad days. Overall, yes, I am happy. Are you not?” It was obvious we were about to embark on a serious conversation. Stacy looked at me straight in the eyes and I could see she was wrestling with personal demons.

“Lately, I’ve been feeling as though I made the wrong choice with surgery.” The tone of her voice revealed deep ambivalence and concern.

I had heard others make similar statements before. There was Andy, the neurosurgery resident with whom I worked during my internship who made a comment about quitting just about every day. This was different though. It was obvious that Stacy was having serious doubts. I felt obliged to dig deeper and try to help in any way I could.

“What exactly is the problem, Stace? We all have bad days. Have you suddenly realized that you don’t like surgery?”

“Not at all. See, that’s the thing…I love surgery. It is just that the rest of my life sucks.” Stacy proceeded to list her complaints, which were numerous: “I don’t have time to work-out anymore… I spend my whole life in the hospital… I don’t have time for a personal life.”

Once the flood gates opened, it seemed that there were an endless number of complaints. Finally, she summed up her bleak reality: “I hate coming to work every day, from the moment that

I get into the elevator until the moment that I walk out the door."

This last statement drove home to me the seriousness of the situation. This went beyond the usual complaining that I was used to hearing from my fellow residents on a regular basis. We all did that, and it was more about letting off steam than anything else. We talked about our problems, but never seriously considered quitting. It was obvious that Stacy was having a really tough time. It was then that I realized and feared that she was now beyond the psychological threshold of giving serious consideration to leaving the program.

"What are you saying, Stace? Are you telling me that you are going to quit?"

"No, I just feel like crap and don't know how to fix the problem." She seemed hopeless and this realization made my feelings go out to her.

In the limited amount of time available, I did everything possible to help. I tried to put things in perspective for her, and I emphasized that things would improve with time. It was to be expected that her personal time would be extremely limited during her junior resident years. I stressed that things would improve as we advanced in seniority. At that time, I had no way of knowing that it would actually be the opposite. It was naïve of me to think otherwise. My time for dinner was running out, and I felt guilty leaving her there alone. I volunteered to be available should she ever want to reach out and discuss these issues further.

"Thank you. I'll take you up on that," she said. But she never did.

Our paths did cross again a few days later in the hallway. Upon inquiring how she was doing, she smiled and told me she was feeling better. It was not more than two weeks later that Chad Yarborough told me Stacy had put in her resignation.

"I think we should talk to her, Chad. Maybe there is still time to get her to change her mind."

"No," He said. "I've already tried multiple times. This has been going on for some time already and she has made a final decision."

"Did you know about this from before?" I knew that Chad and Stacy were a lot closer than she and I, and that they spoke on a regular basis.

"Yes, I did," Chad said flatly.

"I wish you would have told me. We could have done something."

"She made me promise not to tell anyone." Chad seemed sad; a feeling we both shared.

Stacy stayed through the end of the second year. During the last few months with the program, it was awkward for me to deal with her. I never knew what to say. On the one hand, it was my nature to try to convince her to stay. On the other, it was my obligation as her friend to accept her decision and support her as best I could. It was difficult to see her go. After a while, it became evident that Stacy had made peace with her decision and was actually looking forward to her new life. We were all sad at seeing her go but at the same time were happy for her.

After Stacy made her decision known, the only question remaining was, who would replace her? Although we had several preliminary residents working with us during the previous two years, by this time there were only two in real contention: Rick and Ray. I did not have a strong preference either way, but I was aware that this was going to be a hard decision to make as they were both excellent residents and both deserved the shot. Thankfully, it was not a decision for me to make. The opinion of the residents was never sought. In the end, it was Ray who got the nod. Rick was extremely disappointed; we all felt terrible for him. At the last minute, he was able to secure another second-year preliminary position at another program. Although it meant that he would have to repeat the second year, and still with no guarantee that he would be able to continue after that, it did keep his dream of becoming a surgeon alive. My path would cross with Rick's again, in what would turn out to be an exceedingly challenging case that I had to face during my fourth year.

Stacy ended up going to a pathology residency up north. She and I never kept in touch, but through Chad I found out later that she was much happier since she had left surgery. She got married two years later, and the last information that we had on her was that she lived in the northeast and was incredibly happy with her life. My heart always goes out to her when I think of how difficult it must have been to struggle with making the decision to give up what at one point had been her dream of becoming a surgeon.

At the beginning of my third year, I had the opportunity to pose such a question to our program director, Dr. Jason Gottlieb, as we happened to walk together to a conference one day. He was in his seventies and had been involved in the training of surgical residents for decades. He had dealt with the issue of residents quitting before and his perspective was of particular interest to me. "I have found that the difficulty comes in the process of arriving at the decision to quit," he said. "It is that process that is heart-wrenching. Once a resident finally makes the decision to quit, however, usually he/she ends up being quite happy. It is the process of making the decision that is difficult." These wise words proved to be true in Stacy's case.

CIR

It is a great day indeed when medical students find out that they have been accepted to their chosen residencies. "Match Day," as it is called, takes place sometime in the spring of the last year of medical school. Usually there is a gathering of the entire senior class where each student is given an envelope containing the information about the specialty and residency program in which that student will spend the next few years of his/her educational path.

Each school runs this ceremony differently but most often the students are expected to open their envelope upon receiving it and announce to their entire class and sometimes family members present where they ended up matching. For most students this is an extremely happy day indeed. For a few it is a sad day if they fail to match in their desired program or even more tragic, in their chosen specialty. For the overwhelming majority, however, there is great happiness, excitement, and enthusiasm; little thought is given to issues like salary, working hours, or conditions. More important concerns include the reputation of the program, the quality of teaching and training, and the opportunity for research activities. This is particularly true in surgery, as surgeons are indoctrinated early in their training to be proud of hard work, and to equate working long hours during residency with better training.

Soon after training commences, the residents begin to experience the 100 plus-hour workweeks and thirty-six-hour days and the toll that this schedule can take. Often this occurs while struggling to pay their bills with salaries that are borderline at best, especially when taking into consideration the number of hours that residents are expected to work. Most medical students live on loans and financial help from family members. For many, the start of residency is the first time that they earn a paycheck. They are happy to earn any money at all, but they are soon faced with the reality that the salaries they make barely pay their living expenses and fall way short when residents have families to support. Before long, some of the more imaginative residents begin to calculate their hourly income and are shocked that typically residents make much less than minimum wage. This does not sit well after spending four years in college and four more years in medical school, and especially after taking on debt all the while. Although these issues are not enough to deter the passion that residents feel for their jobs, it does chip away at their enthusiasm.

It was in this environment during the end of my first year of residency that I heard rumblings that the Committee of Interns and Residents (CIR), a national resident's union, was going to try to organize the residents of Jackson Memorial Hospital. CIR is a union started in New York City hospitals that represents interns, residents, and fellows. They negotiate with hospitals for resident workhours, salaries, working conditions, etc. Without the union, hospital administrations set the resident salaries, schedules, and benefits unilaterally, taking into consideration regional averages on salaries and living expenses.

CIR is usually not welcomed by hospital administrators, and Jackson Memorial Hospital was no different. The hospital administration's first response to the efforts of CIR at our institution was to take the union to court on the basis that residents were students and not employees, and thus did not have the right to collective bargaining. After this strategy failed, the hospital had no alternative but to agree to a vote by the residents as to whether they wanted to unionize or not. This process took almost an entire year and occurred during my second year of training. The issues raised during this ordeal brought to light many interesting issues that pertain to resident education and resident compensation. It also showed a stark contrast as to how different specialties and different residents reconciled the concepts of medical education and training with the realities of the economic needs of young physicians as they enter the work force.

Since for most of us residency was our first job, unions were an unfamiliar concept. Although many residents were intrigued at the possibility that our salaries and working conditions might improve, there were some with serious concerns about the potential negative impact that a resident's union might have on their training. In an attempt to inform the residents, both the union and the hospital administration organized meetings on the subject of unionization and collective bargaining. Unfortunately, these meetings were extremely difficult for most of the surgery residents to attend, as they took place in the middle of the afternoon when we were in the OR or working on the wards.

One particular afternoon, I found myself with some quiet time in the middle of the day and by chance happened to walk in on one of these meetings. I initially thought this was an educational conference for one of the medical services. In truth, I entered the room because coffee and cookies were prominently displayed on a table at the back of the room. As I was helping myself to the treats, I became aware that this was one of the union meetings and decided to sit in for a bit.

There were two people at the front of the room. One was a woman wearing a lab coat with the hospital resident ID, and the other was an older gentleman wearing a suit, who I discovered later to be one of the representatives from union headquarters. The resident was doing most of the talking. Apparently, she had been one of the residents elected to negotiate the future contract with the hospital should the union be voted in.

She listed some of the items recently negotiated in New York City, which she hoped would also be part of the Jackson Memorial Hospital resident's contract. They included salary that was close to double what we were making at Jackson (I assumed that most of this was due to the difference in living expenses between the two cities), a limit on work hours to eighty hours a week on the average, one free day per week without having to come to the hospital, and the ability to go home after twenty-four-hour calls. Although she mentioned other items, these four were more than enough for me. At that meeting, the items being discussed seemed to me more like a fantasy rather than anything resembling what might one day become reality.

Putting the salary issue aside, I was working thirty-six-hour shifts two to three times per week, and I was working regularly more than 100-hour weeks. Moreover, I knew that in my subsequent residency years I would have rotations of up to two months without a single day off. What the CIR was proposing seemed almost unrealistic to achieve and too good to be true. In addition, other desirable items for the future negotiations were brought up. Some of the residents spoke about better call rooms, more ancillary staff, and protected study time. It was obvious that most, if not all of the residents in the room were sold on the idea of the union. I, however, was still undecided despite the many potential perks being promised.

By this time, some of the residents in the room had begun to notice me sitting in the back. Most of them knew that I was from surgery, and some looked genuinely surprised to see me there. Looking around the room, I confirmed that I was the only surgery resident present. As if on cue, the union organizer began to discuss the members of the negotiation committee. He pointed to a list on the board that included some names next to the different services that the residents belonged to.

"We do not have any residents from surgery. Does anyone know of someone in surgery who might want to get involved?"

No one said a word, but some of the residents looked my way. The union representative did not notice the attention now being placed on me. I looked over the list of names on the board. There were several residents from medicine, a couple from psychiatry, one from obstetrics. From some of the looks I received, it was quite obvious that some of the residents looking my way had expected or at least hoped that I would volunteer to participate right then and there. I began to feel uncomfortable from the obvious expectations being placed on me and felt out of place. After several minutes, I looked at my pager pretending that I had received a page, and promptly walked out of the room.

The surgery residents were not talking about the union much, as many of them did not really understand what it was all about. During lunch one day with several of my surgery colleagues, I ventured to initiate a conversation on the subject.

"What do you guys think about this union thing? I walked in to one of their meetings the other day and there were some interesting things said."

"Terrible idea." This came from Tony Cicilio, a resident in my year who was known for being extremely hardworking.

"How come? Don't you want more money?" I joked.

"I can always use more money, but I don't want anyone telling me how many hours I can work. What are you supposed to do if you are taking care of a sick patient and your limit is up? Are you supposed to leave?"

"The surgery department will never stand for it." This retort from a second resident. "If they have us working like dogs and we barely make do, what are they going to do if they have to send us home?"

I could not argue with this logic. It seemed that we were barely able to make the department function with all of us working awfully long hours. We scarcely had enough residents to cover all the cases, the emergency rooms, and take care of all the consults and patients on the floor. When one of us went on vacation, the rest would be pushed past the limit to try to make up for the missing resident. How could the hospital make things work if we had fewer hours and went home after being on call? Some of us thought that perhaps if the hospital could hire more ancillary staff, this would greatly ameliorate the situation. As we discussed this, I thought of how often I had been asked to do things that were not necessarily the responsibility of the residents. I thought back as to how many times I had been asked to help transport patients to radiology, carry vials of blood to the laboratory, etc. I also thought about my VA rotation, and how Nurse Colon had made it a point to tell me all the things that nurses did not do there, and that by default, were my responsibility. I wondered if performing some of those tasks was enhancing my surgical education in any way. Then again, there was always the lack of funds. The hospital administration was constantly harping on this and used it as an excuse as to why they could not hire any more ancillary staff. If the resident salaries were to be increased, would this not leave even less money for hiring other staff? Some of these questions were obviously beyond my pay grade and the inability to answer them led to my indecisiveness regarding the union despite the potential obvious benefits.

The first official meeting that we had with the department of surgery regarding the union issue took place with the chairman of surgery and the residents in one of the trauma conference rooms. Dr. Fred Schammel was the chairman of the department at the time and the person who had interviewed me and ultimately accepted me for the position of categorical resident in general surgery. I always felt a great deal of gratitude and respect for him. A nice fatherly figure, he seemed to be dedicated to the training program and was quite concerned with resident education. I looked forward to hearing what he had to say.

From the moment he began speaking, I sensed that Dr. Schammel was walking a thin line. It was obvious that he was sensitive to the administration's wishes to try to keep the union out, while at the same time I sensed that from a personal perspective, he understood how the union might make the life of the residents better. He gave what I thought was a fair and honest presentation. He expressed his feelings regarding union rules which might end up limiting the time the residents could spend in the OR or at work learning the vital skills necessary for becoming competent professionals. He discussed how some of the benefits that the surgery residents enjoyed (such as paid conferences during the senior years) might be discontinued if the negotiated contract stipulated that resident benefits had to be uniform across all departments. He further stressed that the hospital administration intended to increase resident salaries in the near future, although this promise was made with few details.

Overall, his presentation was balanced as he discussed the pros and cons of the issue. He stated that he wanted us to have as much information as possible in order to make the best and most informed decision. He answered questions from the residents to the best of his ability. Some of his answers were vague, and he admitted that he would not know the answers to all of the questions until a contract was negotiated.

When Dr. Schammel left the room, most residents stayed behind for a while to talk about the union among themselves. It was difficult to judge the consensus in the room. By and large, most of the surgery residents seemed confused. The anticipated benefits such as increased salary and reduction in working hours were welcomed by all. However, some of the residents were deeply concerned about any mandatory restrictions in their work hours as they feared this would have a negative impact on their training. This particular meeting was informative, but not decisive in any way.

Several weeks later the union vote came up during one of the interdisciplinary conferences at the VA hospital. This conference took place with the joint attendance of the surgical and internal medicine services. Cases that pertained to both areas of medicine were discussed. The conversation started a few minutes before the conference was to begin. By then, several of the residents and attendings were already present. The discussion was illustrative of the philosophical divide between the medical (nonsurgical) and surgical specialties.

While sitting in the back of the room reading, I overheard one of the medicine senior residents bring up the subject of the union. It was the almost unanimous opinion of the internal medicine residents in the room that the union should be voted in. During the discussion, the opinion offered by one of the senior surgery residents after being asked made his bias clear, just as it revealed his lack of tact and judgment. "It is well known that internal medicine residents want the union in, but it is different for us in surgery. We like to work hard. We like to take care of patients."

It was difficult for me to believe that the senior surgery resident would make this statement in mixed company without realizing that it was demeaning and insulting to our medical colleagues. By this time I had realized that this attitude did not represent pride or conceit, but a deeply held belief by most surgeons that at the end of the day, it is they, more than any other specialty, who work the hardest and longest hours and are the most committed to their patients. Perhaps this was not the case universally, but right or wrong, it was part of the surgeon's creed. Having a limit set as to how many hours they could work was offensive to some surgeons.

The perspective of the senior attending staff in our program was on full display during the second official meeting. This meeting took place in one of the main auditoriums. Not only were residents and medical students present, but almost all of the attendings in the department as well. The chief hospital administrator gave a few remarks at the beginning. His presentation had an anti-union sentiment, and it revolved around financial challenges that a resident union would present for the hospital and the individual departments. His message was mostly financial in nature, and it did not pertain to the residents, let alone address any of our concerns. It seemed that he was mostly directing his remarks to the attendings present in the hope that they would be able to talk some sense into the residents. He ended with a vague promise to look into salary increases for the residents at some point in the future.

After the hospital administrator finished his speech and left the room, Dr. Schammel opened the floor to questions and comments by the attending staff. Most of the attending in the room had been trained at the University of Miami and represented different epochs of the evolution of the training program there.

"I don't know why residents complain so much these days." This was the contribution by one of the more senior attendings. "I remember when we literally lived in the hospital and none of us complained."

"True," one of the other senior attendings concurred, "and if we dared to complain, we risked being fired on the spot."

"Who is going to help us take care of the patients?" a third senior attending chimed in.

One of the trauma surgeons expressed an argument that struck a chord with most residents in the room: "Residents complain today for being on call every three days. I remember how we complained when we went from being on call every day to being on call every other day. Our concern then was that we would miss half the cases."

In response to this statement, one of the chief residents ventured the only resident comment of the meeting: "That statement would be true if all residents did was operate. We all know they are being asked to do tasks that are not really their responsibility and should be taken care of by other hospital personnel. Resident labor should not be used as a way to deal with a budget shortfall."

The chairman attempted to explain to the attendings that things were somewhat different now. Residents could no longer be fired on a whim or treated like indentured servants. There were stringent rules in place regarding resident performance, and due process was to be followed before residents could be disciplined or fired. He mentioned how the old patriarchal model was no longer the norm in residency training. He further discussed how applications to general surgery programs across the country were declining, and perhaps better working conditions might reverse this trend.

Responses from the more senior attendings made it seem like they had endured even rougher working conditions than the ones we toiled under. It seemed that the more senior attendings had bought into an unspoken but universal understanding about residency training. Attendings who at one time had been worked extremely hard during their training expected that future generations of trainees should endure the same treatment. It was almost as if they believed that an unspoken pact had been somehow struck between them and future generations of surgeons, that if they'd had to go through it, future generations should be willing to endure it too. In the opinion of some of the attendings present, bringing the union into the institution threatened to undo this grand bargain, although they did not quite express it as such. I got the impression that most attendings were looking at the issue from the perspective of what was best for the patients and for resident training, but there were certainly a few who were looking at it from the perspective of self-interest and were perturbed at the possibility of having diminished resident help. This attitude was disappointing and diminished the respect that some of us held for the attendings who espoused it.

The general consensus among the attending staff at that meeting seemed to be that the union was a bad idea for the residency, the educational program, and, I suspected, for them. Sitting in the back and taking it all in, I wondered whether any other resident would venture an opinion. None of us did despite several attempts by Dr. Schammel to elicit it. I could not ascertain if this came from the residents feeling intimidated or from confusion. I knew it was not from lack of interest.

There was no suspense or surprise when the vote was finally tallied. In the end, I voted for the union, as did over eighty-five percent of the more than 1,000 residents that train at Jackson Memorial Hospital. Some positive changes followed that vote, including a significant increase in resident salaries. Furthermore, over the course of the next couple of years, most of the regulations that pertain to limitation on work hours were put into effect. This was achieved by shifting some of the workload from the more junior residents to the senior residents. Unfortunately, my class and especially the class behind mine shouldered the burden of this shift. We worked extremely hard as junior residents only to find ourselves working even harder as senior residents so as to ensure that our junior colleagues could work fewer hours and meet the work limit requirements. Currently, most of these rules are universally accepted across the country, and union representation for residents is the norm.

It was not until two years later that the first surgery resident was elected as a representative to CIR. Currently, resident working conditions are much improved and the feared dire consequences on surgical training have not materialized, although some do differ from this view. The attending and administrative staff at Jackson should be commended for ultimately making the system work and improving the lives of many future surgical residents. It is hoped that these changes will make surgery a more attractive option for medical students in the future and will prevent residents who love surgery from quitting due to unnecessarily harsh working conditions. I have often wondered if Dr. Stacy Stiles would be a surgeon today if CIR rules had been implemented at Jackson Memorial Hospital a couple of years earlier. We will never know.

THE THIRD YEAR:

Transition (Junior/ Senior) Year

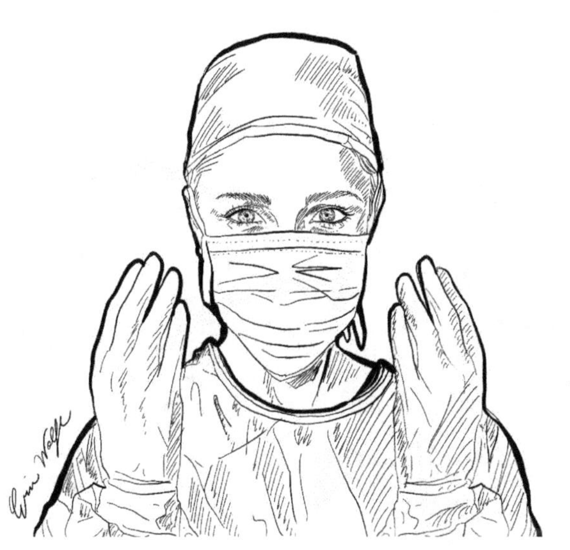

The Ultimate Gift

The third year in general surgery residency is a transition year. Although not yet officially a "senior" resident, some services that do not normally have an official senior or chief resident rotation allow the third-year resident to assume all of the responsibilities and function as a senior resident. In some rotations the third-year resident works under the supervision of a fellow or chief resident; in other rotations, the third-year resident is on his/her own and functions as the senior resident. As with the second residency year, all the rotations were scheduled in two-month blocks; six rotations per year would be the norm over the ensuing three years until graduation.

I was looking forward to finally beginning my third year. It promised greater responsibility, and most importantly much more operating room time. On the other hand, the pressure was exponentially more than in prior years, and the third year included some of the more difficult rotations of the residency program. The transplant surgery service at Jackson was one of them.

The transplant service has two main components, the liver transplant service and the kidney/pancreas service. Third-year residents rotate on the kidney service. The team is composed of an intern, the third-year resident, and one or two transplant fellows. Occasionally, one of the fourth-year residents from the urology service rotates on the kidney/pancreas transplant service as well. They were always welcomed on the team, as having an extra person is a godsend on one of the busiest services in the hospital.

My first encounter with this service occurred during my internship rotation. It was without a doubt the worst rotation of the first year. The amount of work was incredible. My pager never stopped going off. There were the usual large number of patients on the regular floor, patients who needed to be admitted and worked up for the possibility that they were rejecting their transplanted organs, and then of course, there were the transplants. It seemed that transplants never took place during regular working hours. It was always in the middle of the night, which made it that much more difficult for the intern to complete all the preoperative work-up that these patients needed prior to going to the operating room.

Interns worked on a twenty-four-hour, every-other-day schedule, alternating with a "transplant surgery pre-training fellow." These were usually foreign medical school graduates who took on the position for one year while they were applying for admittance to a residency program. Although most of them wanted to do surgery, not all of them did. Some were extremely hardworking and conscientious, and some were less so. I was lucky to be paired with a capable and hardworking intern. Some of my co-residents were not as fortunate.

I had chosen transplant as the first service of the third year for personal reasons. I had befriended a medical student from Spain during my second-year rotation in the cardiothoracic surgery service. Rachel and I had stayed in touch after she finished her one-month rotation at Jackson. Several months later, Rachel secured a one-year position as the transplant "PA" or intern. I had vouched for her for the job, and as such I felt personally responsible for her and wanted to make sure she did well. I chose the transplant service as my first rotation so that I could work with her and teach her as much as I could for the two months I would be on the service.

I brought my call bag with me on July first and took the first call with her. Normally a third-year resident would take the call from home if there were no cases going on or other emergencies, but I stayed in the senior on-call room just in case she needed help. As she was to take call every other day, I fully expected to be able to go home at least on the even days. Unfortunately, that month was extremely busy on the transplant service. We ended up doing transplants almost every night for the first couple of weeks. If not doing a transplant, I was staying on call with Rachel. I did not leave the hospital to go home for the first time until the morning of July ninth. I ate, showered, and slept in the hospital for eight days straight.

Besides the difficulty of the service, the complexity of the cases, and the amount of work involved, the transplant service also had some of the most eccentric attendings in the entire department of surgery. They were hardworking and dedicated, that is true. They were just a little different.

Dr. Ernest Bradley was the previous chief of the service and had been a transplant surgeon at Jackson for many years. Although he only did kidney transplants, he had accumulated many patients over the years. He was a caring physician who was committed to his patients. He worked hard and came to rounds every single day, including weekends and holidays. Furthermore, each night, even when traveling, Dr. Bradley called the intern at eleven p.m. to discuss his patients on the floor. The intern had to gather all the charts of Dr. Bradley's patients and sit in a quiet place to speak with him. These calls took anywhere from fifteen to forty-five minutes depending on the number of patients, and at the end the intern had a long list of things to do. I remember talking with Dr. Bradley while he was traveling all over the world. Without fail, the call would always come in exactly at eleven p.m. Miami local time.

Every morning, Dr. Bradley would show up on the floor promptly at seven a.m. with the ever-present cup of coffee in his hand. He did rounds with the team on his patients only but in the process generated a "to-do list" twice as long as the other attendings who had far more patients on the floor. Unfortunately for the Jackson residents, Dr. Bradley never relied much on the fellows or the residents from other services. He always looked for either the intern or the third-year resident from Jackson to get him the information he wanted, or to solve any problem that his patients might be having. He was also prone to raising his voice and making a scene over the slightest incident or mistake.

This made the rotation stressful for the intern and third-year resident from Jackson, while the other residents and fellows remained somewhat immune to his wrath. His temper was legendary at Jackson, and there were all sorts of stories and myths about his younger days. Of course, these stories were used strategically by the senior residents to put the fear of God in the junior residents and interns. My favorite revolved around a patient of Dr. Bradley's who had been admitted with a fever. Apparently, Dr. Bradley was sure that the patient had an infection, but all the cultures kept coming back negative. The story goes that one day during rounds Dr. Bradley asked the intern what the latest culture results were on his patient. The intern told him that he had just checked that morning before rounds, and the cultures were still not growing anything. Irate and frustrated, Dr. Bradley reportedly grabbed the intern by the neck, threw him against the wall, and yelled, "Well go back down to the lab and stay there until something does grow!" Although I was sure most of these stories were highly exaggerated and some of them were outright fabrications, they did give Dr. Bradley a reputation as someone to be feared.

I will admit that at times the aggravation got the best of me; nevertheless, I had a great deal of respect for him. The dedication he had to his patients was unparalleled, and he welcomed my calls at any time of day or night when I had a question. There were days when I must have called him several times per night. He preferred to be called directly at his cell or home rather than being paged. He always answered on the first ring, he always sounded awake no matter what time of night, and he never seemed annoyed at being called. He did get annoyed rather easily though if you could not answer his request for information, made a mistake, or took too long to get the tests he wanted done.

In fact, because his reputation was known around the hospital, I would often use this when scheduling tests to make sure they were done promptly. "This kidney ultrasound is being ordered STAT by Dr. Bradley," I would say. "And you know how mad he gets if the test gets delayed. I would hate for him to come down here and yell at you." This strategy always worked like a charm.

When he asked you to do something, he expected it done well and quickly. One night I had admitted one of his patients at about three a.m. with a distended abdomen, nausea, and vomiting. We had discussed the patient over the phone, and my impression was that he might be suffering from a gastrointestinal infection. I told Dr. Bradley that I wanted to place a nasogastric tube to relieve his abdominal distention and get some labs. We agreed that this was a good plan, and he asked me to call him as soon as the labs came back. A nasogastric tube is one that is placed through the nose all the way into the stomach, and it employs suction in order to evacuate all the fluid that has backed up into the stomach. Although the tube usually helps immediately with the symptoms of bloating, nausea, and vomiting that these patients get, putting in the tube can be somewhat uncomfortable, and some patients do not tolerate the procedure well. This patient happened to be one of them, and he immediately began gagging, coughing, and spitting to the point that it was difficult for me to get him to follow directions. It took me all of forty-five minutes after a great deal of coaxing and multiple attempts to insert the tube. I then attempted to check the tube position by listening with a stethoscope over the stomach as I forcibly pushed some air with a syringe into the tube. I did not hear the gurgling sound that usually indicates the tube is in the right position. The next step to confirm placement of the tube is to order an X-ray to check tube position. Checking the X-ray after it was done, it was easy for me to see why the sounds were not heard—the tube was short and its end rested on the esophagus, needing to be pushed another five or so inches to make it into the stomach. This required another thirty minutes of manipulation of the tube and all the patience I could muster to finally get it right. I checked with the stethoscope and double-checked by ordering another X-ray. I then walked down with the technician and checked the X-ray, arriving just as it had been developed.

Upon returning to the floor I was surprised to see Dr. Bradley outside the patient's room. It was 5:45 a.m. Apparently, he had called the floor looking for me to give him the result of the labs since I had taken too long to call him back. As the nasogastric tube and other floor issues had diverted my attention momentarily, he had grown impatient and decided to check for himself.

"I think he has an abscess around the newly transplanted kidney," he said sternly. Then he followed with, "And another thing, when you put an NG tube in, PUT IT ALL THE WAY IN," yelling this last part at the top of his lungs right there in the middle of the hall, while most patients were still asleep. Apparently, Dr. Bradley had stopped by radiology and seen the first X-ray that I had ordered. Not seeing the second, he assumed that I had placed the nasogastric tube short and had decided to leave it that way. I will admit that I did take some pleasure in correcting his misconception.

The other two attending surgeons on the kidney service worked in tandem with one another. They alternated call on a weekly basis and covered all the patients on the kidney transplant service that were not Dr. Bradley's patients. On their week off, they were involved in clinical research, as both of them were true surgeon-scientists. Dr. Steve Cosio was in his mid-forties and was extremely quiet and low-key. He was one of the best overall physicians that I've ever met, and the residents loved working with him. He won several awards from the residents for his teaching prowess while I was a resident at Jackson. During rounds, he was methodical, deliberate, and insightful. He spent a significant amount of time teaching, and was fond of quoting from *The House of God*, a book written in the 1970s that was later made into a movie and depicted the life of medical interns at a hospital in the northeast.

In the operating room, Dr. Cosio listened to soft music and was a master of the art. He was extremely good at setting up the case and making any resident look like a great surgeon. He was precise in his surgical teaching, spent all the time required, and allowed residents to do most of the work while he closely supervised every step. During emergencies in the operating room, he was just as controlled and in command. It was with him that I did my first start-to-finish kidney transplant—a truly memorable experience.

Dr. Silvio Sanmartino was Dr. Cosio's partner and was the complete opposite. A urologist by training, he had decided to pursue a career in transplant and was reputed to be one of the hardest working residents that Jackson Memorial had ever seen. He had a distinct combination Spanish/Italian accent and an extremely volatile personality. During rounds, Silvio, as he insisted on being called, would fly off the handle at the slightest provocation and start yelling at the top of his lungs. One always knew when he was covering the service, as the screaming was evident from the moment one stepped off the elevator on the fifteenth (transplant) floor.

In the operating room, Silvio was a master surgeon. He had the best set of hands that I've ever seen. Operating with him, though, was like doing rounds with him. At the slightest mistake he would start screaming at the top of his lungs. This would have the effect of making most residents scared and overly cautious while operating. One of my most vivid memories of operating with him was finishing a kidney transplant on a Saturday night at about two a.m.. Thankfully, things had gone extremely well, and we had completed all the vascular connections and had just finished suturing the ureter to the bladder. The transplanted kidney was producing plenty of urine and we were all pleased. I was particularly satisfied because my hands had worked well that day and Silvio had not screamed much through the entire case. I was looking forward to the closure and thanked my lucky stars that I had been spared a yelling session. I was a bit premature, though. Silvio asked the nurse to play a CD of Andrea Bocelli that he had in his bag. For the remainder of the case, I had to close while listening to Silvio sing at the top of his lungs in Italian. I felt as if I was part of a kidney transplant opera. But at least his "yelling" was not directed at me.

Transplant patients are unique in medicine. Their management is complex, and their care falls outside the scope of the practice of most physicians. Thus, transplant surgeons are in a way more like family physicians than any other surgical specialty. They take care of almost all the medical needs of their transplant patients, as the most innocent of infections or disease processes can rapidly become life-threatening in these patients. Moreover, they are on chronic immunosuppressive therapy, and most physicians do not feel comfortable managing them. This results in a unique situation where the surgeon takes care of most of these patients' medical issues, from the common cold to the rejection of the transplanted organ. Furthermore, the slightest change in their health is taken quite seriously, as it could always be the sentinel signal for an impending organ rejection.

The medical problems that arise in transplant patients can be surgical or non-surgical, but the transplant surgeon is always involved. With time, this fosters a close patient-doctor relationship. Most of these patients are truly in awe of their surgeons, and the majority would not let any other doctor treat them. This perspective is understandable as transplant surgery is life-transforming. In kidney transplants for example, they eliminate the need for three to four days per week of dialysis sessions that keeps these patients chained to a machine for several hours per day, and severely limits their quality of life. When the pancreas is transplanted in diabetic patients, it eliminates the need for daily insulin injections. A successful operation can make a drastic difference in these patients' health and lives, for which they are forever grateful.

For all the work that I had to do during that rotation, I did get to experience this special relationship between the surgeon and the transplant patient, albeit for a limited amount of time. I had already been involved in several transplants when, toward the end of my rotation, I had the chance to meet a brother and sister who had come in for a living-related kidney transplant. This is when the kidney of a matched live donor, usually a relative, is transplanted into a recipient. These were my favorite transplants. They were elective cases, and they were done during regular working hours. As there was plenty of time to do the preoperative work-up, the residents were not under the gun to get all the preoperative work done.

I had participated in living-related transplants before, but I had always been on the harvest team. It was my job to go in and harvest the kidney, which was then transplanted into the recipient who usually was being operated on in an adjacent room. Although the harvest surgery was great, the transplant surgery was much better. Between the third-year resident and the fellow on the service, we alternated surgeon positions on the transplants. This time, it was my turn in the transplant room, and most importantly, I was with Dr. Cosio. It was to be a great day.

I met Veronica and her brother Steve the morning of the operation. During the preoperative interview it was easy to see the deep love and respect between brother and sister. Having a sister myself, I could relate to this personally. Veronica was a woman in her late twenties. She was thin, had shoulder-length brown hair, and exceptionally fine features. She was not only pretty but had an air of elegance about her. While examining her prior to surgery, I noticed the multiple irregularities and scars on both of her arms, the result of multiple fistulas and grafts that are necessary for dialysis. She seemed self-conscious about these and had a way of keeping her arms bent at the elbows and close to her body at all times in an attempt to keep her forearms concealed from view.

She told me how her kidney failure had destroyed her life, including a very promising career as a journalist. Although she still did some writing, having to go to the dialysis center for four-hour sessions three times per week had kept her from continuing her job as an investigative journalist, her life passion. This had affected her more than the multiple medical appointments, operations, and the never-ending dialysis sessions. She was really looking forward to the possibility of never having to have dialysis again. Having her own working kidney again seemed like a fantasy to her, and she was in awe of the possibility that her life was about to change drastically for the better.

Her brother Steve was a man in his late thirties. He seemed in excellent health, he had an athletic physique, and his demeanor was friendly. He had traveled from Maine in order to donate his kidney, and he spoke eloquently of how thankful he was to be able to help his sister in such a significant and meaningful way. "Whatever she needs," he said. It was moving to see how he was looking forward to making his sister's life better. Such a generous gesture from a loved one was truly inspiring. After talking to both of them for several minutes, I was empathetic to their situation and felt that somehow, we had established an emotional connection. Moreover, I walked away hoping I would be willing to donate a kidney to my sister with as much enthusiasm as Steve.

The living-related transplant cases were done in adjacent rooms on the main operating floor at Jackson. The cases usually start simultaneously, and one team harvests the organ while the other team is preparing the recipient to receive the transplant. Although kidney transplantation has a good success rate, there is always the possibility that the transplanted kidney will not work. This can be devastating enough for the patient and surgeon when the kidney comes from a cadaveric donor; when it comes from a living relative, the tragedy is much worse as not only is the recipient affected, but the donor has undergone an operation and given up a kidney for naught. Although I had not been sensitive to this before, I was definitely experiencing more pressure on this case than in the other cadaveric transplants I had done. The fact that I had made such an emotional connection with Veronica and Steve during the preoperative visit did not make matters easier.

As I reached for the knife to start the operation, my hand shook slightly. The shaking got worse the closer the knife came to skin. The steady voice of Dr. Cosio coming from across the operating room table brought me back to the present task. I made a curvilinear incision on the lower right-hand quadrant of the abdomen and started the dissection. As we approached the external iliac vessels, my mind wandered to the adjacent room and the scene that was unfolding there. The team in that room would have gotten started a bit ahead of ours; the patient lying on his side, exposing the flank where the incision would have been made by Dr. Bradley. He performed most of the operations himself, allowing only a minimal amount of involvement by the resident or fellow other than assisting. I knew this firsthand, as I had already been involved in several of these harvests with him. The environment in the room would be tense, as Dr. Bradley was prone to getting impatient and upset while operating.

In our room the environment was calm and controlled. Dr. Cosio was a master at making any resident feel relaxed during surgeries. He would assist beautifully, exposing the surgical field and setting up the next step in the operation to allow for easy execution. We had exposed the external iliac artery and vein as well as the bladder wall when we got word from the other room. The kidney had been harvested and would be brought to us within the next several minutes. The door then opened, and it was Dr. Bradley himself, carrying the metal canister containing the kidney as if it were a newborn baby. He walked over to Dr. Cosio and seemed pleased with the harvested organ, which was resting in an iced-saline solution. They both talked while inspecting the kidney while I made the final preparations in the surgical field for the rest of the operation.

Finally, we were all ready. We clamped the iliac artery, made a longitudinal cut in the anterior wall, and proceeded to connect the artery from the donor kidney to the patient's native artery. Looking through my surgical loops, the light positioned exactly right, the anatomy was clear—as if in a surgical textbook. Under Dr. Cosio's guidance and expert assistance, I was performing at optimal level. The stitches were falling right where they should, and upon completion of the anastomosis (connection between the vessels), I took a second to inspect my work. The environment was relaxed, enjoyable, and I was happy with my performance. We were doing something special. There was pleasure in the act of doing the operation, but there was a deeper and more profound realization that what we were doing was actually going to make a huge difference in someone's life. I was pleased and proud.

We then unclamped the artery and saw the rush of blood fill the kidney, which in turn rapidly changed from a pale to a pink hue. I held my breath as the blood rushed past the connection in the artery that I had just completed. The suture line held; there was no leak. "Textbook," Dr. Cosio looked at me as he spoke. "Good job." I smiled under my mask and thanked him. We then proceeded with the vein and ureter connections, which turned out as successfully as the arterial one. Soon after the blood was allowed to perfuse the kidney, it began making urine. Dr. Cosio and I were both extremely happy. For him, seeing the urine dripping from the ureter was routine and expected; for me it was a thrill.

"It is like liquid gold, isn't it?" The voice was that of the kidney transplant fellow. We were in the ICU later that afternoon. During the middle of rounds, I had wandered off and had come down to the ICU to see if Veronica was awake so that I could talk to her. I had been to see her twice earlier in the afternoon and she had been heavily sedated. I had told her the operation had gone well but was not sure if she heard or understood me. Now I had just finished speaking with her and informed her that all was well. Her smile said it all. I was holding the clear Foley tube connecting her bladder to the reservoir bag, and I was inspecting the flow of clear amber urine. The rest of the residents had continued with rounds and had caught up with me. They were all standing behind me. It was easy to see what the fellow meant comparing urine to liquid gold. It was indeed a marvelous sight to see the urine flow from the bladder, through the Foley catheter tube and into the reservoir bag. It meant the kidney was working. It meant that the operation had been a success. It meant that Veronica would not have to undergo dialysis anymore and could go back to her old life. It was an awesome feeling.

Driving home that night I felt tired, but extremely satisfied. With my hands and a bit of help, I had performed a flawless operation. And by all indications, it had been a success. That evening I was not on call, so I was anticipating a well-deserved night of uninterrupted and peaceful sleep. It was about eleven p.m. and I was dozing off while watching TV when the phone rang. It was the intern.

"Just to let you know about the living-related patient. Her urine output has been decreasing over the last three to four hours."

"How can that be?" I said. "I just left there after seven p.m. and she was still peeing like a horse."

"Her urine output started dropping off after you left. The last hour she only put out 10cc."

This was extremely concerning at it could potentially mean that there was something wrong with the transplanted kidney. For some reason or another it was failing, and it was my job to find out why. "Did you check the Foley catheter?" I asked the intern. "Sometimes it gets clogged or kinked."

"First thing I did," he said. "I flushed and even changed it, but it has not made a difference."

This was a problem. There had been a precipitous drop in the urine output despite the patient being given plenty of fluids and remaining with stable vital signs. We had to find out the reason why, for if it was a mechanical reason, such as a kinked ureter or a leak in the vascular connections, the patient would need emergency surgery to fix the problem. I gave the intern a list of things to do: repeat labs, get an ultrasound of the transplanted kidney to see if the ureter was kinked or if the vascular connections had leaked, give the patient medications that would stimulate the kidney to make urine, etc. "And most importantly," I added, "make sure you keep in touch with me and let me know what is going on."

Although technically still a junior resident, I had been functioning as a senior resident on the transplant service for a little less than two months. I was soon feeling the increased pressure that came with that responsibility. During the first two years, residents rarely make independent decisions on patients. They follow the orders of the senior residents, who are the ones ultimately responsible. Interns and junior residents take their call in the hospital. When they are not on call, however, they go home and are off the pager, without any hospital responsibilities. All residents look forward to the day when they do not have to take in-house calls anymore. The grass is not always greener on the other side though, as the senior resident becomes the responsible party and needs to always be available. What this actually means is lost on junior residents who dream of the day when they no longer have to stay at the hospital overnight.

As a senior resident, most of the calls are taken from home. At first, this appears to the junior resident like a highly desirable option leading to an improved quality of life. The senior resident soon finds out, however, that taking calls from home is actually much worse in several ways. First, just because you go home, it does not mean that you can disconnect from what is going on with your patients. The senior resident still has ultimate responsibility, often for extended periods of time that can last from several days to several weeks before getting a day off. In some rotations, the senior resident must be available and is responsible for the service every day for the entire two months of the rotation. Every single day the senior resident must be available to the junior residents for questions, consults, guidance, and to solve any problems that come up no matter what time, day or night. Furthermore, there is a tricky issue of deciding which issues can be delegated to the intern, and which issues must be handled by the senior resident in person. This is compounded by the constant worry as to which intern and junior resident are trustworthy and responsible enough to follow through on what is being asked of them. There is also the issue as to whether or not they have the judgment to make the right decision. This part of serving as a senior resident was new to me, and I was struggling with it.

I was fully awake now after the phone call and felt I had covered all the bases. There was an issue with the kidney that needed to be addressed quickly. I had impressed upon the intern the importance of the tasks I'd given him, and I told him that he must not be distracted from these tasks by less important floor issues. He seemed to understand and told me he would call as soon as he had further information.

Lying in bed, my mind went back to the operation, and I tried to remember any possible mistakes that had been made which could account for the kidney not making enough urine now. My euphoria from earlier that day was rapidly turning into despair. There was nothing to be done until further information was available from the ultrasound, labs, response to medications, etc. Then I began thinking of the intern: Could I trust him? Did he know how to change a Foley catheter properly? Did he really check that the patient was getting adequate amounts of intravenous fluids? After a few minutes of this contemplation, I could not take it anymore. I got up, dressed, and headed for the hospital.

Veronica seemed surprised to see me.

"Something wrong?" she asked. I told her that there had been a decline in the function of the kidney, and we were investigating the cause. I tried to smile and put on my most confident air as I told her this. "I trust you," she simply said with a smile.

"Please don't, none of my girlfriends do," I joked and tried to seem relaxed and in control.

"I bet," she said. She was smiling again.

I reviewed the chart and confirmed the decline in urine output, replaced the Foley catheter one more time, checked the chart and with the nurse that the patient was getting the medications to stimulate urine output as indicated, checked with the radiology technician that the ultrasound was ordered as an emergency, and did everything else that came to mind. I paged the intern and again told him to make sure to call me as soon as he had any more information. He promised he would.

In the on-call room now, attempting to sleep was useless. It was not going to happen that night. Finally, the intern called; the ultrasound was normal. Neither the ureter nor the kidney showed any signs of dilation, which would indicate an obstruction to urine flow. There was no fluid collection around the kidney.

"Normal, as per the radiologist," he said. He further informed me that the urine output had not increased.

I had done all I knew to do. It was time to ask for help. Dr. Cosio called me right back after being paged. We discussed the case after I explained to him what was happening. We discussed adjustments in the medications and fluids. He complimented me on my management: Everything that needed to be done had been done.

"Now we just have to wait," he said. "Sometimes the kidney is stunned from the lack of blood during the transplant. We just have to hope that it can recover. Time will tell. Sometimes this is the most difficult time of transplant surgery, waiting to see if the operation worked."

Time is hard to endure when there is so much riding on the final outcome. The waiting was exasperating. It was impossible for me to get any sleep that night. This was my case. I had performed the operation start to finish and was solely responsible for the outcome. I found myself praying for the kidney to recover function. After several calls to the ICU to get an update on urine output, the nurse seemed to get a bit aggravated: "I will call you if there is a change in the trend. I promise."

The following morning there was still minimal urine output. Veronica was the first patient I saw that day, even before going up to the floor to start rounds. She had put out an average of less than 10cc of urine per hour almost the entire night, far less than the 30-50cc/hr. that is minimally expected. I tried to sound as confident as possible when I told her that this was just a temporary setback and we needed to wait for the kidney to recover function.

On the floor, Steve was doing great. A young and healthy man, he was responding like one. He had already gotten out of bed that morning and was not having much trouble with pain. "How is my sister?" was one of the first things he asked. I told him about the decrease in kidney function that we were dealing with, but also told him that we anticipated that this was only a temporary setback.

"The kidney will recover, right? The transplant will work, right?" He picked me out of the whole group of residents to direct the question to, but his eyes scanned all the faces in the room as if to gain independent confirmation of my answer from reading the faces of the others. I wondered if I should discuss with him that there was no way that I could guarantee that the kidney was going to recover function, and whether or not to share with him my increasing personal doubts.

"We fully expect the kidney will recover function and the transplant will work," was all I could muster to say.

It was hard to concentrate on my other cases for that day, as Veronica was constantly on my mind. I had gone to see her at the end of my first case and things had not changed. I was becoming more disheartened by the minute, especially since she was always so hopeful and cheerful every time I went to see her. By this time, I was beginning to think about how to break the news to her and her brother that the operation had been a failure.

It was late in the afternoon when a call came into the operating room from the transplant fellow and the message was relayed to me by the nurse. Over the past two hours, Veronica's kidney function had improved, and she was now producing more than 30cc per hour. I breathed a great sigh of relief. The curt thank-you that I gave the nurse did not reflect the exhilaration that I felt. An overwhelming feeling of confidence suddenly came over me. This kidney was going to work; I could feel it. Veronica was going to be free of dialysis, once and for all.

Veronica's transplanted kidney did rally, and progressively improved in function over the next couple of days. It was with great happiness that I went to her brother and told him that his kidney was working beautifully. His sister would now be free to lead a normal life, free of dialysis. "I am grateful to be able to do this for her," he said. His smile was contagious.

Steve was out of the hospital in three days. Veronica stayed a little longer and this gave me a chance to interact more with her. It was obvious that she was extremely grateful to her brother, to all of us on the medical team, and especially to Dr. Cosio and me. The way our operation had changed her life was ever-present on her mind. She was excited and hopeful about her future now, as was I.

During the morning rounds on the day she was to be discharged, I took great pleasure in informing Veronica that she was to go home that day. She was extremely happy and jovial, already making plans for the upcoming days.

"I am very grateful to my brother and to you guys for this gift you've given me." Although she looked at the entire team as she said this, her eyes seemed to pause when they met mine. Like her brother, I was grateful to have been able to be there for her. Helping her had been extremely special for me. In my young surgical career, this was the first time that I truly felt like the sole responsible party during the surgical care of a patient. She had indeed received the ultimate gift, but by being my patient and allowing me to care for her, she had given me a wonderful gift in return: the awesome feeling of gratification that comes from being able to make such a positive change in someone's life. Just as she was thankful to her brother for the ultimate gift and me for the surgery, I felt just as grateful to her for the gift the opportunity to be her surgeon had bestowed upon me.

LETTING GO

"I am sorry." I really meant it. It had been a long and hard ordeal for her.

"Thank you." Her grief was obvious, but she managed a half-smile. I knew she also meant what she said. A hug seemed awkward, so I reached out and touched her shoulder. Mrs. Swartz gave me a half-smile again, shook her head slightly, turned, and walked away. She was followed by members of her husband's family. My eyes followed her to the point where she turned the corner and was no longer in view. The charge nurse walked up to me with a piece of paper in her hand, and handed it to me as I sat at the desk. Extremely tired and with little enthusiasm, I started to fill out Mr. Swartz's death certificate. Looking at the clock on the wall I realized the reason for my lack of energy. It was 3:55 a.m. and it had been an awfully long day physically and emotionally.

"He held on a lot longer than we thought," said the charge nurse who was standing, looking over my shoulder. She wanted to make sure that the death certificate was completed properly and on time. Making sure all the *i*'s were dotted and the *t*'s were crossed was one of her responsibilities.

"He did," I agreed as I handed her the paper.

Dealing with death is part of any physician's life. It is something that medical students struggle with when they start their clinical rotations but something they need to learn to cope with emotionally, lest they become incapable of performing their responsibilities. In the hospital, death is a fact of daily life and can be encountered anywhere and at any time. The geriatric wards where the elderly are treated, and the medical wards where the chronically ill patients are often at the terminal stage of their disease, are areas of the hospital that deal with death on a regular basis. For surgeons, death can be encountered anywhere—on the wards, in the operating room, and even in the consultation rooms. There is no place, however, where the surgeon is forced to deal with issues of life, death, and quality of life more than in the surgical intensive care unit (ICU).

It is here that the sickest of patients in the hospital are brought for close and around-the-clock monitoring. Although for most patients this is but a temporary stop on their road to recovery, for others it is a final destination prior to dying. For the residents rotating in the ICU, this is the time to take a breather from learning about surgical procedures, and to spend some time learning about the medical management of the critically ill surgical patient. It is also a time to deal with the more spiritual aspects of medicine and ponder on issues that residents seldom think about—when is the time to do everything possible to save a patient's life, and perhaps most importantly, when is the right time to let go.

Jackson Memorial Hospital has many different intensive care units (ICUs). There is the medicine ICU, pediatric ICU, neurosurgery ICU, burn ICU, cardiothoracic ICU, trauma ICU, and the surgical ICU. General surgery residents rotate in the latter five during their training. The third-year rotation is through the surgical ICU, where all the general surgery patients who are critically ill are taken. There are also some overflow patients from the trauma ICU when bed availability is an issue, which is a chronic problem as the trauma unit is always full.

Although the original surgical team still manages the main surgical problems of patients in the intensive care unit, the ICU team manages the rest of the issues that pertain to the overall care of the patients, such as the ventilator settings, nutrition, intravenous lines, treatment of any systemic infections, etc. In theory, there is a coordinated effort between the original service and the ICU team in the management of each patient. This is the desired goal and although it is easily accomplished in some cases, it becomes difficult in other cases as communication between members of the various teams is not always optimal.

The ICU team is usually a large one. One of the general surgery attending surgeons, usually a trauma surgeon who has formal training in critical care, leads the team. These surgeons take turns in the ICU on a weekly basis. Other members of the team include the trauma/critical care fellows, who usually oversee the trauma units and cover the surgical ICU during nights and weekends. The third-year resident rotates as one of the seniors on the ICU and takes call every third day, being responsible overnight for all the patients in the surgical ICU. There are also three interns whose responsibility is the direct hands-on care of the patients including the minor procedures such as intravenous lines, cultures, etc. The two to three hours-long morning rounds include other hospital personnel, such as respiratory technicians, nutritionists, infectious disease nurses, medical students, and the ever-present charge nurse.

During morning rounds each patient is discussed in great detail. The patient is presented by one of the interns and all pertinent information including labs, recent events, studies, and culture results are discussed. Input is sought from and given by all members of the team, and a plan of action is formulated. The attendings and fellows also use this opportunity to teach relevant principles of critical care as they pertain to the particular patient being discussed. At the end of rounds, the team disperses, and each member goes off to complete the tasks assigned to him/her for that day. As events warrant, the particular medical situation of each patient can be reevaluated at any time, and the previously formulated plan of action is adjusted to reflect newly acquired information or changes in the patient's condition. These changes are usually made by the senior residents, often in consultation with the attending in charge.

Surgical residents usually enjoy their stint through the ICU. There is a wealth of vital information and skills to learn, which will serve the residents well as they go forth into their senior years, and eventually into their future surgical careers. Moreover, there is ample time for rounds and teaching conferences, as the residents don't have to rush off to the operating room by seven a.m. Although the hours are long, they are fixed, and the residents know that upon completion of their call day, another team will take over and the residents who are post-call will be able to go home. There is no such thing as getting stuck in the hospital for endless hours on a case or in an emergency admission to the service. Overall, the pace in the ICU is much slower than in any of the surgical services. This is a welcome change in the middle of the third year, when the surgical resident has completely lost the nervous energy and enthusiasm of the junior years and is stuck in the grind of the insurmountable work required during surgical training, with no clear end in sight.

Residents start the ICU anticipating the same level of effort and energy that any other surgical service requires. Soon, however, they realize the inherent slower pace and they adjust physically and mentally to the new circumstances. There is more time for reading, discussions of treatment plans, and yes, introspection. Interestingly, a paradigm shift takes place. The nearly complete focus on learning about disease processes, treatments, and surgical procedures diminishes slightly, and thoughts about the patients themselves and their lives creep into the resident's consciousness. I think this is a combination of the slower pace of the service, which allows time for this, and the extremely sick patients who force the residents to deal with life and death issues on a day-to-day basis.

Being in the unit the whole day rather than in the operating room allows the resident ample exposure to the patient's family members. The dramatic impact that illness can have on family dynamics is fully appreciated as one gets to know and talk to the family members of the ICU patients, some of whom stay in the ICU for extended periods of time—sometimes up to several months. It was during my ICU rotation in the middle of my third year of training that a change took place in me. I began to look at my work in residency in a deeper and more comprehensive way. For better or worse, the work I was involved in was having a significant impact not only on the patient's life, but just as importantly on the patient's family as well. This rotation, more than any other, was responsible for increasing my awareness of these issues, and giving me the emotional tools and understanding to become a more empathetic physician.

"You and I will take care of the open abdomens today." The fellow had directed this comment to me as rounds were breaking up on my first day in the unit. My first call day of the rotation was not until my third day on the service, and I was eager to get involved. He directed me to the bed of a young black woman who was obviously extremely ill. She was intubated, did not respond to any stimuli, and had a multitude of medications hung on her intravenous lines (drips) that were helping maintain her blood pressure. She was also connected to a dialysis machine. As I looked into her face while waiting for instructions from the fellow, I noticed that she could not be any older than her mid-twenties. Younger than me, and lying here in the ICU, at the precipice of death.

It did not take long for the fellow to tell me her story. She had been given a general anesthetic called halothane in a hospital in the Bahamas for an elective C-section for her first pregnancy. Everything went well with the surgery, but shortly thereafter she had experienced one of the potential complications to halothane, liver failure. Halothane is no longer used in the United States for adult anesthesia due to this complication. The liver failure had caused a depletion of the proteins in the blood that help with coagulation, as they are manufactured in the liver, and she experienced severe intra-abdominal bleeding on the fourth postoperative day. The bleeding required emergency surgery. Surgery stopped the bleeding, but due to the amount of swelling of her intestines, the surgeons were unable to close the abdominal wall, thus leaving her with what is commonly referred to in surgery as an "open abdomen." Soon thereafter, she had been transferred to Jackson so that her open abdomen could be managed, and she could potentially receive a life-saving liver transplant. She had been in the ICU for approximately two weeks and had experienced further complications including kidney failure. Her prognosis was extremely poor.

"Gown-up," said the fellow who was handing me a sterile gown as he pointed to the bedside table that contained the caps and masks. We both quickly put on our gowns while the nurse opened a large sterile pack on a table that had been placed at the foot of the bed. The curtains were then drawn around the bed, and the nurse proceeded to remove the patient's abdominal dressing. Staring at me was a bloated abdomen which was opened from the xyphoid (right below the chest) to the pubis. The skin margins were wide apart and between them was protruding a large mass of matted intestines, stomach, and the lower edge of the liver. The sight was striking and gruesome for those uninitiated in the care of the "open abdomen," such as me.

"Pour," said the fellow as he pointed to the container of sterile saline (water) which the nurse had placed on the side table. I poured the warm, sterile water onto the open belly as the fellow immersed his hands in it and tried to clean the exposed organs by gently rubbing them with his gloved hands.

"You must make sure to clean in all the recesses." His hands pulled one of the skin edges aside and his hand slipped into the recess up to mid-forearm. With this maneuver, a significant amount of bloody, murky fluid emanated from the hidden space. I continued to pour water while he continued to clean. As the water accumulated and filled up the abdominal space, he would then suction it. Then we would repeat the process. With each washing, the suctioned water became cleaner and cleaner. When the fellow was satisfied that we had done enough, he proceeded to show me how to apply a dressing to an open abdominal wound. This was an elaborate process that took close to fifteen minutes. While doing the dressing, I took a second to straighten my back and glanced at the patient's face. She was serene and did not seem to be in any pain. I pondered on the dramatic change in her circumstances. A couple of weeks before she had gone to sleep thinking that in a matter of a couple of hours, she would wake up from surgery with her baby in her arms to start her new life as a mother. Two weeks later, she was separated from her baby and would have little in the way of hope if she were conscious of her situation. Mercifully, she was not aware of her present circumstances; she was in a sustained coma, either from her disease or the medications she was being given.

Upon finishing with the dressing, I was promptly informed by the fellow that we had two more of these open abdomens to do. I was happy to help and was interested in learning the procedure and how to do the dressings, but I was silently hoping that the fellow was not designating me the "open abdomen" resident. Doing three of these dressings every day would take a lot of time and effort, which would detract from the many other things I had to learn during that rotation. As if reading my mind, the fellow soon informed me that he was taking me through the dressings in order to teach me how to do them. Starting the following day, the senior residents would take turns doing the dressings on a rotating daily basis. Each senior resident would do the dressings with one of the interns, teaching him or her in turn what I had just been taught. It seemed that the fellow was ready henceforth to delegate this daily activity to others.

The two other patients with the open abdomens had tragic stories similar to the first. One was a man in his mid-forties who had been involved in a motor vehicle accident and had sustained severe intra-abdominal bleeding from liver and spleen lacerations. His life had been saved during the initial operation, but the swelling of the intestines that resulted did not permit the surgeons to close his abdomen at that original, life-saving intervention. This particular situation is not uncommon in trauma patients who as a result of their injuries require abdominal surgery and lose a lot of blood and thus require transfusion of large amounts of blood and fluids in a short period of time in an attempt to save their lives. Trauma patients normally go to the trauma ICU; however, that unit was full on the day of his admission, so the patient had been brought to the surgical ICU until a bed became available in the trauma unit.

The second patient was a young, healthy man in his thirties who had suddenly developed a swelling of his pancreas, a disease called pancreatitis. Although this condition can be linked to such causes as gallstones, alcohol abuse, scorpion bites, et al., the reason for this man's pancreatitis had not been discovered. Just the same, the devastating sequelae of this condition was the same. His condition worsened to the point where emergency surgery was needed to clean out all the dead and inflamed tissue around his pancreas, the result of the pancreatic enzymes that had leaked into his abdominal cavity. This open abdomen was slightly different from the other two. Whereas the first two patients' abdomens were open in a vertical direction, the incision on this abdomen was horizontal, approximately below the ribs on both sides. The skin of the lower half of the abdomen was pushed into the wound and it seemed as if it was secured with sutures to some structure deep in the abdomen. There were also large drains sticking out from either side of the man's abdomen, which were continuously irrigated with sterile saline solution.

As we did the dressing on this man, the fellow explained to me what a devastating and life-threatening disease pancreatitis is, something I was soon to learn in my other experiences of the third and fourth year. The pancreas releases insulin, as well as a multitude of digestive enzymes that are responsible for the breakdown of foods that are ingested. These digestive enzymes are released into the gastrointestinal (GI) tract via the pancreatic duct. The GI tract has a special epithelium—lining—which is designed to resist these enzymes. However, when the enzymes leak into the abdominal cavity proper, as in cases of pancreatitis—inflammation of the pancreas—the body in essence begins to eat itself and aggressive tissue destruction and inflammation ensues. Constantly irrigating the pancreatic enzymes from the abdominal cavity with the saline drains, and mechanically removing all the necrotic (dead) tissue from the abdominal wound, was sometimes the only thing that would save the patient's life. As opposed to the first two patients who were intubated and unresponsive, this particular patient, although intubated, was awake and was able to follow commands and answer questions with gestures. We had to sedate him before embarking on our washout procedure so as to ameliorate the pain.

"What ends up happening with these patients?" I asked. After doing three of these washouts in one day, I was curious to know how long these patients stayed like this, and what was the ultimate outcome of this condition. The fellow rolled his eyes before answering.

"This is a long, long process...which sometimes takes up to months." The fellow explained that after many days of these washouts, and like with any other open wound, the abdominal wound slowly contracts over time and a layer of healing tissue called granulation tissue then covers the exposed bowels until finally, patients end up with a large open wound. The matted intestines and internal organs are covered by a thin layer of granulation tissue with the remaining skin of the abdominal wall around the periphery. Since the abdominal wall also contracts, it is almost always impossible to close the abdominal wall, and the usual treatment is to place a skin graft over the healing bed of the open wound. While trying to imagine what that would look or feel like, the fellow seemed to read my mind. "Don't fret; you will take care of plenty of these patients at all stages during your trauma rotation." In this he was right, as I indeed took care of many patients with open abdomens during my trauma rotations as a senior and chief resident.

Although I knew who Dr. Gerald Wodicka was, up to that time my personal interaction with him had been minimal. Being the program director, he was in charge of all the surgical residents. His popularity among the senior residents was known, but the first- and second-year residents did not work with him enough to have an opinion of him one way or the other. My first interactions with him were in my ICU rotation. Ultimately this was the start of a great friendship with someone I liked and came to admire, which continues to the present day. Even though he was only in his early to mid-forties, he was considered a senior attending as he had been teaching at the university for several years. Moreover, he had recently been promoted to co-program director and was being groomed to eventually take that position. An extremely versatile and smart surgeon, he was involved in the trauma service, the hepatobiliary service (Elective 2 or E2), and was also one of the surgical ICU attendings. I soon learned that he took care of all the pancreatitics in the hospital who required surgery. Thus, his interest in our patient was due to the fact that he had operated on him several times already.

A caring man, Dr. Wodicka was exemplary in the way he took care of his patients. Rather than leave most of the routine management decisions to the fellows and residents, Dr. Wodicka insisted on being personally involved. He had two distinctive qualities. One was that when worried about a patient, he would tend to pace and linger somewhere close to the patient's bedside, as if trying to work himself up to being able to handle potentially bad news. When ready, he would then approach the fellow or resident taking care of his patient and inquire as to how the patient was doing. The other feature was extremely unique and almost made for a bad start between the two of us. This feature was his voice. His voice was low-pitched and had a rasping quality which seemed comical, and often elicited a chuckle from those who had never heard him speak. His voice had that effect on me, and I caught myself laughing during rounds the first time I heard it, the day he took over as the ICU attending for the second week I was there.

One night during a phone conversation in which we were discussing a recent admission to the unit of an unstable patient, his distinctive voice was clear through the receiver:

"Joe, if she looks at you the wrong way, Swan her." He meant that if the patient deteriorated in any way during the night, I should place a special catheter that travels from the large veins of the chest or neck through the heart into the vessels that go from the heart to the lungs (pulmonary artery). This catheter would allow us to take pressure measurements and give us a better picture of the intravascular volume of the patient and help us work through the different reasons the patient might have low blood pressure. This catheter was often referred to as a "Swan" stemming from its name Swan-Ganz catheter. The patient's condition having deteriorated overnight necessitated the placement of a Swan-Ganz catheter, which I performed in the middle of the night. During rounds the following morning, after noticing that the patient had the catheter placed, Dr. Wodicka asked, "Joe, why did you Swan her?"

I could not resist, and in my best imitation of his voice I responded, "Because she looked at me the wrong way."

My answer elicited a chuckle from several of those present at rounds, but Dr. Wodicka gave me a look that let me know he did not appreciate the joke. I occasionally tell that story to people now when I talk about Dr. Wodicka, but in retrospect I have always felt guilty at my attempt at humor at his expense, which might have had the unintended consequence of offending such a great man. It is a testament to the person he is that he forgave me for my lapse in judgment. Although I understood by his reaction that the joke registered with him, he has never held it against me. We have since become friends and have had great interactions together in and out of the operating room.

"What is the plan with this man?" Dr. Wodicka was now discussing Mr. Swartz, one of the many liver transplant patients that were in the ICU at any one time. To be honest, I had not thought much of the plan for Mr. Swartz as his condition had not changed dramatically over the week and a half that I had spent in the ICU. His story, as I had been told, was that he was a man in his late fifties who had contracted hepatitis C through a prior blood transfusion. The disease had finally ravaged his liver and he had undergone a transplant about two weeks prior to the start of my rotation. Although his operation had gone uneventfully, he had developed postoperative complications not the least of which was pneumonia, which had prevented his extubation and led to a worsening course and several related complications since then.

When I arrived in the unit, he was intubated and was receiving antibiotics for his pneumonia. Over the course of my short ICU stay, his condition had not changed dramatically in either direction. Dr. Wodicka was obviously concerned that his condition had not improved despite aggressive antibiotic therapy. We discussed this patient in detail, and further cultures and diagnostic studies were ordered. As this patient was a typical ICU patient (sick, intubated, on antibiotics and nutritional supplementation), he had not made an impression on me the short time I was there. Dr. Wodicka's special interest in this patient brought him more into focus.

We arrived at an overall plan that included feedback from the liver transplant service as to why they thought the patient was not improving despite what seemed to be optimal therapy. Communicating with the liver service was to be my responsibility for that day. Upon completion of rounds that morning, I immediately paged the liver service. The intern who answered was not much help but promised me that he would deliver the message to the fellow in charge of the service as soon as he got out of the operating room to contact me regarding this patient. The call came in late that afternoon.

"We don't think there is anything special with him," the voice of the fellow seemed tired. There was a foreign accent, which I could not place. "The liver is working fine, and it is just a matter of treating his sepsis with antibiotics."

I had learned by now that it was a futile effort to argue with other services regarding the management of their patients. It was much more effective to attempt gentle persuasion in order to get your point across. "The ICU team is concerned because despite what we think is optimal care, Mr. Swartz's condition has not improved. We are wondering if there is something else going on, perhaps an intra-abdominal process like a leak or dead bowel."

"Unlikely," the fellow seemed self-assured, "he would have been much sicker if that was the case."

"Agreed." I answered. "Please discuss him in detail with your attending during rounds and call us back with some suggestions. We need some help with this one." I hoped my tactfulness would lead to some positive results.

In the meantime, I set out to do some of my own investigative work. As Dr. Wodicka had unofficially put me in charge of this patient, I thought the least I could do was my own independent evaluation of the patient's situation to see if it led to any ideas as to why he was not getting better. Looking through the patient's chart and through multiple lab and culture results, I could find no answer there. His pneumonia and sepsis were being treated with the appropriate antibiotics as per the lab results. All organisms that had grown from his cultures of sputum (lung and pharyngeal secretions), blood, and the tips of catheters that had been removed (central lines) had proven sensitive to the antibiotics he was receiving. As of the previous week, even antifungal therapy had been started in case his condition was due to an overwhelming fungal infection, which are notorious for not showing up on cultures. I then did a detailed physical exam on the patient looking for hidden sources of infection. I looked at the venous catheter sites and all extremities looking for abscesses, did a rectal exam looking for a hidden perirectal abscess, and checked to make sure that all venous lines were new, thus reducing the possibility that they were the source of the infection. After spending three hours studying the patient in detail, I was no closer to the answer than when I started. Everything seemed to be in order, yet the patient was not responding as he should. When all else fails, surgeons immediately start thinking of a possible intra-abdominal process, such as an abscess, intestinal leak, or dead bowel. These possibilities can only truly be ruled out by an exploratory laparotomy, where the surgeons open the abdomen and search for potential issues. It was now my job to try to convince the liver team to perform such a procedure. It was not going to be an easy task, as taking unstable patients to the operating room often presents its own unique set of risks.

While still at the patient's bedside doing my investigative work, suddenly a swarm of visitors entered the unit. I always found it difficult to perform patient care during visiting hours. As I turned from the bedside in an attempt to make my escape before the family arrived, an obviously concerned woman in her fifties approached me.

"Hi, I am Mrs. Swartz. Are you his doctor?" She smiled as she spoke, but her voice showed a mixture of sadness and concern. I had noticed her before while doing work in the unit during visiting hours, but this was the first time that I had dealt with her one-on-one. From what I had seen to that point, she seemed devoted to her husband and never failed to be present during every visiting hour. Sometimes there were others with her, but most of the time she was alone. As she had mostly dealt with the members of the liver team, I had not up to that point spoken to her about her husband's condition. It was an uncomfortable position to be in, as I had no good news to offer her.

"I am Dr. Garri, one of the doctors in the ICU team." While saying this, my mind was racing for the answer to the question that was sure to come next.

"How is he doing today?"

"Well," I said, buying time. "His condition has not really changed; we are in the process of trying to figure out why he is not getting better."

"I thought it was pneumonia. That's what the liver team told us."

For me this has always been one of the more delicate parts of talking to a patient's family member who deal with more than one doctor or team of doctors—to make sure that what you say does not in any way confuse the family members by appearing contradictory to what they may have been told by others.

"It is pneumonia, but we want to make sure there is nothing else."

"What do you mean—nothing else?" She seemed slightly distressed now.

In an attempt to salvage a situation that seemed to be slipping, I made my best effort to seem confident. "Nothing really. It is just that when we have a patient with an infection, we routinely search for all other causes that might be contributing to it. In his case, we have not found anything else wrong. So far it seems that it is just the pneumonia."

She did not seem completely convinced by my statement and still had a quizzical look on her face. I thought it best to limit my losses and quickly excused myself. As I walked away from her, I felt terrible about the encounter and hoped that the conversation had not added to her worries, but it appeared that it had.

The next morning, I made a point to be at bedside when the liver transplant team came for rounds. At first it was the intern taking some notes, and finally the whole team arrived. The fellow in charge was discussing the patient with the team when he noticed me standing by the group. He smiled and extended his hand, which I shook and introduced myself.

"Any ideas?" My question was an opening for him to share the discussions he had with his attending since yesterday's conversation.

"We don't think there is anything going on in the belly. The patient had a chest and abdomen CT scan just over a week ago and nothing was found except for the pneumonia. The antibiotic therapy and bronchoscopies should make him come around."

I had been on the receiving end of these conversations before, where the ICU team had its theories and wanted the primary surgeon to follow a certain course of treatment. It was an uncomfortable position to be in for everyone involved. I empathized with the fellow having to relay and defend his attending's decisions to the ICU team. Trying to avoid having the two of us become the middlemen between the attendings, I suggested that he have his attending call Dr. Wodicka directly so that they can discuss the case. The fellow promised me he would relay the message.

Over the course of the next few days, however, Mr. Swartz did not improve. Indeed, he deteriorated rather significantly. One of the clinical pictures seen in sepsis or generalized infection is that the capillary beds in the body become leaky and allow the fluid normally contained in the arteries and veins to shift to the tissues. This results in less blood volume, which in turn results in a drop in blood pressure. In order to treat this condition, besides the antibiotics or the treatment of the cause of the sepsis, large amounts of fluid must be given to the patient in order to replace the lost volume in the vascular space. As this fluid continues to shift into the tissue spaces, the patient becomes swollen. The fluid that leaks into the tissues in the lung makes the patient difficult to ventilate, a conditioned called by the acronym ARDS—Acute Respiratory Distress Syndrome. In order to treat this condition, the ventilator settings must be changed so as to increase the concentration of oxygen given and the pressure in which it is delivered in an attempt to overcome this decrease in the ability of the oxygen to be exchanged in the lung's capillary beds. ARDS is a particularly challenging condition to treat and often proves fatal unless the reason for it, which is often an overwhelming systemic infection called sepsis, is treated effectively in a timely manner. With each and every day that passed, Mr. Swartz was spiraling down this well-known path, ultimately leading to death.

A little over a week had gone by since Dr. Wodicka first made his comment during rounds, and Mr. Swartz's condition had greatly deteriorated since then. He was bloated and the ICU team was fighting a losing battle trying to ventilate him and keep his blood pressure up. His blood pressure was no longer responding to fluid infusions and medications were being given to maintain it at a normal level. These medications, commonly referred to as "vasopressors" or "pressors," are often a last-ditch effort that signal a deteriorating and final stage of sepsis.

One afternoon while walking through the ICU, I saw the liver transplant attending by the patient's bedside looking over the chart and I decided to venture a conversation. I introduced myself not knowing what response I might receive, as there was by now some tension between the ICU team and this attending concerning the patient.

"Hey Joe," he responded in a friendlier tone that I was expecting.

"What do you think?" My statement was an invitation for the attending to share his plans.

"I guess we will take a look, but I am sure there is nothing going on in the abdomen. The fellow will come and make the arrangements. Please have the patient ready."

Finally, the decision had been made, and I quickly let Dr. Wodicka know. He seemed pleased. The patient did not make it to the operating room until late that evening, and we were all disappointed during rounds the next day when we learned that the exploratory surgery had not revealed the cause of the patient's deterioration. The abdominal exploration had been completely normal.

"Sorry to hear that." Dr. Wodicka's words conveyed his utter disappointment. It was obvious that he genuinely believed that finding something in the patient's abdomen and treating it was the only chance that Mr. Swartz had. "We need to start talking to the family." Dr. Wodicka's statement had obvious implications, but none of us on the team thought that all was lost for Mr. Swartz. He was fairly healthy, young, and with the right antibiotic treatment and some time, his condition should surely turn around.

Dr. Wodicka had rotated in the unit a full two weeks by now, one more week than the usual stint, but eventually his time came to an end and he was replaced by Dr. Vignona, one of the trauma attendings with whom I had worked very little. He was of the same opinion as Dr. Wodicka, and he had extraordinarily little hope for Mr. Swartz. During rounds on the first day of Dr. Vignona's rotation, it was obvious that he was well-versed in Mr. Swartz's hospital course. He already knew of and did not seem interested in most of the details, but quickly inquired as to whether the liver transplant service had conveyed to the patient's family the gravity of the patient's condition. He seemed to direct his question toward me.

"To be honest with you, sir, I am not aware of what conversations the transplant team is having with Mr. Swartz's family."

"Well…what have you told the family?"

"I've told the wife that he is not improving but I have not discussed his condition in great detail out of respect for the primary team."

Dr. Vignona looked up from the patient's chart and in the calm voice that was his normal tone said, "Well, you better start talking to her. We are reaching a point of futility here and we need to get the family ready. Talk to the transplant people and find out their thoughts on this."

From previous comments by Dr. Wodicka and the daily deterioration of Mr. Swartz, the possibility of the demise of this patient was becoming more real by the day. It was something that most of us in the ICU team thought privately but did not express to one another. Now the issue had been brought out in the open, and it became real for the first time right then and there, upon Dr. Vignona uttering those words.

I was having problems dealing with this new reality regarding Mr. Swartz. Why now? Why him and not another patient in a similar situation? It was obvious that Mr. Swartz was extremely ill, and that despite our best efforts his condition was worsening. But at the same time there did not seem to be an obvious irreversible condition. If we could get over this episode of sepsis somehow, he could potentially come back. In my estimation all hope was not lost, but I was fully aware that my opinion conflicted with that of people who had been doing this kind of work for years, and who had worlds of experience over me.

When Mrs. Swartz visited her husband that morning, I decided to get a sense of how she felt in regard to the conversations she was having with the liver team. My pretense was to come to look at the chart and engage in conversation. She already knew me from our numerous interactions, and it was my sense that she liked me. Moreover, she seemed thankful for the work all of us were putting into her husband's care. After she inquired about her husband, however, and I told her that he seemed to be getting slightly worse, her response took me a bit by surprise. "Yes, I can't wait until we get over this infection." It was obvious to me that she did not appreciate the full extent of her husband's condition and that she was nowhere near ready to consider discontinuation of care.

"You gotta get all that fluid out." The liver transplant attending had been visiting the patient's bedside another late evening several days later. I made an attempt to impress upon him the ICU team's negative prognosis for this patient—a conviction that by now had become mine as well. My discussions with the transplant fellow had not gotten me anywhere in this regard, but I was sure he was just regurgitating his attending's opinion.

In the most respectful way possible, my response was a synopsis of the frustrating aspect of taking care of this patient: "We are trying, as it is getting more and more difficult for him to breathe, but the minute we try to get some fluid off, his blood pressure bottoms out. He just can't take it. We are giving him multiple pressors all at maximum dose and we can barely keep his pressure up." The pressors were medications like epinephrine and norepinephrine, which cause the patient's heart to contract harder, while at the same time causing the peripheral blood vessels to constrict, the combination leading to an increase in the patient's blood pressure to normal levels. The problem with these medications is that they can be detrimental if used in high doses or for long periods of time.

"You must keep trying. If you get all this fluid out of his lungs, he will breathe easier and he will turn around."

"We are trying our best, but he is just not tolerating it. The ICU team feels it is time to talk to the family about discontinuing his care." I interjected this last sentence in as nonthreatening a manner as possible.

"Absolutely out of the question. We are not giving up on him." The attending's answer did not leave any room to maneuver.

This situation represented for me a true dilemma. Here were experienced surgeons on both sides of this issue, and I was in the middle. The entire ICU team including attendings, fellows, and residents seemed ready to give up on Mr. Swartz, while his primary surgeon was not. Who was right? Who should prevail in this issue? How is one to decide in these matters?

While having dinner at the hospital cafeteria a couple of days later, I shared my ambivalence with one of the chief residents who was now rotating in another service. He told me a story about that particular liver attending which he thought might provide me with some perspective on the attending's point of view. It involved a patient dying in the operating room while he was performing an operation. He immediately started doing CPR and attempting by all means to resuscitate the patient. After a while, it had been the consensus in the room of all doctors present both in the surgical and anesthesia team, that it had been too long, and it was time to stop attempts at resuscitation. This particular surgeon disagreed, however, and insisted the efforts continue, which they did for close to one hour. Although that amount of time is most likely an exaggeration, the gist of the story was that the attending had refused to give up and the patient finally recovered and eventually walked out of the hospital.

"That's why he never gives up," the chief resident concluded.

"It is hard to argue with success, but what is right for this patient and his family?" My question came truly from the heart. I was living each and every day with the struggle of how hard it was to find the answer to that question.

"I am going to speak to him today, and then we are going to have a family meeting," said Dr. Vignona, his patience exhausted, and he'd had enough of communicating through me to the family and the liver team. It was time for him to argue his position with the liver transplant attending personally. Looking at Mr. Swartz, I concurred. He was extremely bloated now, an unrecognizable figure from what he had been when admitted. His facial features were obscured by all the edema. His extremities were three times the size of what they had been. We had switched him to a ventilator called the jet ventilator—a last-ditch effort to ventilate his lungs despite all the accumulated fluid. I wondered what his wife was thinking every time she visited him now. I felt sorry for her. She had been there by his side for nearly two months.

When I walked in for rounds a couple of days later, the charge nurse informed me that we were having a meeting with the family that morning. This meant only one thing: Dr. Vignona had persuaded the liver transplant attending, and the discussion with the family was finally going to take place. As it was a situation that I had never encountered before, I was eager to know how Dr. Vignona was going to approach it.

The family, which now included Mrs. Swartz and her sister, was brought into a small room adjoining the ICU. The charge nurse then called for Dr. Vignona and me and we all walked into the room together. Mrs. Swartz looked up at me and our eyes met. She forced a smile of recognition. Dr. Vignona and the charge nurse sat immediately in front of Mrs. Swartz and her sister; I chose one of the empty chairs on the wall of the room, directly to the side of the group.

Dr. Vignona spoke first, and after exchanging small talk he proceeded: "What is your understanding of your husband's condition?"

Mrs. Swartz was holding her sister's hand as if expecting bad news. Her voice trembled as she spoke. "I know he is being treated for a systemic infection which started in his lungs. I also know that he is very ill."

"He is terribly ill, and unfortunately we have reached the point where we all feel that there is not much else we can do for him. We have discussed his condition with the liver service, and we all feel the same way." The words hung in the air for a moment as Dr. Vignona had intended them to. He said nothing else.

"What do you mean?" Mrs. Swartz seemed somewhat surprised. "Are you giving up?"

From the side of the room, I now felt somewhat guilty about being present in this conversation. This seemed like such a private moment for Mr. Swartz's family, and I felt I was intruding, as I truly had little to contribute. Since I was there already, it was impossible to leave. I found myself unable to look at Mrs. Swartz directly; my gaze drifted to the floor in a feeble attempt to offer her some privacy.

"We would never give up if we thought we could do some good. But in medicine sometimes we reach a point where we know we can no longer help the patient. At that point, our thoughts turn to the patient's wishes and about letting the patient die with all the human dignity that he or she deserves." Dr. Vignona's words were delivered slowly and calmly, knowing the recipient needed time to take their meaning in. My eyes were still focused on the floor and on the periphery when I saw Dr. Vignona reach out to Mrs. Swartz's hand.

"You know him best, what would he want us to do at a time like this?"

Mrs. Swartz did not say a word, but her sobbing was audible. I looked up to see tears on her face and her sister gently stroking her hair. No one uttered a word for a few minutes as the moment lingered. Dr. Vignona was the next to speak: "Take all the time you need to think about this. I want you to know that we are all here to help you in any way we can. Please feel free to call on us any time you wish." Mrs. Swartz sat looking at the floor now and did not seem to want to say anything else. Dr. Vignona sat for a few seconds longer and then slowly stood up. He looked my way and shook his head slightly. I took his lead and followed him out of the room, leaving the two women and the charge nurse behind.

Later that afternoon, I saw Mrs. Swartz at her husband's bedside well after visiting hours were over. Obviously, she was being given plenty of leeway as she struggled with an exceedingly difficult decision. Our eyes met briefly but neither of us spoke. Later that day I heard from the charge nurse that Mrs. Swartz had advised her that she was ready to discontinue care. She had called for Mr. Swartz's parents to come down from Ohio, and they were expected the next day at noon.

It just so happened that the next day I was on call. Mr. Swartz's parents had been delayed and did not arrive until after four p.m. The entire family had been shown to the bedside by the charge nurse, who then pulled the curtain around the bed to give them some privacy. About two hours later while I was admitting a new patient to the unit, the charge nurse came up to me and informed me that she was going to discontinue life support for Mr. Swartz. She would have me sign the orders later. I saw her disappear behind the patient's curtain to discontinue the pressors and place the patient on a morphine drip in order that he not suffer any pain. In such situations, the ventilator is always left on, as well as the EKG machine to monitor the patient's heartbeat, the absence of which would alert us to his death. As she went behind the curtain, I went back to my work.

As my new admission had been somewhat complicated, I lost track of what was happening with Mr. Swartz. Several times while in the unit doing something else, my eyes would glance at the pulled curtain of Mr. Swartz's bed, and I would inquire of the charge nurse. "Not yet," she would say.

It was way past three a.m. now, and I was in the middle of my sixth admission for that day. It had been a busy call night and my focus on other patients had taken my mind off thinking about Mr. Swartz. I was sitting at a small desk by the nurses' station writing orders when the charge nurse finally came up to me and grabbed my shoulder. When I looked up at her she turned her head slightly in the direction of Mr. Swartz and softly said,

"It won't be long now…he is in agonal rhythm." This is an abnormal heart rhythm that heralds impending death.

It suddenly occurred to me that we had stopped his medications at around six p.m., and he was still alive. He was a fighter. Having completed my admission orders on the patient who had just arrived, I handed them to the nurse. I still had several things to do but felt obliged to be around for Mrs. Swartz. I felt I owed her and her husband that much. I leaned over on the desk, put my head in my arms, and waited for Mr. Swartz to die.

FOR LIFE AND LIMB

The vascular surgery service was reputed to be one of the worst rotations in the entire residency when it came to the amount of work involved. There were usually three residents assigned to the service, including a chief resident, a third-year resident, and an intern. Perhaps even more frustrating was the fact that medical students did not rotate through the vascular surgery service, as this was not one of their core rotations. By now I had been in the game long enough to realize how much medical students helped with the more mundane and tedious chores of running a service, like writing daily progress notes, collecting lab values, calling in consults, etc. I was paired with an orthopedic intern who always seemed to find the time during working hours to get in his daily workout at the university gym on campus but yet never got his work done, leaving me to finish the task. Thus, I easily became overwhelmed within a few of days of being on the service.

It soon became my mission to try to recruit a medical student to come help me. I knew recruiting medical students from the University of Miami (UM) was futile, as they were not allowed to rotate on vascular surgery. However, there were always numerous foreign medical school students doing core and elective rotations at the hospital. They had much more flexibility as to which rotation they wanted to take, particularly during their final year when they were allowed to take electives. I thought perhaps one of them could be enticed to join the cause.

One day while in the elevator during my second week on the service, I noticed one of the foreign medical students leaning against the back wall. Since we were alone in the elevator, I decided to make an attempt at recruiting him. Ramiro Beguiristain was in his late twenties or maybe early thirties, of medium height, and somewhat heavy-set in appearance. Upon striking up a conversation with him, I learned that he was a third-year medical student going to school in Grenada and was about to start his nephrology rotation the following week.

"Nephrology?" I said. "Why are you doing that?"

"Because I want to learn about the kidney…" He could have easily ended that sentence by saying, "Duh!"

"But why? That's boring. Don't you like surgery?"

He suddenly had a huge smile on his face. "I love surgery. As a matter of fact, I used to be a scrub tech before going to medical school. It is my plan to be a surgeon."

This was all I needed to hear. "Would you not rather do a surgery rotation instead?"

He seemed terribly disappointed. "I would love to, but they are all taken by the UM students. We are not allowed." This was the opening I needed and was waiting for.

"Not vascular surgery. We don't have any students rotating on the service currently. I can promise you plenty of operating room time; you just need to help me with some of the work on the floor." Ramiro looked at me suspiciously, but I could see the possibility intrigued him. After all, how passionate can one be about the kidney?

I decided to add further enticement. "By the way, I also happen to have plenty of leftover meal tickets. I will be happy to share them with you." I knew that medical students, even more than residents, were always tight on cash. The promise of a free lunch on a regular basis was always a great fringe benefit of any rotation. By this point, I was ready to offer him whatever was left in my checking account if he would agree to come help me with some of my floor work.

To seal the deal, I invited him to join me in the cafeteria for lunch and promptly paid for his food with my meal tickets. While eating, I told him a bit about the service, and I explained to him all he needed to do was to contact the foreign medical student liaison's office and advise them that he wanted to change his elective rotation from nephrology to vascular surgery. I would take care of the rest and deal with the attending surgeons on my end. He did not commit right then but told me he would think about it. When Monday morning of the following week came around, I saw him sitting in the nurses' station on the ninth floor as I walked in for rounds. He told me he was in, and I could not have been happier.

After Ramiro came on board, things got much easier. He turned out to be a great guy and we became good friends. Moreover, I found him to have an excellent work ethic. He was motivated and enthusiastic and had great technical skills. Due to his previous job as a surgical tech, he was familiar with surgical procedures and became invaluable to me on the floor and even in the operating room.

The vascular surgery service at that time had two main attending surgeons. One happened to be the son of a classmate of my father's during medical school. He was a true clinician and had little interest in academics or research. He had excellent hands and was fearless in the operating room. After our first case together, I dubbed Dr. Albert Perez a "Master Samurai."

Then, there was Dr. Rafael Ogle, the chief of the vascular surgery service. Dr. Ogle had been recruited to Jackson Memorial Hospital about one year before I rotated on the service. He was in his early forties, was extremely smart, and the opposite of Master Samurai in that he was more of an academician and researcher than a clinician. His vascular surgery knowledge base was encyclopedic; it was easy to see how he had quickly ascended the academic ranks. For every particular case we discussed, he would offer a verbose dissertation on all pertinent research that had been done for that particular problem or malady, and would then offer his assessment of how well or poorly the research had been done. It was rumored that one of the reasons he had been highly recruited for the program was that he brought with him large research grants. Bringing your own war chest for research is a great advantage when seeking academic jobs.

Dr. Ogle's main research interest was the development of minimally invasive techniques for the treatment of aneurysms of the great vessels. Aneurysms are dilations of the arterial wall that are prone to rupture after they reach a certain size, at which point they can be life-threatening. He was working on techniques with the use of stents that were deployed inside the vessels in the area of the aneurysm to reinforce the weakened arterial wall from the inside. Some of those techniques are standard practice today, and the commercial stents and delivery mechanisms have been fine-tuned to the point of routine use. When I rotated through vascular surgery as a third-year resident, this subspecialty was at its inception and Dr. Ogle was one of the surgeon-scientists developing the equipment and techniques that would someday become routine.

Back then, commercial products like stents for large vessels such as the aorta were not available, as this technology was relatively new. Instead, the stents were crudely fabricated on a back table by the surgeon during the case. Furthermore, the delivery systems were also custom-made and did not always work smoothly. Dr. Ogle was at the forefront of that research and had taken the technology to the patient human testing phase under protocol at the university.

Prior to starting my rotation, I had heard horror stories from the other residents as to how much work these cases entailed and how stressful they were. Surgeons were not used to working with these aneurysms without first having great surgical exposure and controlling the vessel at either end, in order to arrest blood flow so that the surgeon could repair the vessel with minimal risk of bleeding. When performing these endovascular techniques—as they would come to be called—stents were deployed through access at a distant vessel like the groin (femoral) artery. If things did not go well and bleeding ensued, the surgery team would have to scramble under extreme pressure to gain open access to the vessel involved. If the vessel happened to be the aorta (main vessel that runs from the heart to the rest of the body), the amount of time required for exposure and control was several minutes at best, allowing for the real possibility that it would take too long to stop exsanguination, resulting in death. The chief resident rotating with me on the service at that time did not have the appetite for such stress and had already told me she had no interest in working with Dr. Ogle. She made it clear to me that I was to scrub on all his cases while she worked exclusively with Master Samurai. This was her prerogative; I had no choice but to accept and comply with her wishes.

My first interaction with Dr. Ogle was interesting, to say the least. On the first day of the rotation, I was consulted by the medicine service on a patient they had admitted to the ward with uncontrolled diabetes and fever. They attributed this to gangrene on her right big toe. They were concerned that it was the gangrene that was causing her illness, and they wanted the toe amputated as soon as possible. Mrs. Johnson was a lady in her late sixties, somewhat thin and emaciated, who seemed not at her best. Nevertheless, she did not appear in any distress when I first met her. She was sleeping; four family members were at her bedside. After reading her chart and studying her lab values, I came into the hospital room to examine her. The right big toe was completely black all the way to where it joined the foot proper. It looked very much like the toe of a mummy you see in museums and had a sharp area of demarcation between the affected (black) skin and the healthy appearing skin. The toe appeared desiccated and did not have drainage of any kind, nor was the surrounding viable tissue either red or inflamed. The presentation was clinically consistent with what is called dry (uninfected) gangrene. I discussed the case with the senior resident on the medicine service and told him that the gangrenous toe did not appear infected, and I thought they should continue to work-up the patient for another source of the fever and the uncontrolled diabetes. He informed me that the attending on their team was insistent that this was the cause of the problem and that they wanted the toe amputated as soon as possible. They had actually kept the patient NPO (without eating or drinking) in the hope that we would take her to the operating room that same day.

Before calling Dr. Ogle to discuss the case, I inquired with the operating room about the possibility of taking the patient for the amputation that day. I was promptly told that they had a long list of waiting emergency cases and could not get me on the schedule that afternoon or evening. I was advised to add Mrs. Johnson to our elective schedule for the next day.

It was already late afternoon by the time I called Dr. Ogle to discuss the case. "Joe, that case does not warrant a trip to the operating room. I do think the toe needs to come off; just go ahead and cut it off now at bedside." As he was saying this, my mind conjured a macabre scene where the patient would be screaming at the top of her lungs in excruciating pain as I cut her toe off right there on her bed.

I explained to Dr. Ogle that I had never done a bedside amputation before, and I thought the patient would be better served by a trip to the operating room where she would be more comfortable after being put to sleep or at least sedated. Besides, I told him I did not think the source of infection was the toe and thus we could afford to wait and put her on our elective schedule over the next couple of days, whenever feasible. "Joe, the toe is already dead. Get a knife and borrow a rongeurs (an instrument that cuts bone) from the operating room and take it off already. Trust me, she is not going to feel it."

As I had never done any kind of amputation on an awake patient, this request from Dr. Ogle seemed highly unusual and I diplomatically declined to follow his request. Frustrated, he asked where my chief resident was. I told him she was scrubbed in on a long case with Dr. Perez and would not be out for several hours. I again suggested that we book the patient on our next day's schedule. The exasperation in his voice became obvious.

"Our schedule tomorrow is packed, and we simply can't fit her in. Get the stuff we need ready; I will meet you at bedside in one hour."

Aggravated, I took care of all the required paperwork (consents), and then walked to the operating room. After some difficulty and admonition from the nursing staff, I borrowed a small amputation tray and gathered all the other supplies I thought necessary for the procedure. After placing the supplies at the patient's bedside, I sat at the nurses' station checking on some labs and waited for Dr. Ogle to arrive.

Although I knew who he was and had spoken to him on the phone, we had not formally met. Dr. Ogle walked up to the nurses' station and, upon seeing me there, without much ceremony asked me to direct him to the patient. We walked into the patient's room together and I promptly asked the patient's family to please wait outside and directed them to wait by the door in the hallway.

By the time I walked back into the room after closing the door, Dr. Ogle had already placed a sterile drape under the patient's foot, had placed betadine all over the foot, and was opening the sterile tray by the patient's bedside. He took a surgical knife and cut circumferentially around the patient's toe about a millimeter beyond the area of demarcation. The cut was deep, all the way to the bone, yet there was no bleeding. He then took the rongeurs (an instrument that looks a lot like pliers but with sharp, cutting prongs) and inserted the sharp blade into the cut he had just made and engaged the bone. He squeezed and I easily heard the crunchy sound of the bone giving way. He then twisted the instrument a bit and the toe promptly came off. The patient lay in bed and looked at us all the while, without saying a word or expressing the slightest concern or discomfort. Dr. Ogle placed the toe on the drape by the patient's foot, looked up at me, and as if to prove his point, said, "Send this toe to path and dress the wound."

He got up, took off his gloves, washed his hands, and walked out of the room without saying another word. Point made!

Dr. Ogle seemed to be from the old school of surgical training, and always felt it within his purview to have you at his disposal whenever he needed you. The fact that you were off duty never seemed to bother him when he needed you to do something. Thus, it was not a surprise during my second week on the rotation that my pager went off at 11:30 p.m. on a day on which I was not on call. I heard Dr. Ogle's voice when I called the number on the pager. "Joe, I need you to come in and help me with an emergency case. The senior on call tonight has been working nonstop and is very tired."

Through my mind flashed thoughts of the many reasons why his request was wrong and should not have been made. First of all, I was not on call that day, but I was going to be on call the following day. Secondly, there was a senior resident already on call and whether that resident was tired or not, he/she was the one who was at the hospital specifically assigned to help with emergency cases. Lastly, no one ever seemed to care when I was on call whether I was tired or not. I wondered why Dr. Ogle had become so caring all of a sudden, especially since his sensitivity and caring were to my detriment. I surmised that the issue was that he either did not trust the other resident or had not yet worked with him/her before and felt this was not the time to break in someone new. The union had been voted in by the residents at that point, but the rules and contract relating to resident work hours had not yet been finalized and ratified, so although I thought about it, I could not use this as an excuse to refuse Dr. Ogle's request.

"I will be right there." I wanted to kick myself as I heard the words come out of my mouth.

Walking into the operating room, it was easy to see why Dr. Ogle felt compelled to call for help.

"This is a bad one," he said as soon as he saw me. Dr. Ogle and one of the interns on call that night had already opened the patient's abdomen, mobilized and retracted the patient's colon on the left side, and had exposed a very large abdominal aortic aneurysm (a large bulging of the aorta—the large artery that carries the blood supply from the heart to the organs of the chest and abdominal cavities, and ultimately to the lower extremities). When the dilated arterial wall becomes sufficiently weak, it can perforate and leak blood, a condition that can rapidly become fatal if not addressed promptly. This was the story with Mr. Juan Fernandez, the patient currently on the operating room table.

I quickly scrubbed, gowned, and approached the table. Dr. Ogle was placing the clamp on the normal aorta above the level of the aneurysm in order to disrupt the blood supply to the affected area so that we could perform the repair. Shortly after, he placed a clamp below the level of the aneurysm as well. He then proceeded to cut the aneurismal wall longitudinally along its length and opened the arterial walls like a book, exposing the internal contents of the vessel. These consisted of a thick mixture of blood and a material (clot) with the consistency of coffee grounds that coated the entire inner aspect of the walls of the aneurysm. After resecting this deceased segment of the aorta, Dr. Ogle requested a Dacron graft. The graft looked like a cylinder made of a soft cloth-like material that had the approximate diameter of the patient's normal aorta. Dr. Ogle adjusted the length by cutting one of the ends and proceeded to suture the top part of the graft to the superior end of the aorta in a circumferential fashion. He allowed me to suture the inferior end of the graft in the same way as he had done the upper end. It was with great excitement that I saw the blood resume its course down the now reconstructed aorta once the clamps were removed. There were no significant leaks of blood; our (interpositional) graft held and our suture lines were true.

It was evident that Dr. Ogle was relieved as well. After washing out the area and the rest of the abdomen with warm saline solution, we proceeded with the abdominal closure. "He is a very lucky man," Dr. Ogle offered as he began to close the deeper layer of the abdominal wall with a large nylon suture. "We were almost too late in getting to him, as he was already ruptured. Furthermore, he is not out of the woods yet, as he has a similar aneurysm in his thoracic aorta." I knew this was bad news. Aneurysms of the abdominal aorta are difficult to treat, but aneurysms of the thoracic (chest) aorta are even more so. I was just thankful for the patient (and me) that the thoracic aneurysm had not decided to rupture that day as well. I was extremely tired when we finally got done with the case, and I sat down to write the postoperative orders. It was close to four a.m., and my workday was to begin in less than two hours. There had been no sleep for me this night, and as I was on call that day, there was little chance I'd get any sleep on the following night. I also realized I had come to the hospital without my overnight bag, which carried my toiletries and a change of clothes. This was not starting out as a good day.

Mr. Fernandez did extremely well after his operation. He was in the intensive care unit for three days, was then transferred to the regular floor, and just a little over a week after his surgery he was sent home. During rounds on Mr. Fernandez while he was still in the ICU one morning, I inquired of Dr. Ogle whether he wanted me to consult thoracic surgery regarding Mr. Fernandez's thoracic aortic aneurysm. "No." Dr. Ogle was firm in his response. "We are going to give him a few weeks, and then we are going to stent him."

This answer was not what I wanted to hear. Before coming to the rotation, I had been warned of Dr. Ogle's research and particular interest in the treatment of large-vessel aneurysms through the use of intravascular stents. This was all well and good, except that as this endovascular technique was just being developed, the technique had a high incidence of complications across the board. Some of the senior residents had already warned me as to the high level of stress that these cases placed on Dr. Ogle, and also on the involved residents. Prior to starting on the service, I had hoped that I would not be personally involved in any of those cases during my two-month rotation. Now here I was, just a few days into the rotation, and already there was the potential of at least one of these stent cases in my future. I dreaded the thought that after having saved this man's life, we might end up causing his demise on a subsequent operation. I then remembered the term "MDK" of which I had become aware during the cardiothoracic rotation the year prior, and secretly hoped the case would be scheduled long after I had left the service. That was not to be.

Two weeks before my rotation was to end, I saw that Mr. Fernandez was on the schedule for Dr. Ogle to stent his thoracic aortic aneurysm. It was Dr. Ogle's only case for that day, and of course, I was to be the one helping him. I made sure Ramiro came in to help as well. Dr. Ogle had enlisted for these cases the help of one of the senior interventional radiologists. He would help with the surgery itself, along with the intraoperative radiological imaging necessary to position and deploy the stent in the proper location within the vessel.

The case started smoothly enough, as Dr. Ogle, Ramiro, and I exposed one of the main arteries in the groin of Mr. Fernandez in order to access the aorta from there. Once this step was completed, Ramiro and I remained at the operating room table while Dr. Ogle and the radiologist went to a back table to finalize the fabrication of the stent. As he worked, Dr. Ogle explained that this technique was in its developmental stage, there were no commercial stents yet available, and each stent had to be custom fabricated for each patient.

From the radiological studies performed before the operation, Dr. Ogle had decided on the length and width of the stent. The length would be several centimeters longer than the aneurysm so that it could bridge the affected area of the vessel with a couple of centimeters to spare on either side. After packing the open wound with a moist gauze pack, Ramiro and I came over to the back table where Dr. Ogle was working so that we could watch the stent fabrication up close.

Dr. Ogle had chosen what looked like a metal wire mesh cylinder. This cylinder was collapsible into the shape of a cigar when under pressure but would deploy to about two to three centimeters in diameter when allowed to expand. Once he confirmed that the expansion mechanism of the metal contraption was working to his satisfaction, Dr. Ogle took a cylindrical piece of Dacron, a cloth-like material, and carefully sutured it to the inside and then the outside of the metal cylinder, the sutures being anchored to the metal itself. Once finished, Dr. Ogle tested the contraption by collapsing and allowing it to expand several times. He then inserted the finished stent into one end of a long, flexible plastic sheath, which at the other end had a pushrod-type mechanism consisting of a long, stiffer plastic tube that would be used to deploy the stent within the lumen of the diseased (dilated) segment of the aorta. After working for what seemed close to one hour on building the stent and loading it into the deploying mechanism, Dr. Ogle finally announced that we were ready to proceed.

The entire surgical team returned to the operating room table and stood by the patient's side. Dr. Ogle asked the anesthesiologist to inject some dye through the patient's central line in his chest and then turned on the fluoroscopy radiology unit that had been set up to image the patient's entire torso during the operation. We watched for several seconds as the dye reached the aorta and we were able to visualize the dilation of the aorta within the patient's chest. Satisfied with this, Dr. Ogle announced that we were ready to insert the stent.

Ramiro and I simply stood by as Dr. Ogle inserted the sheath into the arteriotomy (opening) we had previously made in the femoral (groin) artery. He released the clamp that was occluding the vessel, and some blood leaked around the sheath into the surgical field. It was not a large amount, and it lessened as Dr. Ogle began to slowly insert the sheath containing the stent into the vessel.

Once he thought he was deep enough, Dr. Ogle asked again for the fluoroscopy machine to be turned on, and we were then able to visualize the metal component of the stent slowly migrate superiorly along the patient's aorta until it reached the approximate location of the aneurysm up in the chest. I held my breath as I saw the stent travel through the abdominal aorta, as I knew that was the place where we had positioned the Dacron graft a few weeks prior. I was somewhat concerned that manipulating that segment of the aorta might cause some of the fresh sutures to give, thereby causing bleeding that would immediately turn the case into a dire emergency. Thankfully, that didn't happen.

Dye was again injected by the anesthesiologist to aid in visualization of the aneurysm until Dr. Ogle was satisfied that the tip of the stent was a couple of centimeters above the superior extent of the aneurysm. He then began to slowly push the rod while pulling out the sheath, causing the stent to deploy. We clearly saw the stent begin to deploy and slowly expand within the vessel.

Standing there watching the mechanism work as planned, I experienced a sense of confidence that things would turn out as expected and began to wonder what could have possibly gone wrong on some of the previous cases that I had heard about. Things seemed to be progressing extremely well, until all of a sudden, they weren't.

"It is stuck." Dr. Ogle's concerned voice brought my eyes back to the operating room table from the TV monitor where I'd been watching the stent deploy. It became obvious to me that Dr. Ogle was pushing on the rod quite hard, but the stent was no longer deploying. The radiologists offered suggestions on how to fix the problem, and Dr. Ogle began to pull back on the pushrod to ensure it was not kinked or stuck on the sheath in any way. He then tried to re-engage the stent and deploy it again. Nothing worked. The stent was stuck, and it was not budging.

Dr. Ogle asked the nurse to give him a mallet. This is when I began to really worry. He started banging on the pushrod gently at first, but with more and more force as the stent still did not budge. While observing this, a sense of dread began to overtake me. I was fully aware that with the stent half deployed and engaged to the vessel wall it could no longer be pulled back, and yet it was stuck within the sheath and it seemed that we would not be able to deploy it. Furthermore, I knew that if for any reason the metal in the stent were to perforate the aortic wall, the patient would surely bleed to death in seconds, not giving us enough time to enter the patient's chest and place a clamp on the vessel in order to stop the bleeding. With every bang of the mallet, I expected this dreadful possibility to materialize and pandemonium to ensue. I noticed copious perspiration on Dr. Ogle's forehead and saw his surgical glasses fog…a sure sign that he, too, felt the stress of the moment. Moreover, I began to wonder how long it had been since Dr. Ogle had treated a thoracic aortic aneurysm through an open approach, since this was considered mostly within the purview of thoracic surgeons. These thoughts further added to my distress.

At the suggestion of the radiologist, Dr. Ogle ceased banging on the rod and they both took some time to regroup and to discuss and troubleshoot the issue. Ramiro and I looked at each other and I saw him raise his eyebrows. While standing there, I began to wonder what would make someone like Dr. Ogle put himself through this kind of stress. For all intents and purposes, Dr. Ogle was an extraordinarily successful surgeon. He was relatively young in years but considered a senior surgeon in experience and position. He had a prestigious academic position, research grants, and his own laboratory, and yet here he was struggling and trying to develop a new technique in vascular surgery, the process of which had the real potential of harming patients while the technique was being perfected. I wondered what drove surgeons to take that kind of risk personally and on behalf of their patients. Was it the need for recognition? The promise of riches? Intellectual curiosity? Or was it due to entirely altruistic reasons? I hoped it was the latter.

I then thought about all the techniques that were commonplace at that time and how during their development they probably had resulted in harm to some patients, while at the same time bringing great distress to the surgeons who were trying to develop and perfect them. I further pondered that this was a common human struggle, not just in medicine, but in all aspects of human endeavor, such as travel, development of new technology for construction, new materials for manufacturing, et al. In the course of human events sometimes progress is accompanied by pain, suffering, and even death.

Surgeons deal with this type of issue to different degrees in their daily practice. It happens every time a surgeon undertakes a new technique, technology, or treatment modality that promises improved outcomes, but with which the surgeon is not yet completely comfortable. While mastering a new technique, there is the understanding that there will be a learning curve that might temporarily lead to less-than-optimal outcomes while the new technique is being perfected. Sometimes this learning curve leads to increases in complication rates, and although not all of these complications are life-threatening, they are to be taken seriously when a surgeon is considering trying something new. How to balance the potential for improved outcomes in the long run with the potential of inferior outcomes and potential complications during the learning process is something that all surgeons deal with at one time or another during their career.

As a matter of fact, residency training, whether it is in surgery or any other discipline, is a microcosm of this concept. Resident physicians and particularly surgeons, learning to perfect certain skills, are by definition in a position to cause patients harm, as they are not yet proficient in the surgeries and techniques that they undertake as part of their training. Residency programs moderate this risk by providing didactic education, ensuring ideal instruction and proper supervision by more experienced surgeons. However, in the process of becoming surgeons, well intentioned residents will at times harm the patients under their care, a reality that all of us have experienced at one time or another.

Recently, this principle was clearly driven home to me during a particular interaction I had during a case. At the end of a reconstructive operation with a local neurosurgeon, I complimented him on his experience and technical skills. What he told me in response captures the raw reality of this issue when it comes to the practice of surgery: "Joe," he solemnly said, "before I got to this point where I have the knowledge and skills to really help my patients, I had my share of bad outcomes. I hope that when all is said and done, I end up helping many more people than I hurt."

Dr. Ogle, utterly frustrated by this time, resumed his banging with the mallet, as he apparently had decided that this was the only course of action. After a lot more struggling, a bit of cursing, a lot of praying on my part, and a lot more banging with the mallet on his, the obstruction finally gave, and the stent fully deployed within the aorta. As we watched the stent deploy in real-time in the monitor, we all held our collective breath. The patient's vital signs remained stable, indicating that the aortic wall had not been breached and there was no internal bleeding. After some tense seconds of waiting to ensure that all was really well, we all let out a sigh of relief. Afterwards, we took out the sheath and rod from the patient's femoral artery, sutured the arterial opening, and eventually closed the skin incision in layers. The operation had turned out to be a great success, but not one I was keen on repeating anytime soon.

Mr. Fernandez was transferred to the surgical ICU, where I watched him like a hawk over the next few days. I was determined to do anything I could to ensure this trip into uncharted surgical waters was a successful one. It was a happy day for me, and especially for Dr. Ogle, when Mr. Fernandez was discharged home after having been successfully treated for a ruptured abdominal aortic aneurysm (via the open approach), and several weeks later for the thoracic aorta aneurysm (through an endovascular approach). It was a day to be proud indeed, not only for me, but for all of the vascular team, particularly Dr. Ogle.

It turns out that Dr. Ogle's struggle was not in vain, as some of the endovascular techniques that he worked on and helped pioneer during the time I spent with him are commonplace today and have saved the lives of countless patients. I was recently reminded of this particular case with Dr. Ogle and of the overall efficacy of endovascular surgery by the recent travails of one of my plastic-surgery mentors. It seems that while on vacation in South Carolina, he developed a dissecting abdominal aortic aneurysm which threatened his life, followed a week later by a unilateral dissecting external iliac (pelvic artery) aneurysm, compromising the blood supply to his leg. Back-to-back aneurysms put both his life and limb at risk. Both aneurysms were treated successfully with two endovascular stents, each deployed a week apart. Six weeks later, my professor is back to his passion, swimming.

Endovascular surgery has truly arrived and is routinely used today, even more so than open techniques, to treat aneurysms of the large and small vessels. This is due to the efforts of people like Dr. Ogle and many other surgeon-scientists like him who have had the foresight and taken the risks to perfect the techniques in use today. At the end of the day, the techniques they pioneered and perfected have helped many more people than they ever hurt and have indeed saved many lives and countless limbs.

RACHEL

"Is this the heart team?" asked a quiet, feminine voice with a peculiar Spanish accent, in a dialect not quite what I was used to hearing in Miami. Dr. Gregorio Esposito was conducting rounds with the second-year residents (I was one of them). We all turned in unison to look at the person posing the question. Approaching us was a most charming young woman in a white lab coat with the distinctive ID tag of a foreign medical student. After Gregorio acknowledged in the affirmative, she extended her hand to him: "My name is Raquel Garcia, and I am a medical student from Spain (sounded like 'Espain'). I will be rotating with your team for the month."

Gregorio shook her hand as he introduced himself and the rest of the team, each of us shaking her hand in turn, as he called out our names. He asked her to join us and told her he would talk to her in detail about the rotation after rounds. Later that morning Gregorio informed me that he was going to assign the new medical student to me, as I was the only Spanish-speaking member among the three rotating residents.

After rounds, I invited Raquel to breakfast where she proceeded to tell me a bit about herself. She was from Valencia, Spain, and was in the last year of her medical education and doing her elective rotations. She had just finished rotating for several months in Ireland, and since she had relatives in Miami, had decided to come to Jackson to do a month-long cardiothoracic surgery externship. Her English-language skills were not bad but needed some polishing. I realized what made her accent peculiar was that she pronounced the letter "C" with a "TH" sound, a feature of Castilian Spanish. Having lived in Spain for part of my life, I was used to listening to this sound when people spoke Spanish, but I was not used to hearing it when someone spoke English. She pronounced *Garcia* as *Garthia*. Raquel had light eyes, shoulder length auburn hair, was taller than average, and slender. Her two most striking features were how young she looked and her beautiful smile.

Most medical students rotating through the surgical services were in their third or fourth year of medical school and were at least twenty-five or twenty-six years of age. Raquel had just turned twenty-two. When I inquired as to how she was in her last medical school year and yet so young, she explained that in the European system medical school was a five-year program. It commenced upon the completion of high school, and that an abbreviated college education was somehow incorporated into those years. After breakfast, I extended my hand to her once again over the table.

"Welcome to Jackson Memorial Hospital and to America." I smiled at her.

"Thank you." Her smile was contagious.

"Since you are now in America, I think I will call you Rachel Garthia," I jested as I tried to imitate her accent.

"My name is Raquel." She continued to smile but did not seem amused. I've called her Rachel ever since.

We then went upstairs to the floor to start on the many tasks that Gregorio had assigned us. Over the next several days, we followed this routine without change. After rounds, we would go to breakfast and then go up to the floor to do our work. I tried my best to teach her as much as I could, and in turn she proved to be a great help to me in getting my work completed. I found her to have a sound medical knowledge base but was weak in performing the daily tasks that our University of Miami Medical School students routinely performed while on rotations—things like writing progress notes, calling consultants, drawing blood, etc., which she had not yet done much of. I had to take a significant amount of time to teach her how to do these things, but time I spent teaching Rachel was never a burden to me. The other two rotating second-year residents often joked that she followed me like a puppy and that I should share her with them so that she could help them do their work, too. I could do nothing but smile and remind them that Gregorio had assigned her to me. This arrangement between Rachel and me was short-lived, however. One day during the second week of the rotation, Gregorio announced that Rachel had spent enough time learning floor work, and from now on she was to go with him to the operating room. I was sorry to see her go.

Over the next three weeks Rachel and I got to spend time together only after she was done in the operating room and during morning and afternoon rounds. We went to drink coffee several times during the ensuing days, and she seemed eager to know what residency was like, particularly in surgery. While talking over coffee, I learned quite a bit about her. The more I learned, the more enamored I became.

During the last week of our rotation, Gregorio came to afternoon rounds particularly happy about his "stellar" performance on a particularly difficult case and invited Rachel and me for a beer after work to celebrate. It was then that he opened up somewhat and told us a bit about himself and his struggles in coming to America from Italy in order to pursue further training in cardiac surgery. Rachel seemed inspired hearing this story, and later confided in me that she too had the same aspirations of coming to America to become a heart surgeon. I tried to be as encouraging as possible. I told her that if Gregorio had done it, then so could she.

Several days later, one of the other second-year residents, Gregorio, Rachel, and I met at my apartment in South Beach. Gregorio had decided that we should have a small gathering as a way of saying goodbye to Rachel, who was due to travel back to Spain the following Sunday upon the completion of her rotation. Over pizza and beer, we all talked about our experiences in the rotation and how much each of us had learned. When we finished eating, Gregorio, who was now a bit tipsy, insisted that I play some Italian music that he had brought with him on a CD. As the music started to play, he went over to Rachel and asked her to dance.

Gregorio it seems, was fond of ballroom-type dancing, and they made a comical pair as Rachel tried to follow along. In a fitted red dress and high heels, she towered over him and laughed the entire time they danced together, probably more from embarrassment than joy. Watching from the couch, I saw their silhouettes move against the background of the lights of downtown Miami, on the other side of Biscayne Bay directly across from my balcony. I could not help but wish that I was dancing with her, instead of Gregorio. While laughing all the while, she turned her head to glance my way. I was struck by how pretty she was and suddenly admitted to myself how much I liked her. After concluding our festivities, I walked Rachel down to her uncle's car and asked her to go to dinner with me the night before she was due to leave; it happened to be a night when I was not on call. She agreed.

A couple of days later, I picked up Rachel at her uncle's house and took her to the Clevelander, a restaurant/bar in South Beach. We ate and talked about our recent rotation, the good times we had, and what we anticipated in the near future. At one point, our hands inadvertently touched for an instant and I got the sense that she pulled away. I pressed no further. She was nice as always, but her thoughts seemed to be elsewhere. Rachel appeared somewhat melancholic. I thought perhaps this might be because she was sad to leave Miami and would miss her new-found friends. I entertained the thought that perhaps she would miss me as well. The next day she phoned me in the morning to say goodbye and asked me to please call her a cab to take her to the airport. I did as she asked while sitting in my on-call room at the hospital, realizing all the while that I was already missing her.

Over the next several months we kept in touch mostly through email. She told me things were wrapping up for her in medical school, and she was anticipating her graduation. She was then to complete her rural rotation, a year-long rotation in underserved areas that graduating medical students were required to do in Spain prior to applying for residency training in their chosen specialty. She further wrote that she had not forgotten her dream of coming to the United States to pursue surgical training, and that she had already completed the necessary examinations. I read her email early one morning before going to work. In the three-mile drive from my apartment to the hospital, I thought about her email and decided that if it was the last thing I ever did, I was going to help make this happen for her. The only matter remaining was to figure out how.

The answer to that question occurred to me a couple of weeks later when riding down the elevator of the West Wing at Jackson Memorial Hospital. While standing in the back of the elevator with a couple of other residents, the door opened on one of the middle floors and Dr. Ernest Bradley entered. Dr. Bradley was the chief of the kidney transplant service and knew me from my internship rotation on the service. He had liked my performance during that month and had even brought up to me that I should consider a career in transplant surgery—an idea which did not appeal to me in the least.

"Hello Joe," he said as he walked in and noticed me standing in the back. I responded in kind. It suddenly occurred to me that that transplant service had one position for an intern slot that was outside the customary hiring patterns of the residency. The service was so busy that they needed two full-time interns rotating every other day on call. They were only assigned one intern, so they had decided to hire another person outside the normal channels and directly through the transplant service. Technically, they could not offer the position as an official internship, so they called it a physician's assistant (PA) position, except that hiring an "intern" was much cheaper for the department than a real PA. Furthermore, interns were willing to endure atrocious work hours and untold abuse, whereas the average, qualified physician's assistant would not consider putting up with that abuse even for three times the salary. This position was usually taken by a foreign medical graduate who was in the process of getting credentialed in the United States and needed a place to get started in the system in order to eventually land a residency slot. It occurred to me that this position would be perfect for Rachel.

Dr. Bradley got off on the second floor, no doubt to go look at X-rays and ultrasound studies on his patients. Although I was headed elsewhere, I got off the elevator with him as I immediately decided to approach the issue.

"Dr. Bradley," I called out while approaching him from behind.

"Hey, Joe."

"Sir, can I talk to you for a minute?"

"Of course, but only if you walk with me. I am in a hurry." Dr. Bradley was always in a hurry.

When I inquired about the transplant PA position, he told me that they were in the process of interviewing candidates for the position for the upcoming residency year.

"I have someone who is very interested in applying for that position," I ventured.

"Is it a relative?" I don't know what made him ask that, but perhaps he had noticed my eagerness when I brought up the subject.

"Not yet, but I hope someday she will be."

He gave me a knowing smile as he turned his head in my direction and looked at me over his glasses. He drank a sip from his ever-present cup of coffee, perhaps considering what he should say next.

"Is she in Miami? I can't promise you anything, but I will be happy to interview her. Next week maybe? I want to make a decision soon."

"She is," I lied, lest he change his mind when he found out that she was in Europe. "I will make the arrangements for her to come see you next week."

It was a long shot, but it was the best I could come up with. The following day, I woke up at four a.m. to call Rachel during daylight hours her time. I told her of my machinations and asked her if she would be willing to come to the interview. She was incredibly surprised at first because she was not expecting to take the plunge towards a career in the United States this soon. I got the sense from talking to her that she thought I was either joking or crazy. Her plans for coming to train in the US were for the long-term, not for now. She had been planning for her rural year in Spain and was making final decisions as to where she was to go the following academic year, where she was going to live, etc.

"Do you think it's a good idea? Do you know how many people are applying for the job?" I told her I had no idea how many people were applying for the job and that it was a long shot for sure, but that I did think it was a good idea. Moreover, it was the easiest way I knew of getting her into the system so that she could show her abilities as Gregorio Esposito had done.

"I am sure a round-trip ticket to Miami is expensive on short notice."

"I would be more than happy to buy you the ticket." My offer was an empty one, as I was overdrawn on my bank account.

"I wouldn't think of it. Let me ask my parents and I will call you back." She called me back several hours later to say that her parents had agreed to give her the money. She was ready to buy the ticket to Miami as soon as I could arrange the interview. I was extremely happy to hear her say this as it meant I would be seeing her again soon.

The following week I met Rachel at Jackson Memorial Hospital and walked her to Dr. Bradley's office. Upon seeing her, I was again struck at how young she looked. As I dropped her off, I wondered if she had a chance with Dr. Bradley. I began to feel guilty for persuading her to come all the way to Miami and spend a significant amount of money in what I now feared might be a futile effort. I was sure Dr. Bradley, a senior surgeon at Jackson who was now in his late sixties, would have a hard time trusting a recent medical school graduate with little experience and who looked like a teenager. But I underestimated him…and her.

Later that day while walking on the first floor of the hospital, I saw Rachel standing outside the house-staff administrative office, which was located on the ground floor of the Center Building.

"What happened?" I tried to figure out how to console her after she told me about what I expected to be a negative outcome. "You did not call me after the interview."

"I got the job!" She was beaming as she came over to hug me. "He gave me the job on the spot, and I've been at the house-staff office all day trying to get my paperwork done. I wanted to surprise you by bringing you my new Jackson ID."

I was surprised indeed…and extremely happy. Rachel was to start at Jackson in the transplant service in a mere six weeks. I never did formally thank Dr. Bradley, but I will forever be grateful to him for the decision he made to give Rachel this opportunity. We went out to dinner again before Rachel returned to Spain to prepare for her move to Miami. It was easy to tell that she was extremely happy, but there was that hint of melancholy again. This time I did not flatter myself in thinking that it had anything to do with me but wondered if she was leaving someone behind in Europe. If she were, I knew he would be sorry to see her go.

The next few weeks were a blur as I negotiated with my co-residents to change the schedule so that I could have the transplant rotation first. I wanted to be on the service when Rachel started her new job so that I could teach her the ropes and make sure she started off on good footing. I knew the year she spent on the transplant service would be pivotal in her future aspirations. She had to do a good job and show the surgeons on that service and the rest of the department her determination and capabilities. Her future hopes and aspirations all rested on how she would perform throughout the upcoming year.

Rachel arrived one week early in Miami and settled at her uncle's house in Coconut Grove. We had several study sessions where I tried to prepare her for what was to come. As she was inexperienced in the protocols and paperwork involved in being an intern, I took a significant amount of time explaining to her the different chart entries she would be expected to make, what each of them meant, and how to properly write them. She paid close attention as we generated templates for her to memorize and follow.

She never acted discouraged, although one day, upon realizing the amount of work involved, she looked a little scared: "This is quite a lot. I hope I can do this."

"Don't worry. I've made arrangements to start as the senior on transplant for the first two months and I will be there with you until you can fly solo." I further promised that for the first few times she was on call, I would stay and sleep in the on-call room on the transplant floor so that she could reach out to me in case she needed help, or if she had any questions or patient issues she could not handle on her own. My promise to be there seemed to allay her fears a bit.

My plan was to start with Rachel on the service, make sure to teach her what to do, and back her up when she needed help. I knew the first few times she stayed on call would be the scariest, like they had been for me as an intern, as she would be on the floor alone with all the senior residents and the attending at home. Having me there on the floor during those first call nights would give her an added sense of security and comfort. The transplant service was one of those rotations where the third-year resident acted in the capacity of senior resident, and therefore was allowed to take call from home. The trade-off was that the senior resident had to be available at all times for surgery no matter what time of day or night. The transplant service was remarkably busy, and surgeries were performed around the clock and could come up at any time. The only saving grace for the third-year resident was that he/she did not have to go on organ retrievals. That duty was assigned to the transplant fellows and/or junior attendings. I figured that I would act as a senior on the service, as was my role, and then stay to sleep in the hospital on odd-numbered days, which were to be Rachel's on-call days. The plan worked well in theory, but not so well in practice. I walked in with Rachel on July first with my call bag containing a couple of sets of underwear and socks. I did not leave the hospital until July ninth.

For those first eight days, I was either in the hospital taking call with Rachel or operating around the clock. It seemed every single time Rachel was not on call and I thought I was going to get to go home, even for a few hours, either we had a really sick patient who needed my attention, or one of the attendings would announce that we had a kidney coming in and we had to get ready for surgery. After several days, I was working on fumes. I took showers in the hospital and changed from one set of scrubs to the next. After a couple of days, I stopped wearing socks or underwear because I did not have clean ones available.

During call nights with Rachel, I spent a lot of time teaching her how to do such things as admissions, fever workups, and procedures such as IVs and central lines. She was a quick study, and after my two months were up and I was ready to move to my next rotation, I felt comfortable that she had gained the experience and confidence to fend for herself. That feeling of responsibility for her never left me, however. I still felt compelled to talk to the third-year resident who was to replace me. I asked him to look out for her and to make sure to cover her back. She eventually found out that I had done this and although appreciative, let me know she was not happy about it. Rachel was fiercely independent and wanted to make her own way in the world.

One day towards the end of my rotation, I was sitting on the desk in the on-call room talking to the OR nurse in order to schedule an emergency case. From the corner of my eye, I noticed that Rachel walked into the room to pick up her on-call bag. I smiled and nodded at her while still talking on the phone as she waved goodbye as she walked out the door. What happened next was utterly unexpected. Approximately thirty seconds later, I saw the door of the room open and I saw Rachel walking back in. As I was still on the phone, I assumed she had forgotten something and was coming back to retrieve it. I did not notice at first, however, that she walked straight towards me. When I looked up towards her inquisitively, she bent over and kissed me. The kiss took several seconds while the OR desk personnel could be heard through the phone asking if I was still there. Without saying a word, Rachel then turned right around and walked out of the room. I quickly completed the call and walked out after her, but by this time she had already taken the elevator and was gone. That afternoon after surgery I called her. She made it clear that she had developed feelings for me. Her words filled my heart with unimaginable joy because by then, I knew I loved her. We became inseparable after that, at least as inseparable as two people in surgical training can be.

Rachel rented an apartment in South Beach not far from mine. We worked together and also spent a lot of our free time together. Over the next two years we tried to coordinate our vacations and traveled to Kentucky, New Orleans, New York, and we took several trips to Key West. I genuinely enjoyed our friendship and was happy to see how she matured as a resident, and eventually became one of the more respected residents in the program. We were both quite pleased when Rachel was offered a preliminary position as an intern for the following academic year. At the end of her intern year, we were extremely disappointed when a categorical position opened up for the second-year and it was given to another preliminary resident. The day when she found out, I remember taking her call in the trauma resus area. Her disappointment was evident in her voice. I was incredibly sad for her.

Upon hanging up the phone with her, I felt compelled to call Dr. Henry Willoughby who was by then the chairman of the department of surgery, but with whom I had not really interacted directly since my first hernia case during my internship year. I made the call instinctively without formulating a definite plan. I intended to leave a message for him to call me back, but when his secretary put my call right through, I suddenly realized I did not know what to say.

"Dr. Willoughby, I don't know if you remember me, but I am one of the fourth-year residents…"

"Don't be silly, Joe. You are one of my residents. Of course, I know who you are." I was trying to think of what to say next, when he surmised the reason for the call. "I assume you are calling me about your girlfriend, Raquel. Look, we are sorry that she did not get the position this time, but we all feel that she is a great resident. Tell her to continue to work as hard as she is, and I am sure she will end up securing a categorical spot—if not here, then somewhere else."

I never told Rachel about the call because I did not know how she would react. She wanted to accomplish her goal on her own merit, and she probably would not have appreciated my meddling. It was difficult for me to resist, however, as I always felt this sense of protection towards her. I was compelled to do whatever possible to make her dream become a reality; by then, helping her realize her dream had become my dream. After all, I was the one responsible for her coming to Miami with my far-fetched plan, and it would break my heart if all the sacrifices she had made turned out to be for naught.

One day during the beginning of my chief resident year while walking through the trauma resus area, I saw the bricks (emergency communications radios) sitting on the counter unattended as an ambulance was putting in a call to the trauma center. I heard the call come in unanswered for the third time when I saw Rachel come from behind a curtained partition where she had been tending to a patient.

"Rachel, you can't leave the bricks unattended." My voice reflected my frustration.

"Listen dude, you are my boyfriend, not my chief resident, so you can't tell me what to do." Her response caught me a bit by surprise. I guess Rachel had grown in confidence to the point she was ready to assert herself against anyone telling her how to do her job, and that included me. She felt that she no longer needed my help and was poised to make it on her own.

Make it on her own she did. Rachel went on to eventually secure a categorical spot in our program. She graduated from general surgery, had a change of heart about heart surgery, and went on to pursue a fellowship in transplant surgery, of all things. After spending a couple of years in Spain for visa reasons, she eventually returned to the United States. She now lives and works in Chicago where she got married and became a "mum," as she puts it.

Before she returned to Spain, Rachel and I had slowly grown apart. Sometime during the middle of my chief year, she invited me over to dinner at her apartment and told me that she thought we should go our separate ways. Although it was somewhat expected, it still hurt and made me extremely sad. The exact time and reasons why our paths diverged have always been unclear to me, but some of it might have had to do with the paternal feelings I always had towards her, and her eventual resentment of it. I could not help myself because I felt responsible for bringing her to Miami, and I felt compelled to push her so that she would succeed in her quest. She had an extraordinarily strong independent streak and always resented being told what to do, even if it only related to her work, and no matter how pure my motives. As far as break-ups go, this was the easiest I have ever lived through thus far. It was "easy-peasy" as she often liked to say. Although she made it clear that she did not want to be my girlfriend any longer, Rachel remained my friend and was sure to answer my calls whenever I felt lonely or needed to speak to her. She called often to see how I was getting along.

After our break-up, I experienced two contemporary, very telling events related to Rachel. The first occurred towards the end of my chief resident year when Dr. Gerald Wodicka called me one afternoon to tell me that he had to send the trauma chief resident home because he was ill, and he needed me to cover the rest of his call. Although I had reached the point where I detested taking in-house call, it was hard to refuse Dr.

Wodicka, and I told him I would be happy to help. He then told me to head to the trauma OR, where I was to run the second-year resident through her first appendectomy. It turned out that resident was Rachel.

While scrubbing, it occurred to me that Rachel and I had never operated together. We faced each other across the patient on the OR table; she did not seem nervous at all. I was. After collecting my thoughts, I asked her several questions regarding this particular operation, this being my usual routine every time I took a junior resident through a case. The questions pertained to things such as surgical anatomy, where to make the incision, tissue layers we would be traversing, etc., and she was on-point on all of them. It was very obvious that she had been studying diligently. She took the marking pen and showed me where she was to make her incision. I told her to proceed. Watching her work, I noticed her hands like I had never noticed them before, despite the fact that I had held them in mine countless times. Her fingers were long and thin and moved with grace and precision. They were the hands of a surgeon, a good one at that, as it was obvious that she had the innate ability that comes naturally to only a few lucky practitioners of the art. The rest of us learn to hone our skills to that level only through a great deal of effort and practice.

Once Rachel had dissected down into the abdominal cavity, I explained to her how to insert her finger, hook it, and rotate it in such a way as to deliver the appendix into the wound. I then watched in astonishment as she quickly did as instructed and as if by magic, the appendix suddenly appeared in the wound. I thought back to my first appendectomy and how difficult it had been for me to deliver the appendix. The resident running me through the case had to finally help me in order to get it done. Rachel proceeded to tie off the base of the appendix, sever it, and then wash, close, and dress the wound. All too soon we were done. I left her to write her notes and postoperative orders, but as I walked out of the operating room, I felt a great sense of pride. Rachel was becoming an amazing surgeon.

The second event took place two years later while I was rotating as a plastic surgery fellow at Mt. Sinai Hospital on Miami Beach. While in the surgeon's lounge one day, I struck up a conversation with the OBGYN surgeon who was in charge of the rotating general surgery residents from Jackson. When I asked who was rotating with him at the time, he told me it was a resident named Raquel. "Joe," he said, "I have always thought you guys from Jackson are great residents, but she has the best hands I've seen in any of the residents from Jackson...yourself included." Yes indeed, Rachel had made her own mark after all.

Not long ago I had another incident somewhat related to Rachel that reminded me how old habits die hard. She had come to town for a wedding and called me out of the blue to tell me she was in Miami overnight and suggested that perhaps we could meet after the ceremony to catch up, as we had not seen each other in years. It just so happens that I was at home sick with a terrible cold and did not think it was a good idea for me to come and meet her, thereby risking that she might get sick as well. I was sorry to have missed her.

The following day, I had the urge to do a search online to see what she had been up to for the last several years. During my search, I came upon a short promotional video from the institution she worked at which depicted a story of a patient on whom she had performed a pancreas transplant. The video showed segments with both the patient and Rachel talking about the surgery. In one of the clips, Rachel made a comment as to how the patient "was enjoying his organ." I chuckled at the comment and my first instinct was to get on the phone and tell her that in the future she should phrase that differently and say something like "Mr. So and So is enjoying his new life/his new pancreas/his transplanted pancreas," etc. But then I thought better of it. After so many years, I was not sure how Rachel would take my meddling, no matter how pure the motives. After all, this irresistible protective instinct I've always had toward her is one of my least redeemable qualities in her eyes.

Only Rachel truly knows of her feelings for me and whether she ever loved me like I loved her. No matter what those feelings might have been, I am sure they were mixed with a certain sense of gratitude for helping her reach her lifelong dream of becoming a surgeon. I myself have had others help me throughout my career in many different ways, and I will forever be grateful to each and every one of them for their efforts. Although my reasons for helping her might not have been completely altruistic, I will forever be glad and proud for whatever my contribution was toward the achievement of her goals. Not only was she truly deserving, but through her knowledge and surgical skills, she has undoubtedly helped many patients up to this point, and she is sure to help many more for years to come.

Whenever my mind wanders back to my residency years, those thoughts are always intertwined with Rachel. Getting to know her and being her friend will always be one of the highlights of my life. Although we were no longer together, when she eventfully finished her residency training at Jackson Memorial Hospital and went off to complete her transplant fellowship elsewhere, I was very saddened to see her go.

The Worst Rotation

From what I had surmised, the third-year burn rotation was supposed to be a slow one. The team consisted of two burn attendings, one third-year general surgery resident rotating as a senior, and two interns alternating call every other day. All members of the team would take call from home, but the third-year resident was on perpetual call straight for the two months of the rotation, without a single day off. Moreover, he/she had to be available to come into the hospital at any time for new burn admissions, or any other reason that required his/her presence. The team took care of their admitted patients both on the floor and in the ICU, although the trauma fellow covered the ICU burn patients at night for their routine issues. This, in turn, gave the senior resident some reprieve from the multiple calls from nurses that ICU burn patients generated nightly.

My first day on the rotation was a clinic day, and after morning rounds and taking care of the clinic patients, I sat down for a strategy session with the two interns. Once all that was done, I was on my way home before five p.m., which was almost unheard-of during residency. The two interns seemed nice enough; one was a preliminary resident from orthopedics, and the other was a preliminary unassigned resident. The latter turned out to be incapable of waking up early in the morning and showing up for rounds on time at six a.m. I soon realized that there was no way I was going to get him to wake up on time, so I came up with a strategy of staggering the interns. The orthopedic resident, Andrea, would show up at six a.m.

for rounds but would get to go home no later than three in the afternoon. The general surgery resident, Eddy, would show up at eleven a.m. but would have to stay around the hospital finishing up the daily scut-work and could not leave earlier than eight in the evening. This system was not optimal, as I had to take extra time to get the late resident up to date on patient issues. Nevertheless, it gave me the flexibility of having an intern in the hospital for almost the entire day. This freed me up a bit, as I could call the late intern from home and get him to handle routine issues that came up later in the day.

It turned out that Rachel was not on call that first day. She had to house-sit for her uncle and aunt who were away on vacation. We thought it would be a great idea to grab some pizza and eat it at their house by the pool. It was a cool night, and I was looking forward to a nice, relaxing evening and perhaps a midnight swim. I hoped that the first day of the rotation would be an indication of my two months on the service. My rotation months did not include potentially high admission days such as the July Fourth holiday or New Year's Eve, where the use of celebratory fireworks usually meant increased admissions to the burn service. At around eleven p.m., however, the beeper went off. I expected it to be a routine floor call, but when I looked at the pager, I suddenly realized that my night of relaxation was going to abruptly come to an end. Two burn victims were on their way to trauma resus via helicopter.

After bidding Rachel goodbye, I headed for the hospital. As I was in Coconut Grove, it took me a good thirty minutes to get to the trauma resus area. I was relieved to see Andrea was already there attending to the two patients, John and Sara. After a brief glance at each of the patients, I realized that these were profoundly serious burns. John was burned on about seventy percent of his body, mostly second-degree. Sara had burns to almost forty percent of her body, mostly to her back, the back of her neck and scalp, and scattered areas in the back of both legs. Her burns, however, were deeper and a great portion of her back sustained third-degree burns.

The damage to the skin and deeper tissues from burns is classified in terms of degrees. A first-degree burn is a very superficial injury to the outer layer of the skin (epidermis) which usually heals within a few days, an example being the typical sunburn. A second-degree burn causes tissue damage into the deeper layer of the skin called the dermis. Although these burns can sometimes heal by themselves, at times this healing process takes too long, and skin grafts are used to expedite the process. As a general rule, second-degree burns that may take longer than two weeks to heal are skin grafted. A third-degree burn is one in which the tissue injury extends full thickness through all layers of the skin (epidermis and dermis) and reaches the fat layer that exists below the skin. These burns never heal on their own, and the treatment requires the complete removal of the entire skin with the underlying fat layer and the application of skin grafts to the underlying fascia and muscle tissue. Fourth-degree burns involve injury to muscle tissue and/or bone, and sometimes are the result of lightning strikes, electrical burns, or prolonged exposure to flames.

Burns are particularly dangerous because they interfere with body temperature regulation and the ability of the body to fight infections. Burns affect the protective functions of the skin that keep bodily fluids within the body, and the barrier function of the skin that guards against potential invasion by microorganisms, be it bacterial, viral, or fungal. Thus, when a significant portion of the surface area of the skin is burnt, the victims can experience severe metabolic derangements, loss of bodily fluids, and are particularly prone to infections. Another mechanism of injury that the burn victim can present with is tissue damage to the lining of the respiratory tree (trachea, bronchi, and lungs), which happens when the victim inhales smoke or other toxic fumes. This type of injury (inhalation injury) can be life-threatening, as it prevents the free exchange of oxygen from the lungs to the blood.

From the moment I first saw John and Sara in the trauma resus area, I was keenly aware that they were both in trouble, as their burns were severe and the tarry material they were coughing up and the poor oxygen saturation of their blood indicated that they had both sustained a significant inhalation injury. After fully assessing them both, I knew I was not going to be able to leave the hospital anytime soon. As patients with inhalation injury require significant ventilatory support, I had anesthesia intubate both John and Sara right there in the trauma resus area. After sedating them heavily, we then proceeded to do the initial debridement (cleaning) of the involved areas.

When patients come with significant burns, the initial care they receive in the emergency room or trauma resus area involves removing all of the damaged burnt skin and the application of an antibacterial cream called Silvadene. As this process is accompanied by significant pain, patients often get large doses of pain medications, such as morphine, prior to this initial process and then on subsequent dressing changes.

Once the morphine had been given, and having employed strict sterile technique, Andrea and I gowned, gloved, and proceeded to use wet gauze pads to remove all of the dead skin in the burnt areas. This burnt skin peels off rather easily, similar to how sunburn skin comes off, leaving a bright red surface that indicates the burn is a second-degree with underlying viable dermis. After we removed all the skin, we proceeded to apply the Silvadene and dress the wounds. This white cream, which is remarkably similar in appearance and consistency to whipped cream, is a powerful antibacterial agent containing a silver-based compound that is commonly used on burns to prevent skin pathogens from causing infection. It is difficult to explain, but the initial process of cleaning the burn wound and the application of Silvadene is reminiscent of cooking, and in an odd way it is a very enjoyable process for the person doing it. The victim, however, has a vastly different experience, as burnt skin is exquisitely tender and the debridement process can cause excruciating pain.

Since John had the largest burn, we started with him and then moved on to Sara. In her case, however, almost her entire back was third-degree burns. Such deep burns involve all layers of the skin and cause the skin to appear white. This burnt, dead skin does not easily come off and removing it has to be done in the operating room. We debrided her second-degree burns the same way we did for John and applied the Silvadene cream to all the burnt areas and dressed them with gauze padding and wrap. After a couple of hours, we were done with this process; I started to make arrangements to have both John and Sara transferred up to the burn ICU.

Once in the ICU, I proceeded to give the respiratory technician the vent settings, insert central intravenous lines (through which they would receive fluids and medications), and insert Foley catheters in their bladder so that we could measure their urine output in order to assess their hydration status and the response to the fluids we were infusing through their IV lines. Finally, I wrote their admission orders while Andrea wrote their admission history and physical. We finally got done just in time to go to the third floor to start morning rounds. We did not even have time to wash up or go for a quick breakfast.

My first night on the burn service was a harbinger of things to come: The two months that I rotated through the service turned out to be the busiest two months on the burn service for that entire year and indeed, many years prior and since. It seemed as if Miami had caught fire and people were getting severe burns almost on a daily basis. After a while, I started sleeping more often at the hospital than at home. It was a great dismay that I showed up at my call room—a converted patient room on the burn floor—one night only to find out that the charge nurse had commandeered it so that she had a place to put a new burn admission to the floor. There were simply no empty burn beds. From that day on and for the next month of my rotation, I was forced to sleep in a recliner in a corner of the burn ICU. The aching muscles and back pain that I experienced every time I slept on that chair made the long operating room sessions that much more grueling.

John and Sara's story came into focus over the next few days and it came in pieces, first from the police and then from their relatives. It seems that John and Sara had been together for less than a year. He was twenty-nine, she was twenty-two, and they were both from upstate New York. They had recently moved to Miami where Sara was pursuing a career in modeling. They had moved into a small house in the west part of the city, which was the house that caught fire. Arson was suspected and Sara's old boyfriend was the prime suspect. Neighbors described how John had initially come out of the house with minimal burns, but when he realized that Sara was still inside, he had gone in to find her and get her out. I admired his unselfish act and hoped that faced with a similar situation, I would have the courage to do the same. My intentions were to tell him how I felt about his heroic act the first chance I had to talk with him. That conversation never took place.

Both John and Sara were facing a tough road ahead, including a prolonged ICU stay, multiple trips to the operating room, and finally a prolonged stay on the regular floor and months of rehabilitation—but only if they were lucky enough to survive their initial injuries. It turned out that Sara did, but John did not. He fought hard though and did not succumb until about four weeks into his ICU stay.

Operating on burn patients is a much different experience than operating on the average general surgery patient. For one thing, burn surgery is essentially a skin operation where the dead, burnt skin is removed and replaced with skin grafts taken from unaffected areas of the body. If the burn is second-degree, the dead skin is removed using a special instrument such as a Humby knife, a long surgical knife with a very sharp blade with a mechanism that is set on the knife in order to only remove the desired depth of skin, and thereby not remove the viable deeper layers of skin that are necessary to sustain the skin graft. The knife is used on the dominant hand of the surgeon, and after engaging the knife on the skin it is advanced while moving it back and forth in order to slice off the dead skin in a fashion somewhat similar to how one would carve a turkey for Thanksgiving dinner.

If the burn happens to be third-degree, then the entire layer of skin including the subcutaneous fat is removed down to a layer of connective tissue which covers the muscles called fascia. This full-thickness skin removal is usually done with a Bovie, a surgical cautery instrument that allows for cutting and cauterization at the same time, thus minimizing bleeding during the procedure. Once the necrotic (dead) skin is removed, it is covered with a skin graft harvested from an unaffected area on the patient. This skin is usually harvested with a dermatome, an electric instrument that also has a very sharp blade and depth settings. These are set depending on how thin or thick the surgeon wants the graft to be (usually between 10/1000th and 16/1000th of an inch). Once the skin is engaged, the electric blade vibrates back and forth as the surgeon slowly advances the instrument. The harvested skin is then put through a "mesher," which opens perforations on the skin and allows it to stretch in order to increase its surface area. Although areas of normal skin can be harvested multiple times after the site has had a chance to heal, one of the challenges of treating patients with large surface area burns is that there is often not enough normal skin to harvest in order to cover all the burnt areas. The meshing of the skin allows for the skin grafts to expand to three or four times their original surface area, thereby allowing coverage of much more surface area than that which is harvested.

Burn patients present two significant challenges in the operating room, specifically related to the mechanism of the burn injury: loss of body heat (hypothermia) and blood loss. The skin is an organ system adept at regulating body temperature. This is physiologically accomplished by a large plexus (network) of blood vessels located in the layer just under the skin, which dilates and contracts depending on whether heat contained in the body needs to be dissipated or maintained. Sweating and the heat loss caused by the evaporation of sweat from the skin is another important mechanism by which the body controls its core temperature.

When the skin is burnt, this entire mechanism of body temperature regulation is lost, and loss of body heat can occur to dangerous levels, especially when the patient is exposed, as in the operating room. In order to ameliorate this, the temperature in the operating rooms when burn patients are being treated are set quite high, thereby causing utter misery to the surgical team members, who not only have to wear their scrubs, but also surgical gowns, masks, hats, and gloves. Operating on burn patients is akin to operating in a sauna, where profuse sweating is experienced throughout the entire procedure. Although "cooling vests" exist that circulate cool water through the lining on the vest, thereby keeping the surgeon wearing it cooler during the operation, neither residents nor attendings at Jackson Memorial Hospital were afforded this luxury.

After finishing each of these cases, my immediate reaction was to go to the locker room and take a shower and cool off. Not having enough time for this, I usually had to settle for quick trips to the locker room to dry off and change scrubs. On several occasions I had to excuse myself for a few minutes in order to rehydrate, as the intense heat and sweating in the operating room at times made me a little lightheaded from dehydration.

Another challenge faced in operating on burn patients is loss of blood. In order to remove the dead skin as previously described, the surgeon must carve or slice off the dead skin down to the level of healthy skin. Clinically one can tell when this level is reached when there is "punctuate" bleeding. As burnt skin is dead, and therefore does not bleed, the surgeon carves off the skin in thin layers until he/she reaches a layer of skin that bleeds. Once this layer is reached, one first sees multiple dots of blood, which soon coalesce into a uniform layer of blood in the surface of the skin being treated. If the surface area of skin to be debrided is large enough, this bleeding can be so severe that it puts the patient into shock. Thus, it is impossible for patients with burns to large surface areas to be completely debrided in only one trip to the operating room. This debridement is usually performed area by area in separate procedures, limited by a total blood loss of less than two liters per trip to the operating room or if the body temperature drops below a certain threshold. Fairly routinely, blood transfusions need to be given while burn patients are being debrided in the operating room.

Many were the days and hours I spent in the operating room during the two months of my rotation. The heat, sweating, and physical exhaustion endured during those many hours were made tolerable by the two burn attending surgeons, both of whom were great teachers and extremely committed to the patients they took care of. One of them in particular, Dr. Philbert Everett, always seemed to have interesting anecdotes that made the time pass more quickly. He even added to my vocabulary in a most unusual way.

Shortly after the start of my rotation I was experiencing the frustration of properly applying Silvadene to burn wounds. This cream has to be applied in a uniform way so as to cover the entire burnt surface of skin. This is easy enough to do when the burnt area is flat and located in the part of the patient that is facing up, such as the abdomen or the chest if the patient is supine—something like putting frosting on a cake. However, when the burns involve the flanks or an extremity, the Silvadene cream easily slides off the glistening, slippery debrided skin. When explaining my frustration with this problem to Dr. Everett one day, he empathized and offered a solution:

"The reason you are having that problem is that you are not using a trellis." He did not elucidate further.

"Of course." I did not want to appear completely ignorant, so I pretended to know what he was talking about. Burn surgery requires instrumentation that is not routinely used in general surgery. By this time in the rotation, I had already suffered enough embarrassment by failing to know the names of these instruments and some of the technical jargon used by the burn attending surgeons. My assumption was that a tralus/trallus/trellis (I did not know how to spell it) was some sort of surgical instrument, and I promptly asked the nurses during my next burn surgery for one. None of them knew what it was or even how to get one. I asked the nurse in the room to please call the nurse supervisor in the operating room and inquire as to how we could get a trellis in the operating room. I was promptly informed that the nurse supervisor had never heard of such an instrument and that I had to offer more information so that she could see about procuring one.

I then went back to Dr. Everett and told him that, unfortunately, the operating room had lost the trellis and they no longer had one; even worse, they did not know where to get a new one. He seemed amused and explained to me that a trellis was another word for a scaffold or a latticework. He explained to me that rather than applying the Silvadene first to the slippery, debrided, burnt skin, it was best to first place or wrap over the skin a single layer of a highly porous gauze dressing called a Kerlix. This would act as a scaffold and hold the Silvadene in place when the cream was subsequently applied. I've never forgotten the meaning of this word, nor the unique way in which I came to learn it. I often use the same trick when teaching young residents how to take care of burn patients.

John and Sara each endured multiple trips to the operating room. Initially just for removal of the dead burnt skin (debridement), and eventually, as the deeper layers of skin became healthy and free of infection, they went for debridement and skin grafting. John and Sara each presented their own different set of challenges due to their burns. On John, his burns were seventy percent of his total body surface area, and the challenge on him was finding enough healthy skin to harvest for his skin grafts. We eventually had to resort to shaving his head and harvesting skin from his scalp, in order to have enough skin to cover the burnt areas. Contrary to what some believe, harvesting skin from the scalp does not affect the hair follicles, which are located in the deep dermis. When skin grafts are harvested, they are taken somewhere at the level of the mid-dermis, thereby allowing for skin regeneration. Harvesting the skin at this level does not in any way affect the hair follicles or sweat glands, which are anatomically located at a deeper level. Once the hair grows back, the scars from the harvesting are completely covered by the hair. Thus, the scalp is actually an excellent donor site for skin, limited only by its small surface area.

Sara, on the other hand, had only forty percent total body surface area burn, so finding enough donor areas on her was not the problem. Her issue was that almost her entire back, the back of her neck, and her posterior scalp were third-degree burns. Thus, we had to debride the entire full thickness of skin down to fascia in these areas. Even on a thin person as she, I was astonished to realize how thick the skin and the underlying fat layers were. Once all her skin was removed and we grafted the thin layer of skin to those areas, there was a huge drop in the contour of her normal skin on her sides and flanks down to the level of the fascia covered with the thin layer of meshed skin. This gave her an unusually odd appearance. She appeared completely normal when viewed from the front, but utterly distorted when viewed from her side and back.

To someone not used to seeing burn patients, something seemed immediately off when the eye followed the contour of her torso. It was as if a part of her was missing. To add to this odd visual effect, Sara had beautiful blonde hair in the front seventy percent of her scalp and was totally bald in the back thirty percent. Upon looking at her, I was reminded of characters from books or movies such as the *Phantom of The Opera*, whose main character's face is half normal while the other half has a grotesque and distorted appearance. Her appearance made me feel extremely sorry for her. I knew the havoc that it would cause to her psyche once she made it through her hospital stay and attempted to return to a "normal" life. Being an aspiring model, she came from a world where physical attributes and beauty were the coin of the realm.

By the time Sara was out of the ICU and had been transferred to the regular floor, I realized for the first time why she was seeking a career in modeling. Sara had beautiful facial features and the tall, thin body of a runway model. Multiple times when visiting her room for rounds, I caught her looking at herself in a hand mirror. One particular day she called my attention to a couple of small areas of superficial second-degree burns on her cheek and neck. These were so superficial that they had not required treatment and had been allowed to heal on their own. Although both of these areas had healed uneventfully, it was easy to see the difference in texture and color between these areas and the surrounding normal skin.

"Do you think these areas will fade? I need to get back to modeling when I leave this place." Her tone of voice conveyed simultaneous hope and despair.

"I think so. You just need to make sure you keep those areas out of the sun to optimize the healing and minimize scarring." As I said this, I wondered if Sara had even looked or was aware of what her back looked like. She never asked me about this area; she seemed to be completely ignoring the back of her body and scalp.

I wondered if this odd behavior was her coping mechanism at work. However, as burn patients often required high doses of narcotics daily in order to manage their pain, especially during dressing changes, I am not sure if the fact that she was medicated had affected her demeanor. Whether it was her coping mechanisms or the powerful narcotics she was being given regularly for pain control, it was obvious to me that the Sara with whom I was now interacting was an altogether different person psychologically from the Sara that existed prior to her injury. It was obvious that she had been damaged in many ways, both physically and emotionally.

Interactions with John at any level were not possible. For the four weeks that I took care of John after his injury, he was in the ICU the entire time, intubated and sedated. John's condition went up and down over those four weeks, and he eventually developed sepsis and ARDS (Acute Respiratory Distress Syndrome). This is a condition in which the lining of the lungs involved in the exchange of oxygen and carbon dioxide between the air and blood become swollen to the point that this exchange was affected and it became impossible to keep his blood oxygenated. This condition can be brought about by sepsis (generalized infection) or direct injury to the lungs (as in inhalation injury). Despite the input of consultants from infectious diseases to help optimize his antibiotic coverage, and multiple manipulation with ventilator settings culminating in the use of the jet ventilator, John was unable to fight this devastating condition and finally succumbed during his fourth week in the ICU.

As John's family was already back in New York, it was my job to call them and let them know. John's death was by this point anticipated, and they took the news as well as could be expected. With the permission of John's family, I also informed Sara's family, who were still in Miami and were kind enough to spare me the job of telling her. Sara never brought up John to me, and I never brought him up to her. She only spoke of John to her family and to the consultant from psychology who was brought in on her case.

My rotation through the burn service taught me that severe burns are a devastating injury and perhaps one of the worst maladies than can befall human beings. Even if the victim survives the initial injury, he/she will then endure a very tedious, painful, and exhausting treatment process followed by months, if not years, of rehabilitation. These patients are often left with permanent disfigurements and disabilities that they must endure and learn to live with for the rest of their lives.

From the standpoint of the amount of work required, my burn service rotation was without a doubt the worst rotation that I endured during my five years of surgical residency and professional life thus far. Prior to my burn rotation, the first nine days of my transplant rotation had been the most intense and exhausting period of time that I experienced during residency. During the burn rotation, however, I had to keep up this level of intensity for an entire two months without a single day off. In time, my efforts were recognized and appreciated.

During the graduation ceremony for the chief residents at the end of that academic year, I along with Tony Cicilio were co-recipients of the Burn Award. This award was given to the third-year resident voted by the attending staff as having had the best performance during the burn rotation for that academic year. The award included a plaque and a $500 gift certificate to the campus bookstore. I bought a five-volume set on surgery of the alimentary (gastrointestinal) tract, and two atlases of general surgery operations. Total purchase price: $498.27. Medical textbooks are extremely expensive. Rachel and I celebrated my award with a dinner at one of my favorite restaurants in South Beach. She would also go on to win this same award three years later after her burn rotation. The pride I felt upon learning of her winning the award far surpassed that which I experienced years earlier for winning it myself.

THE FOURTH YEAR:

SENIOR RESIDENT

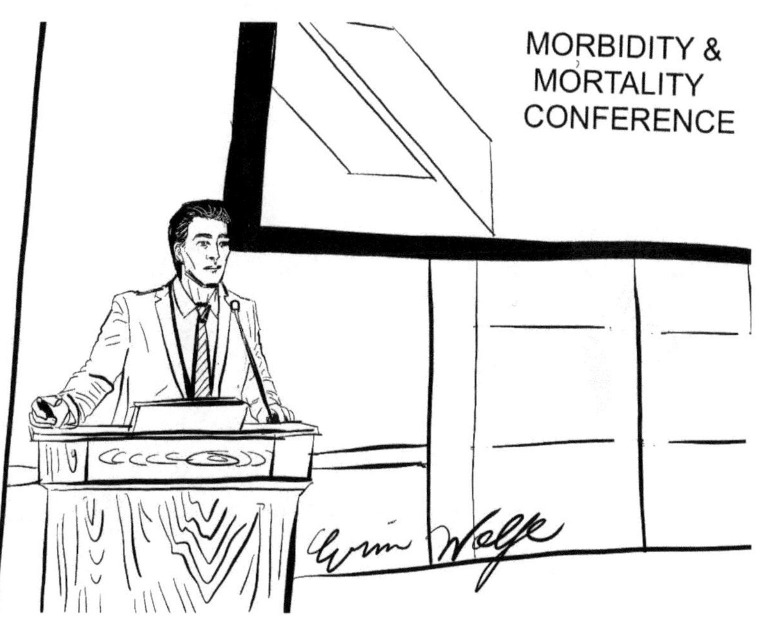

THE FISHBOWL

"I'll meet you at the fishbowl at two p.m. I need your help with a case."

The request had come from Dr. Brad Bustillo who was one of the four pediatric surgery attending surgeons, and the last addition to the group. He was young (late thirties), brilliant, and had just completed his pediatric surgery fellowship at Johns Hopkins. I had been introduced to him several days before, when I had started my fourth-year rotation in pediatric surgery. I was to be the only senior resident on the rotation, as the chief residents did not rotate through this service. This was a good rotation to get introduced to the added responsibilities of a senior resident. The four attendings on the service were protective of their patients, always hovering over the residents to make sure they did the right thing. Thus, I felt I had plenty of support and a good safety net in case I ran into trouble.

During the first week of the rotation, Dr. Bustillo had given the residents and medical students rotating through the service an introductory lecture on the common surgical issues dealt with by pediatric surgeons. As he was new to the hospital, he used the first few minutes of the lecture to introduce himself. A native of Miami, he had decided to return once his long surgical training was over. He seemed quite happy to be back home, and it showed in his demeanor.

"I guess you can say that professionally and personally, I am where I've always wanted to be."

When he finished his introduction with that statement, I felt a certain sense of kinship with him, as his words made me think about what was possible. Most residents labor under a perpetual state of delayed gratification, putting in long, hard years of medical school and surgical training in order to be able to someday live the words that Dr. Bustillo had just uttered. Hearing him say that made me realize there was indeed light at the end of this long tunnel. Moreover, I got a sense that Dr. Bustillo felt that he had "arrived"—not necessarily financially, at least not with his salary as a junior attending surgeon in an academic institution, but in a much deeper and yet meaningful way: He had reached a state of personal fulfillment in seeing his lifelong dreams realized.

I have found through my long years of study and training and now practice, that the feeling in young surgeons of accomplishment at realizing their dreams is almost universal, quite powerful, and rather self-evident. Moreover, it is almost paradoxical because all of a sudden, young surgeons find themselves in a place that for many years seemed impossible to reach. This empowering realization can overcome the stresses (personal, financial, and emotional) of dealing with the many challenges encountered by surgeons starting their careers in an academic or private practice setting, be it with a group practice or as solo practitioners.

The fishbowl was the name given to the neonatal ICU at Jackson Memorial Hospital. Different from the newborn unit, the fishbowl was where the sick newborns were sent. It was a large room located on the second floor of the Center Building at Jackson. This room was surrounded by a large glass partition that allowed doctors, visitors, and family members to stand on one side and not come into close contact that could potentially contaminate the resident patients, many of whom were premature and thus were sick, frail, or both. Inside the room, one could see row after row of small flat "cribs" containing their respective miniature patients, some of whom did not weigh much more than a full can of soda. Hovering over them, like guardian angels, was a whole army of nurses, technicians, pediatricians, neonatologists, and when called into service, pediatric surgeons.

"He has a patent ductus arteriosus, and I need you to help me clip it," Dr. Bustillo said as we stood over the crib of a newborn not much bigger than a large rabbit. The child had been born premature, and his work-up had revealed this condition. An attempt at nonsurgical treatment with the recommended medication regimens had failed. The child was experiencing a lot of physiological and cardiac distress while feeding—which were symptoms of this condition—and pediatric surgery had been consulted in order to surgically address the problem.

The ductus arteriosus is a short vascular connection between the aorta and the pulmonary artery that allows for the blood to bypass the nonfunctioning lungs while the child is in the womb. Shortly after birth, when the lungs fill with air, the pressure differential in the vascular system caused by this lung expansion normally causes this connection to close a couple of days after birth. Sometimes, in premature babies, this physiological process fails to take place and the ductus arteriosus remains open, a condition referred to as "patent ductus arteriosus." Children with this condition are often said to suffer from a "failure to thrive," as this shunting (diversion) of blood leads to the arterial blood being less oxygenated than normal. This, in turn, leads to many physiological derangements, such as problems with feeding, excessive sweating, cardiac distress, and the inability of the child to grow and put on weight, as his/her physiological reserves are limited by the condition.

While having this discussion over the patient's crib, I suddenly realized that Dr. Bustillo and I were no longer alone. The pediatric anesthesiologist and the nursing scrub team from the OR began to arrive and set up a makeshift operating room at the patient's bedside in the fishbowl.

After realizing what we were about to do, my incredulity got the best of me.

"You are going to be doing that . . . here?" After saying it, I immediately caught myself and hoped that Dr. Bustillo did not take offense at my statement. I had assumed that this type of surgery would be done by the pediatric cardiothoracic surgeons in the operating room.

"Yes," he said without appearing to take offense. "We are going to do that, and yes, here. There is no safer place for this child."

During my pediatric surgery rotation, I was to become exposed to the truly wide scope of pediatric surgery as a specialty. In today's world of specialization and subspecialization, pediatric surgeons are the only true general surgeons left. Adult general surgery has been relegated mostly to surgery of the abdominal cavity organs, just as any other anatomical or organ system has its own specialized group of surgeons. This being the case, for example, with thoracic surgeons who operate in the chest, vascular surgeons who treat the diseases and conditions of the arterial and venous system, cardiac surgeons who operate on the heart, etc. In contrast, pediatric surgeons operate on many different organ systems and body cavities—except for niche areas like pediatric neurosurgery and pediatric cardiac surgery. The scope of their specialty is limited only by the fact that they operate on children.

In short order, Dr. Bustillo and I were both scrubbed, gowned, and facing each other across the makeshift OR bed, which was the child's crib. The patient's body was so small that it resembled a small animal more a miniature human. The instruments we used were scaled-down versions of their counterparts used for adults. The whole scene seemed odd and out of place, as operating in the fishbowl was not something that I had anticipated. I wondered how many of these procedures Dr. Bustillo had done, and what would happen if we encountered any intraoperative complications, particularly bleeding.

My apprehension intensified when after marking the placement of the incision on the patient's chest along the top of one of the small, visible ribs, Dr. Bustillo handed me the knife and told me to proceed. My hand trembled a bit while I made my initial cut, a very superficial one at that. The top of my head and the back of my neck felt like they were on fire from the powerful light that we were operating under, intended not only to allow us to see, but it had the secondary function of keeping our patient warm. Loss of body heat is an issue with small premature babies, and powerful lamps stood atop the cribs of many of the babies in the fishbowl. The heat of this lamp along with the portable OR light that had been brought in to illuminate the surgical field combined to create significant heat, which seemed to be wholly concentrated on the back of my neck.

"We need to be very meticulous on this case, as any blood loss on a patient this size could be disastrous." Although his words were calm and confident, this statement by Dr. Bustillo served only to add to my anxiety. I was very aware that children, especially this tiny, have a small blood volume, and bleeding during surgery must be minimized lest the patient go into shock and potentially die from excessive blood loss. Surgical bleeding that is easily tolerated during adult surgery, as when making a skin incision, needs to be carefully attended to when operating in children, particularly newborns. For this case we would be dissecting along two great vessels in the chest. The smallest mishap could injure one of these vessels, and the subsequent bleeding could become life-threatening in a matter of seconds if not properly controlled.

Thus, I was somewhat relieved when, as we entered the chest, Dr. Bustillo began to take over more and more of the case. After placing a retractor between the ribs in order to give us space through which to work, we retracted the lung and after careful dissection eventually reached the location where the aorta and the pulmonary artery abutted, separated only by a small connecting vessel, the ductus arteriosus. Dr. Bustillo's hands were sure and steady as he carefully dissected around the aforementioned vessels and was eventually able to pick up the ductus with forceps to allow a clamp to be inserted behind it. He then asked for a surgical staple and very carefully put two staples on one end of the ductus arteriosus. Following this he handed me the staple-clamp and asked me to do the same on the opposite side as he retracted. I had to use both hands on the clamp in order to steady it as I gently slid one arm of the clamp under the tiny vessel. Once it was stapled, Dr. Bustillo severed the ductus arteriosus in the space between the two sets of staples with fine, blunt-tipped scissors. After placing a small chest tube and closing the incision on the chest, which he let me do, the operation was finally completed. I was quite happy the procedure went well. Adding to my happiness was the fact that I was finally able to get out from under those infernal lights located just above my head.

Our patient did very well in the ensuing days and was eventually transferred out of the fishbowl to the regular floor after several weeks of nutritional support. Seeing the patient eventually go home in the arms of his mother was satisfying and rewarding. After this particular case, I gained a great deal of respect for Dr. Bustillo, which has only increased as I have witnessed him complete many amazing procedures in the operating room in the weeks and years that followed.

The fishbowl was not the only intensive care unit for children at Jackson. There was a large pediatric medical ICU, and even pediatric surgery had a small intensive care unit at one end of the fourth floor of the Center Building. It was there that the pediatric surgery team met for rounds every morning, and where I spent considerable time during that rotation taking care of extremely sick, surgical pediatric patients. The entire team would gather for rounds at seven a.m. and after rounding on all the patients there we proceeded to the fishbowl, and then to the regular floor. Rounds were usually led by the two senior attendings, Dr. Reiss and Dr. Oropeza. Both had been at Jackson for many years. They were excellent surgeons and exemplary teachers. Most striking, however, was the special relationship they seemed to have with the patients we followed in the clinic, as they had cared for most of these patients from the time they were born. Indeed, many of these patients would not be alive if it were not for the efforts of these two surgeons.

One group of patients that were regular customers at the clinic were the so-called "short-gut" patients. These were children who had developed conditions that caused some sort of ischemia (lack of blood supply) eventually leading to gangrene (death) in a portion of their bowel—especially their small intestines—which eventually required resection (removal) of said bowel. The small intestine serves the purpose of allowing the body to absorb from the foods we eat the nutrients needed to maintain bodily functions and enable growth.

Although both adults and children have redundancy in the length of the small bowel, there is a critical point after which resection of the small bowel does not allow for the remaining bowel to be able to absorb enough nutrients. Thus, these patients need to have special diets and supplemental feedings, but some also need to have their nutrition augmented by PPN (partial parenteral nutrition), a liquid containing amino acids, fats, carbohydrates, and vitamins that is injected through a central line—a catheter placed through the skin into the great veins of the chest or neck. These catheters are inserted surgically and are meant to stay in long-term but have the downside of being a potential source of infection. These patients were closely followed by the pediatric surgery team in order to ensure their nutritional regimen allowed them to thrive, and also to pick up early signs of trouble, such as malnutrition or catheter infections. The ultimate solution and hope for these patients was to undergo a small bowel transplant, as this would allow them to be able to absorb all the nutrients they needed from the food they ate, and thereby make them forever independent of their PPN and most importantly, their central line catheters.

The close relationship between the short-gut patients and the two surgeons who had cared for them for years was evident in their interactions. Most children are afraid of doctors or anyone wearing a white coat. These kids, however, were cheerful around these two surgeons and did not seem to exhibit the slightest fear. It was almost as if they instinctively knew that they would not be alive if it were not for the efforts of these two men. Moreover, Drs. Reiss and Oropeza, who were in their late sixties and fifties respectively, seemed to develop a certain child-like playfulness when around these kids, even more so than is customary in healthcare providers who care for children. They had nicknames for most of the children they cared for on a regular basis. There was Rocky the Rocker, Harry the Head-banger, Don Donatello (Ninja Turtle inspired nicknames were a common theme), and many more such nicknames. One of the challenges for the residents and students rotating through the service was to learn all the nicknames and the special, unique jargon that Drs. Reiss and Oropeza had developed over the years.

Enzo (short for Lorenzo) was one of these short-gut patients who had been under the care of the two senior surgeons for most of his six years of life. At about four months of age, his parents had brought Enzo to the emergency room after he had been crying and unwilling to feed for close to twenty-four hours. The parents had initially thought that Enzo was suffering from a common cold or viral infection, but when he developed blood in his stool, the parents became alarmed and were prompted to bring him to the hospital. The work-up done in the emergency room had revealed that Enzo had intussusception, a condition in which one part of the small bowel telescopes inside another piece and often causes intestinal obstruction and edema. If not treated promptly, bowel gangrene and potentially death can follow. Attempts at medical management through a barium enema, which sometimes can resolve this condition, were unsuccessful. Dr. Reiss had been brought in as a consultant to address the issue surgically, after those noninvasive attempts had failed.

By the time Dr. Reiss got Enzo on the operating room table, his condition had deteriorated considerably, and he was extremely sick. Upon opening the abdomen, Dr. Reiss found a large portion of Enzo's small bowel had become gangrenous from a restricted blood supply, and there was nothing left to do but resect it, leaving poor Enzo with only a very short segment of healthy small bowel. This operation saved Enzo's life, but made him a short-gut patient, who would now require PPN to live, until and if he were to ever get a small-bowel transplant. Enzo was at the top of the list for a transplant, but the transplant surgeons wanted him to grow a bit more before they attempted this still-experimental surgery at the time. Over the ensuing years, both Drs. Reiss and Oropeza had treated Enzo for multiple catheter infections. He was a regular not only at the clinic, but at the pediatric surgery ICU as well.

I had met Enzo when he had been at his best and found him to be a friendly and gregarious child. He was extremely intelligent and had a most remarkable vocabulary for a child his age. He seemed to relish in the attention he received as he was not only a favorite of Drs. Reiss and Oropeza, but also of many of the nurses and the clinic staff. For his part, Enzo was quick to offer a great smile and a hug to everyone who greeted him. Upon entering the clinic, he had a habit of going to every staff member he knew and saying hello to them before allowing anyone to direct him into one of the exam rooms. He never showed any fear and would let himself be examined by anyone who wanted to do so.

Thus, when Enzo was bought by his parents to the emergency room with a high fever and lethargy for twenty-four hours, we all knew what the problem was most likely to be; Enzo had yet another catheter infection. I promptly admitted Enzo to our pediatric surgery ICU where Dr. Oropeza and I removed his infected catheter and started a new central line. This was difficult as Enzo had been stuck so many times that he had no venous access on his extremity, and the access to large vessels on his chest and neck was scarred from the many previous catheter placements.

We started Enzo on fluids and antibiotics, and although at first it seemed that he was on his way to a full recovery as with the previous catheter infections, this time he was infected with a bacterial strain highly resistant to antibiotics. We brought in consultants from the infectious diseases service to help us choose the correct antibiotics to treat Enzo's catheter infection, but despite our best efforts he developed severe sepsis. Enzo put up a great fight but eventually his little body gave out and he died at 11:30 one Sunday evening with me at his bedside.

Even though I had not known Enzo for long, I too could see that he was a special little boy; he had a great fighting spirit, and he would be greatly missed. I had to go speak to the family and give them the sad news. The nurse taking care of him that last day came with me. Giving family this kind of news has always been painfully difficult for me and speaking to this family in particular was heartbreaking. They had gone through a lot with Enzo, and their love for him was evident in the way they worried for him and took care of him. Upon hearing the news, the family was utterly devastated to say the least.

On my way back with the nurse to the ICU, it was easy for me to see that she was shaken up too. She had worked in the ICU for many years and had taken care of Enzo multiple times before. Like most of the staff, she had developed a great attachment to him and his family.

"Tough, huh?" I took the liberty of putting my hand on her shoulder.

"Yes, it is." She had tears in her eyes. "Every time I see a child die, I wonder if we have just lost our next Einstein, or Mozart…so much potential lost. It is so sad. No matter how long I work with kids, seeing them die is something I can never get used to." I nodded my head in agreement. There was nothing left to be said.

Operating and taking care of kids is special. Kids, unlike adults, always seem to wear their emotions on their sleeve. When sick, children tend to cry or get cranky. When happy and feeling good, they are all smiles and become joyfully playful. Children can get sick quickly, but can also get better, especially through surgery, even more quickly. Having helped in a child's psychological transformation from being sad to happy, it is easy for the surgeon to get swept up in the euphoria that the child projects. In doing so, the surgeon temporarily forgets his/her own personal problems and challenges.

Operating and taking care of children also has an added dimension. When one makes them whole again and particularly if the child's life is saved, the surgeon has given this child a great gift beyond restoring their physical health. This gift is far more precious and encompasses the promise of a future not yet realized, and the awesome potential of a life not yet lived. This was the sentiment expressed by the nurse as we returned to the ICU after talking to Enzo's family. Having the ability to bestow this gift to another human being, particularly a child, is an awesome thing, and one of the most profound reasons for becoming a surgeon.

I did not become a pediatric surgeon per se, but I did choose to become a plastic surgeon with a subspecialty in craniofacial surgery. A significant part of my practice involves operating and taking care of children with craniofacial anomalies and challenges. Without a doubt, taking care of these children is one of the most rewarding and personally fulfilling aspects of my profession. It will forever be an honor and a privilege to facilitate the ability of children to fulfill their dreams and realize their full potential.

The Visiting Surgeon

Since Jackson Memorial Hospital was affiliated with the University of Miami, ours was an academic general surgery training program. However, most of the residents aspired to end up in private practice after graduation and we were eager to experience the private side of medicine. The opportunity, however, was not to happen for us until the fourth year of residency.

Less than four miles from Jackson across Biscayne Bay sits Mt. Sinai Hospital, a private hospital that serves the residents of Miami Beach. It is there that during the fourth year the residents from Jackson Memorial were sent for a two-month rotation designed to afford them exposure to gynecological (female reproductive tract) surgery. We were also to rotate every third night and serve as senior resident on call for the general surgery service. Mt. Sinai Hospital had its own general surgery residency program as they took two categorical residents per year. Their residents rotated through Jackson as well, in order to gain experience in services that did not exist at Mt. Sinai Hospital, such as transplant and burn surgery.

From the first day of my rotation at Mt. Sinai, some of the differences between the academic and private practice world became apparent, starting with the food. Despite renovations to the cafeteria at Jackson during my first few years of training, the food could not compare to the quality and options available at the Mt. Sinai cafeteria. At the doctor's lounge, they even had metal silverware and cloth napkins. Residents were technically not allowed to eat there, as the doctor's cafeteria was meant for the attendings only, but occasionally we would get invited by one of the attending doctors to get a literal taste of what was to come once we were no longer residents.

Another area of stark difference was the interaction of doctors and nurses. At Jackson, there was an obvious difference in the way nurses treated attending physicians versus residents. The nurses acted more like high school teachers toward the residents and were often very protective of their patients. They feared the patients might suffer from the mistakes resulting from the residents' inexperience. This dynamic often eroded the mutual respect that should be the norm in doctor-nurse interactions. At times, the nurses were quite stern, a posture that caused friction and ruffled the feathers of many a junior resident who often felt that nurses were not showing the proper respect.

At Mt. Sinai Hospital, the residents were few and most nurses dealt directly with the attending staff. As such, there was a certain decorum in the way nurses and physicians acted towards one another and this included the residents as well. The interaction seemed more of a collaborative effort toward the betterment of the patient. This was a welcome experience and gave residents yet another view into the future and how things would, or at least could, be once the process of residency was over.

Surgery training in a private practice setting was a little different, as most of the patient interactions were initiated at the attending level with little resident input. An internist, for example, would consult a surgeon for a particular problem. Most times, the attending surgeon would go see the patient first, make a decision as to what the plan should be, and then contact the resident and tell him/her what was to be done. Often, by the time the resident interacted with the patient for the first time, most decisions had been made at the attending level and the resident was more of a passive observer of the process, rather than an integral member of a team given the opportunity to offer his/her perspective as to the treatment plan and learn from the experience of having to defend it.

Whatever drawbacks the Mt. Sinai program had in terms of the flow of patient interactions, it more than made up for in operating room time for the residents. This point became obvious when I started operating with junior residents from that program. It became clear that their level of manual dexterity and surgical skill was light years ahead of the residents from my program at the same level of training. The reason for this discrepancy in surgical skills soon became clear. As opposed to my training, where I hardly got to go into the operating room during my entire first year, and when I did, it was as the second and even third assistant, the residents from Mt. Sinai were operating from the first day of their residency. It was common for interns and second-year residents to be the only resident operating with an attending surgeon on a multitude of different types of cases, some of which were of such complexity that at Jackson they would have been the sole purview of the senior residents.

Another pleasant surprise during my rotation at Mt. Sinai Hospital was that I got a chance to get reacquainted with Rick Lopez. Rick and I had started as interns together at Jackson, but as he was an undesignated preliminary resident, he unfortunately did not make the cut after the second year and was forced to seek the continuation of his training elsewhere. After much effort, he was lucky to find a preliminary position at Mt. Sinai Hospital with the caveat that he would have to repeat his second year as that was the only position available. When we were reunited during my rotation, Rick was a third-year preliminary surgery resident, now acting as my junior resident. This was somewhat awkward for me, especially since after operating together for the first time, it became obvious that Rick could outperform me easily when it came to surgical skills. He had made particularly good use of his operating room time during the year and a half since we had last seen each other.

For this rotation I was to function as his senior resident, a rather uncomfortable position since we had started together. However, I as the visiting surgeon would be playing on his home turf. For his part, Rick was welcoming, cordial, and helpful in getting me situated to what was to be my home for the next two months. He was popular all over the hospital, particularly with the nurses, and doing rounds with him was always fun. As he had more experience than the typical third-year resident, Rick was able to function fairly independently and would only call me on complicated cases or when patients needed to go to the operating room, as was the existing protocol.

One such occasion occurred during the middle of my rotation. I had just finished having dinner and had retired to my call room to do some reading when Rick called and asked me to meet him in the radiology reading room.

"We have a dissecting triple A (abdominal aortic aneurysm) that is about to blow at any minute."

By this time in my residency, during my vascular surgery rotations with Dr. Ogle, Dr. Perez (Master Samurai), and my prior outside rotation during my fourth year, I had been acquainted with this particular condition and knew firsthand what an ominous diagnosis Rick had just described. I rushed downstairs to meet him.

I walked into the reading room just as the radiologist was reviewing the films with Rick. The CT scans of the patient's abdomen revealed a large mass in the center of it, which displaced the adjacent small intestines and colon. The mass was the dilated aorta which measured close to nine centimeters in diameter at its widest point, more than four times the two centimeters that is considered normal width. The lumen of the aorta was filled with clot, but we could also visualize some of the injected contrast within the lumen. This contrast indicated the areas of the lumen, which was patent for the flow of blood, which was not much. On the right side of the aneurysm, the contrast was extremely close to the weakened wall of the vessel, heralding the possibility of impending leak and rupture.

"If the aneurysm ruptures, it will most likely rupture at this point." The radiologist pointed with his pen to an area where there was visible thinning of the aortic wall.

This particular aneurysm was not only very wide, it was also long in the vertical dimension. It originated far above the level of the arteries that go to the kidneys and extended almost all the way down to the level where the aorta bifurcates into the arteries of the pelvis. After a brief glance at the film, I immediately realized our patient was in trouble.

Aurora Weiss was seventy-eight years of age; she had been visiting her relatives in Miami Beach for the past week. She had gone to bed the night before with some abdominal discomfort that had turned much worse by the time she had woken up that morning. At first, she and her family thought it had been indigestion, but then she began to develop abdominal distention and increased pain. Her family became increasingly concerned and eventually decided to bring her to the emergency room. Since Ms. Weiss did not have a primary care physician in town, the emergency department contacted the on-call resident in order to evaluate her and arrange for the necessary care.

Rick and I walked in to meet the patient together. Ms. Weiss lay on the stretcher surrounded by family members. The grimace on her face and the expressions of her relatives spoke of the seriousness of the situation and the fear they all shared. We were informed that she was fairly healthy for her age and was closely followed in Chicago by her primary care physician. Her high blood pressure and borderline diabetes were well-controlled, and she had a highly active lifestyle for her age.

Ms. Weiss was a thin woman of about five foot six, and her distended abdomen looked out of place on such a frail body. Light palpation of the abdomen revealed a tender, pulsatile mass in its center. The pulses in her lower extremities were not palpable and could barely be heard with a doppler (a device that uses sound waves to detect blood flow). I could not ascertain from the patient nor the family the state of her lower extremity pulses prior to this incident, but very much feared that the dissection of the aneurysm had occluded, or at least greatly diminished the blood flow to her legs. This was a bad sign as it could lead to potential complications for the patient once the blood flow was reestablished to the tissues affected, a condition referred to as reperfusion syndrome.

Once we walked out of the room, Rick and I decided to divide and conquer as we were very much aware that in this particular situation, speed was of the essence. We split up the work necessary to get Ms. Weiss to the operating room as soon as possible. I asked Rick to work on such things as ordering blood, getting the proper intravenous fluids started, and otherwise start getting the patient ready for the OR. Rick stayed at the patient's bedside to oversee the preparations personally, while I immediately put in a call to the vascular surgeon on call for the evening and called the OR desk and anesthesia to book the case.

Things began to progress efficiently and quickly as this case demanded; however, it was not until several minutes later that the OR desk nurse asked me who the attending surgeon was. I realized I had not yet gotten a call back from the vascular surgeon. To make matters worse, Rick came to me and told me that Ms. Weiss was beginning to experience an increase in the intensity of the pain and he was becoming very concerned that the aneurysm could rupture at any minute, right there in the emergency room. I nervously called the hospital operator to confirm that she had put in a call to the attending surgeon, and when she said she had, I asked her to put it in again, this time making sure to let the surgeon's service know that this was an emergency.

Half an hour had now passed since my initial call when I received the return call from the vascular attending on call. Through a nurse, he relayed the message that he was currently scrubbed at another hospital and would return my call as soon as he finished his case, which he guessed would take him another two hours. When I described the situation I was dealing with, he got on the phone himself and suggested I call the attending on second call as he feared he would not be able to finish his case and get there on time. I immediately put in that call and made sure to let the answering service know that this call was an emergency.

In the meantime, I called the OR desk again to ask whether we could start moving the patient to the operating room and was promptly informed by the OR desk nurse that I could not do that until I had a surgeon of record on the case. I did not yet, so for the time being, we were on hold in the emergency room. Rick would continue to come every couple of minutes to keep me abreast of the patient's condition and inform me that things were continuing to deteriorate.

"The family continues to inquire as to when we are going to get her to the OR." Rick was only relaying information, but I could not help but become more stressed and aggravated with him.

"I can't do anything yet, Rick. The second attending has not called in so far and the OR nurse will not let me bring her to the OR."

"Well, then call the chief of surgery if you don't want this lady to die here on us. You need to get someone here now."

The added pressure Rick was putting on me was not helpful although I understood he was doing what he thought was best for the patient. I did not feel comfortable calling the chief of the department of surgery until I gave the second attending on call a few minutes to answer. However, I felt that I had to do something, so I put in a second emergency call to the vascular surgeon and dialed one of the chief residents directly. I was hoping that like a superhero, he would come help me with my present predicament.

"You are the senior on tonight, Joe. You need to get an attending in there ASAP. If the guy on call is not calling you back, you need to call the chairman and let him figure it out." The advice was sound, but I was praying the vascular attending would call me back prior to me having to take this up to the chairman of the department.

As I was hanging up with the chief resident, Rick approached me once again with a frustrated look on his face. "Joe, I ordered a thoracotomy set to be brought down from the OR to the patient's bedside. If the aneurysm ruptures, I am going to crack the chest and clamp the aorta."

These words more than anything else brought my level of stress to a fever pitch. Upon hearing them, I realized the potential ramifications of what he was saying. His words hit me like a freight train. My mind took me back to my intern year when Rio and I performed an emergency room thoracotomy in the resus bay on a patient who had sustained gunshot wounds to the chest. Performing such a high-risk procedure in the emergency room of a community hospital which did not even treat trauma patients and without an attending's permission would be highly risky and controversial, particularly for me as the senior resident present. After all, I was a visiting surgeon from another program. I doubted that the emergency room nurses or attendings working that day would let me do it, even if I wanted to.

"Okay Rick, get the tray ready but look at me..." I paused what I was doing to emphasize the point, "don't you dare do anything without getting my approval first." It felt awkward to give orders to Rick in this way, but since I was the senior, his actions were my responsibility and I would be the one called to account if he were to do something extreme. All the while I prayed I would not be put in a position to have to make that decision either way.

Rick's desire to do something to prevent our patient from dying was understandable, but as a senior and the person ultimately responsible for what took place that day, the decision to take matters into our own hands without the backing of an attending would for better or worse fall solely on me. I dreaded the possibility of being put in a position where I was forced to make that decision. If the aneurysm ruptured, the only way to save the patient's life was for me to go ahead and attempt to clamp the aorta right there in the emergency room, a high-risk, low probability of success maneuver. By this time, the pressure I felt was becoming unbearable.

Out of desperation and out of options, I put in an emergency call to the chairman of surgery and also dialed Dr. Albert Perez (Master Samurai), one of the vascular surgery attendings from Jackson with whom I had recently worked on his service and whose cell phone number I had stored in my phone.

"Dr. Perez, I am rotating at Mt. Sinai and have a big problem I need advice on. I have a seventy-eight-year-old lady with a dissecting aneurysm which is about to rupture, and I'm waiting for the vascular attending to return my call. I'm wondering if I should crack her chest in the ER if the aneurysm ruptures."

Dr. Perez immediately understood the precarious position our patient was in, as well as the serious nature of what I was pondering. The grave tone of his voice showed his concern:

"Joe, you are the one there and I can't make that call for you. You are aware that an ER thoracotomy is a long shot and will be highly controversial if you are to make that decision on your own. Best thing you can do is to make sure that the patient's blood pressure is well controlled (it was) so that the aneurysm does not rupture and get someone in there to help you quick."

As Dr. Perez uttered those words, the name of Dr. Ben Beck came to mind. Dr. Beck was a general surgeon and one of the busiest at Mt. Sinai. He was always a pleasure to work with and was fond of the visiting surgeons from Jackson. By this time of the rotation, I had already scrubbed with him several times and knew him to be a great surgeon and teacher. I suddenly also remembered that he had vascular training and lived close to the hospital. My call to him was answered in less than three minutes. When I explained my predicament, his answer was a breath of fresh air: "Get her to the OR as quickly as you can. I will meet you there in less than ten minutes."

Now with an attending of record, we were set to go. Rick and I had our patient on the OR table and intubated by the time Dr. Beck walked into the room. Seeing him felt like a great weight was taken off my back. I paused to take a deep breath and exhaled slowly, then proceeded to give him the particulars of the case. "Get her prepped. I will go meet and talk to the family and will join you in a few."

Rick and I promptly complied and had everything ready to go by the time Dr. Beck walked back into the OR, now fully scrubbed and ready to go. It was at this time that the OR desk nurse walked into the room to let me know that both the second vascular surgeon on second call and the chairman of the department of surgery were on the phone asking to speak to me. Dr. Beck intervened and asked the nurse to let both gentlemen know that he was on the case now and had everything under control.

As our patient was a very thin woman, we had little difficulty in opening her abdomen, mobilizing the left colon, and exposing the huge aortic aneurysm. The dissection around the aneurysm was a different matter, however, and took considerable time. Although the aneurysm had not yet ruptured, the walls of the dilated vessel seemed extremely thin and calcified. There was an inflammatory reaction around the entire area of the aneurysm making the tissues extremely friable; minimal manipulation of them would result in bleeding. After some time, we were able to get around the normal aorta above and below the level of the aneurysm. Soon thereafter we were able to place clamps on both of these areas, and as a group we took a collective breath and a sigh of relief, knowing that we had averted a rupture.

After longitudinally opening the aorta, we noticed that the large aneurysm was mostly filled with clot and fibrin and had a small lumen. Furthermore, the walls of the artery were very friable and would not hold sutures. This became an issue when we tried to suture the Dacron graft into place. Time and time again the sutures on the arterial wall would pull through, and it would require us to resect another segment of the artery in the hope of finding a section of healthy, non-inflamed arterial wall. This process took several attempts, and the surgery began to take longer than expected. After we released the clamps, there were several areas of significant blood leaks at the interface between the arterial wall and the graft. This required us to re-clamp the vessel and reinforce those areas with more sutures.

Finally, we released the clamps and the entire suture line held. After watching it for several minutes to ensure there were no further leaks, we washed out the area and began our closure. Somewhere in the middle of closing the abdomen, the anesthesiologist alerted us that our patient was becoming unstable. Her blood pressure began to drop, and her blood tests (arterial blood gas) were showing that her blood PH was dropping—becoming more acidic. He pointed as he asked us to look at the patient's urine as it was collecting in the Foley bag and which had turned dark yellow/red. All indications were that our patient was suffering from what is called a reperfusion injury and rhabdomyolysis, a profoundly serious condition indeed.

When tissues, particularly muscle, are deprived of blood (and thus oxygen), they begin to break down. The byproducts of this breakdown create a very acidic environment in the area affected. When the area in question is reperfused (revascularized), as for example after the aorta clamps are removed and blood is allowed to come into the area, the blood washes away all these toxic byproducts and denatured muscle protein back into the systemic circulation. If the amount of these byproducts is significant enough, they can cause metabolic derangements such as acidosis (lowering of the blood PH making it more acidic). In addition, the denatured muscle proteins from muscle breakdown (rhabdomyolysis) can lead to acute kidney failure as they overwhelm the kidney's ability to filtrate them out of the blood. These are metabolic issues that must be addressed promptly before these toxic byproducts and low PH have a deleterious effect on organs such as the heart, which if severe enough, leads to malignant heart rhythms (dysrhythmias) and death. This ominous metabolic derangement is aggressively treated by giving the patient medications that alkalinize (increase the PH) the blood and intravenous fluid so as to dilute the toxin concentration in the intravascular space. This overall metabolic deterioration is referred to as reperfusion injury or reperfusion syndrome and it is entirely a medical diagnosis, as there is not much the surgeon can do to treat it, other than to make sure there is access to the patient's circulatory system through adequate IV catheter or central line access through which the necessary fluids and medications can be given.

Despite the efforts of the anesthesia team in instituting all recommended modalities, the follow-up blood tests (blood gasses) did not improve significantly, and the patient began to develop heart rhythm abnormalities. As surgeons, we could not do much except try to finish the closure as soon as possible in order to get the patient off the OR table and into the ICU where she could be warmed, monitored, and medically optimized. While in the middle of the abdominal closure, the patient developed ventricular fibrillation. We started CPR and were successful in converting this malignant heart rhythm initially after two consecutive electric shocks to the heart with chest paddles as per ACLS protocol. When she developed the same heart rhythm several minutes later as we were putting on the dressing, she would not convert despite our best efforts. Ms. Weiss unfortunately expired several minutes later while still on the operating room table.

We had all been at this for over five hours by now, and it was disheartening to suddenly realize that our hopes of saving our patient were not to be realized. It had been a long shot at best, but for a time we thought we would be able to pull her through. After several moments of silence, Dr. Beck asked Rick and me to wrap things up in the OR. He was going to talk to the family. This was another difference between Jackson and this hospital. Here most of the family discussions, especially of this kind, were handled by the attending surgeons directly and the residents were seldom involved. I did not envy Dr. Beck and felt relief that it would be he who would have the uncomfortable talk with the family, rather than me.

Rick and I finished the dressing and headed to the recovery room to write our notes and complete the necessary paperwork.

We were both exhausted. I could tell he was disappointed. We both wondered if we could have done anything different to change the outcome. Perhaps if the family had brought her in sooner, or we had gotten her to the operating room a little earlier, or if we had given her more fluids before the operation… or perhaps if the arterial wall had been healthier allowing us to suture the graft in a much shorter time. As in most cases that did not end well, there were always plenty of unanswered ifs. Rick and I did not have the luxury to ponder on the case for too long, as by now there were several other consults waiting for us in the emergency room.

The rest of my rotation at Mt. Sinai went pretty smoothly. The two outside rotations during my fourth year gave me a good idea of what life in private practice was like. Despite having to make certain adjustments regarding the logistics of patient care, the rotations were extremely educational, rewarding, and insightful in many ways. I was always made to feel at home at both of the institutions by the attendings, residents, nurses, and ancillary staff alike. I very much liked the experience and looked forward to the time when I would be in a similar environment as a practicing surgeon.

Rick and I got to work together several more times on call and in the operating room. We always maintained a cordial and friendly relationship after sharing that mutual experience. I was happy to learn that he eventually secured a categorical spot in general surgery and went on to practice general and trauma surgery. He became an excellent clinician and a great innovator and has developed certain laparoscopic techniques to treat difficult general surgery problems such as large abdominal wall hernias and challenging abdominal wall reconstruction. Moreover, I've been privileged to attend some of his lectures where he presented some of these techniques.

Sitting in those lectures, I found myself in awe of how Rick—who had struggled to secure a categorical spot—had transformed himself into an expert in the field and had matured into a recognized figure in his specialty. I pondered as to how he, as well as people like Gregorio Esposito and Rachel, were a great testament to how drive, determination, and perseverance are essential ingredients to the achievement of success.

THE LORD

I first heard about Dr. Zach Wolfe in passing while still in medical school during my residency interview at Jackson Memorial Hospital. While getting a tour of the hospital by one of the chief residents, he directed our group of seven interviewees into one of the trauma center elevators as he was going to show us the ICU on the second floor. Being one of the last in the group to enter the elevator, I stood next to the chief resident by the elevator doors. Before the doors closed, another resident rushed in at the last minute and stood by the chief resident alongside me.

This newcomer looked disheveled, with his hair uncombed and his lab coat appearing slept-in.

"How is it going?" the chief resident inquired.

"E2," came the reply. I saw the resident raise his eyebrows and take on a look of pity as he answered the chief resident.

"Ah! The Lord. Hang in there, it will eventually end."

Just as those words were uttered, the elevator door opened, and we all filed out into the trauma ICU. The unhappy resident was the first to exit, and he hurried down the hallway toward the main hospital. I was immediately curious about this unusual exchange and the comment pertaining to "The Lord," but I thought it better not to ask. Besides, the chief resident was already talking enthusiastically about what he wanted to show us in this area of the hospital. Come to think of it, although I eventually became aware of whom that most peculiar nickname referred to, I never learned the origin of the nickname nor what might have been done to earn it.

I soon forgot this short elevator conversation, only to be reminded of it close to a year and a half later while I was an intern rotating through the anesthesia service. On one particular day, I had been assigned to the liver room along with one of the second-year anesthesia residents (she was to act as my mentor and supervisor during the case). The procedure to be performed was a "Whipple," an extraordinarily complex operation for resection of tumors of the head of the pancreas and/or bile ducts.

Due to the complex anatomy of the area, this operation is extremely challenging technically, and it is usually undertaken by oncological and general surgeons who are experienced and proficient at it. This operation, which can last anywhere from four to six hours, requires intense concentration on the part of the surgeon, as well as the entire operating room team. Dr. Zach Wolfe was the attending surgeon of record, and the operation was scheduled to start at 7:30 a.m. Getting ready for the case that morning, it all seemed routine to me, and the name of the attending surgeon did not ring any special bells. Unknown to me at the time was that it had been Dr. Wolfe whom the chief resident had referred to as "The Lord" in the elevator during my residency interview. I was soon to learn the reason why the E2 (Elective 2 or Hepatobiliary) service, of which Dr. Wolfe was the chief, is the most feared rotation of the general surgery residency.

The surgery senior resident had been in the room when we put the patient to sleep. I did not know him but noted that he seemed like an affable guy and was friendly enough to the anesthesia team. He glanced at my badge and nodded as he seemed to recognize me as one of the surgery interns. After the patient was asleep, he went outside the room to scrub for the procedure, and shortly thereafter Dr. Wolfe and the resident walked together into the room ready to begin. By this time during my anesthesia rotation I was used to the lull in cases between the time of induction where patients were intubated, and the end of the case when they were extubated. The anesthesia team had to monitor the patient throughout the procedure and ensure that all vital signs remained stable, but during the middle of the case if all was stable there was certainly time to ponder on other things. I had decided to spend time watching surgeons at work, not necessarily the technical aspects of the surgery, but rather the way they behaved and acted during surgery. This particular operation turned out to be a great case study.

The yelling started almost immediately after the commencement of the procedure, and it did not abate for the entire six-hour case. I remember that right after he cut skin, Dr. Wolfe started asking the resident about the patients on the floor. He wanted to know how the patient was doing overall, and about specific lab values and test results. Every time the resident hesitated or did not know a particular piece of information that Dr. Wolfe wanted, the resident had to endure a barrage of complaints and criticism expressed in a loud, whining, and high-pitched voice. Once this grilling session was over, I mistakenly thought that perhaps the yelling would cease, but it did not. The yelling then was elicited by mistakes the resident was making in the surgery.

"Suction here! NOOO, HERE! HELP ME! PLEASE HELP ME!" And so, on and on it went as the resident repeatedly meekly apologized.

From my unique vantage point behind the "blood-brain barrier," the scene was somewhat surreal as Dr. Wolfe appeared very much at ease and methodical in everything he was doing, except for his continuous yelling that seemed to focus entirely on the senior resident. He was cordial to the nurses, and even to the anesthesia team (at first), but it seemed that the resident could not do anything right. I began to feel rather uncomfortable after a while, and a couple of times when my eyes met those of the resident, I evaded his glance.

Eventually, even the anesthesia team—of which I was a member—was not spared Dr. Wolfe's wrath when he had some difficulty closing the patient's abdomen, due to what he surmised was not enough muscle relaxation. I anxiously watched as the anesthesia resident reacted to Dr. Wolfe's yelling at us by quickly injecting paralytic agents into the patient's intravenous line. Her nervousness was revealed by the tremor of her hands as she performed this task. Once finished with the surgery, Dr. Wolfe walked out of the room, leaving the resident to finish dressing the wound prior to meeting upstairs with the team for rounds. As soon as Dr. Wolfe walked out of the room, the resident pulled down his mask, took a deep breath, and let it out quite slowly. The tension he was under was easy to read in his body language. He looked toward me, and after catching my glance he gave me a tired look: "This will be you in four years." At the time, four years seemed like an eternity, as I could not think beyond the next rotation.

I sure hope not, I thought to myself, hoping that Dr. Wolfe would retire by the time I became a senior resident.

Over the next few years, I saw Dr. Zach Wolfe only at conferences such as Grand Rounds where the entire surgical department gathered for weekly lectures, usually from visiting professors. I never spoke nor interacted with him in any way, but always remembered that particular day during my intern anesthesia rotation. Before I knew it, however, the end of my third year approached, and with it the impending fourth year E2 rotation. I was very much aware that Dr. Wolfe had not yet retired and that I would soon be up on the docket. Nevertheless, I still had some maneuvering to do. When it came time to sit down with the other third-year residents to plan our fourth-year schedule, I managed to get myself assigned to E2 as my last rotation of the fourth year. I figured this way, I would give Dr. Wolfe almost another year to ponder retirement (unlikely), and if that did not work, I would at least get to that particular rotation with the most training and experience of all my co-residents, as I would have had all of my other fourth-year rotations by the time I got to E2. I was hoping I would thus be more prepared for the rotation than the rest of my cohorts.

My anxiety over this rotation intensified over the course of the fourth year as I kept hearing wild stories of residents in prior years having nervous breakdowns during the rotation. There was even a story of a resident who reportedly vomited into his mask during surgery due to the stress he was under. I never found out the veracity of these stories, but I had a feeling there was more than a grain of truth to them.

I checked in often with my fellow residents vis-à-vis on the different rotations, and I paid particular attention to the thoughts of those residents who were rotating through the E2 service. It was universal that it was a grueling rotation, not only in the amount of work, but also in the amount of stress. The patients were all sick, the surgeries were complex, long, and required great concentration in the operating room. Moreover, a great amount of time had to be devoted to the patient's post-operative care. Most of the residents felt that Dr. Wolfe was very demanding and expected nothing less than optimal performance at all times. As the residents related their unique stories of Dr. Wolfe, I noticed a recurrent theme. He seemed to ask the same questions during surgery from each of the residents. Although the questions he asked were many, and varied dependent on the procedure being performed, there was certainly a set of "most favorites."

After asking several residents to describe what their first Whipple with Dr. Wolfe was like, most said that things started to go bad when upon lifting the head of the pancreas, Dr. Wolfe pointed to a vein emanating from the anterior aspect of the IVC (inferior vena cava)—the main vein returning blood from the body to the heart—and running inferiorly and slightly to the right. All the residents were stumped and could not identify what this vein was, even after looking at anatomy books after the surgery. Dr. Wolfe, after expressing disappointment and admonishing the residents to study more, then would divulge the name of the vessel in question.

It turns out that the vein in question was the right gonadal vein, which drains the blood coming from the right testicle in males, or the ovary in females, into the IVC. Surgeons are known for their expertise in anatomy. Not only do they study it from the first year of medical school, but more than other medical specialties, they continuously review it time and time again in preparation for their surgical cases. The fact that most fourth-year surgery residents were not able to identify such a large and prominent vein was notable, and due to a thought distortion of the way we all conceptualized the location of this vein. Of course, we all knew that there is a right gonadal vein, and we knew that it drained into the IVC. However, since it is routed from the testicle or ovary (pelvis), we all assumed that it would drain into the IVC much lower in the abdomen and insert from the side, rather than insert in the front as high as the mid to upper level of the abdomen where the pancreas sits.

In any case, this was one of Wolfe's "most favorite" questions that stumped most if not all the residents, and I took note of it. Soon, I learned that there were several other favorites, like when he would ask the resident if he/she had given the patient Aquamephyton. This question would throw the residents into a panic before realizing that it is another name for intravenous vitamin K, which is routinely given to patients who undergo liver surgery to help with blood coagulation. After I detected this recurrent pattern in the questions Dr. Wolfe liked to ask, I began to write them all down, and I made sure to look up the correct answers. Before the start of my rotation, my compilation of these questions with their respective answers grew to more than a few typed pages.

As the last two months of my fourth (senior) year approached, the realization sunk in that Dr. Wolfe was not to retire before my rotation after all, and that in the end I would have to endure what many residents of our program had endured before me. The day before my rotation was due to start, I called the resident who was to give me the report on the service. Nadya Miocevic called me late in the evening for what I anticipated was going to be a long conversation in which we would go over in detail each of the patients on the service. Nadya was the current chief resident on the service and from whom I was to get sign-out. For most of the evening I had been anticipating her phone call. However, as it got later and later in the evening, I began to get nervous as I wanted to make sure to go early to bed on the eve of what I anticipated was going to be a brutal rotation.

When the phone finally rang at 9:30 p.m., it was obvious that Nadya was tired and was not in the mood for much talking. It turned out she had been operating with Dr. Wolfe all day and was just finishing rounds. She called from the hospital and it became evident that she did not intend for our conversation to keep her from going home. She was eager to pass the "hot potato" to the next person in line. She briefly gave me an overview of the patients on the service, what was to be done over the next couple of days with each of them, and then she spent a little more time telling me about the two patients on whom Dr. Wolfe and I were to operate the next day. Two cases were on the docket, one of which was a Whipple.

"Sleep tight," she said. "It will be a long first day."

The next morning, I was promptly on the floor by 5:30 a.m. and took the first thirty minutes to read over the charts of Dr. Wolfe's patients before meeting the new interns on the team. After rounding on all the patients, I headed down to the operating room. Once I had all the paperwork ready for the patient to undergo the first surgery, I sat outside the operating room and attempted to memorize the pertinent lab values of Dr. Wolfe's patients, as I knew he would expect me to know them by heart. As I was extremely stressed and nervous, this exercise proved quite difficult.

By 7:30 a.m. the patient had been brought into the room, intubated, and given anesthesia. As I finished prepping the patient, I saw through the glass window in the OR Dr. Wolfe approach the sink and start to scrub. I rushed out to meet him and formally introduced myself.

"Hello, Dr. Wolfe. I am Joe Garri, and I will be the senior resident on your service starting today."

Dr. Wolfe looked up toward me, but with his mask on I could not read his facial expression.

"Hello, Joe."

I proceeded to start telling him about his patients while looking at the notes I had taken during rounds, but he stopped me with a wave of his soap-soaked hand. "That's okay. Let's talk while we work."

Dr. Wolfe and I then proceeded to drape the patient. He had a particular way he liked the towels and drapes placed on the patient, a technique that I use to this day. A few minutes later he proceeded to make the skin incision along the midline of the abdomen from right under the chest bone (sternum) to a few inches below the belly button (umbilicus). Just as he gave the knife back to the nurse upon completing his incision the dreaded questions started: "So how is Mr. Platt?"

I took a deep breath and started to regurgitate everything I remembered about each of the patients he asked about including the pertinent lab data I had memorized right before the case. I anticipated the screaming was about to begin at any moment and psychologically braced myself for it. To my amazement, however, that first day Dr. Wolfe did not raise his voice through the first two cases. The only hint of frustration I noted was when I gave him wrong lab values, he looked toward me and repeated them as if asking a question. That prompted me to realize the numbers were wrong. I got the sense that Dr. Wolfe already knew most if not all the information he was asking me about the patients. It dawned on me that the point of his questioning was to see if I knew it.

"So, what do you know about this patient?" This last question came after we had fully discussed all his patients on the service. I proceeded to tell him what I had learned about Ms. Singleton (the patient on whom we were operating) from reading her chart, my interview with her prior to the surgery, and my conversation with Nadya from the night before. "That's all you know? Did Nadya not give you her chart?"

Dr. Wolfe went on to inform me that in the future, his office would make available to me a copy of the medical records for all the patients we were going to be operating on. He made it clear to me that he expected me to intensively study those records and completely familiarize myself with all the patients. Since it was obvious that I was not fully familiar with the details of the case, he volunteered some pertinent information.

"Ms. Singleton is sixty-seven years old and as you can tell extremely thin and frail but is otherwise extremely healthy and active. She was diagnosed with this pancreatic mass three weeks ago and since her metastatic and other work-up has been negative, she has requested that we attempt a curative resection. That is the reason why we are doing this Whipple today."

Just as he said this, he raised the head of the pancreas and right behind it, there was a large, long vein running obliquely superiorly almost parallel to the inferior vena cava and inserting into its anterior surface. "What's this structure?" he asked while pointing to it with the dissecting scissors.

I could not help but smile under my mask. "The right gonadal vein." While still looking at the operating field, I felt Dr. Wolfe's gaze. I pretended not to notice. He said nothing and did not ask another question for several long minutes after that.

The pancreaticoduodenectomy (Whipple) procedure is one of the more intricate procedures in general surgery. It is performed to resect tumors (particularly malignant) of the head of the pancreas and sometimes bile ducts. Since the blood supply to the head of the pancreas is shared with the first portion of the small bowel (the duodenum), the procedure involves the resection of this part of the bowel as well. This was to be my first Whipple, and even with my high level of stress and anxiety, I was still very thankful that I would be assisting a surgeon with so much experience in performing this operation. I knew it was going to be a great learning experience.

Dr. Wolfe did not disappoint me. I was in awe watching him work. His ability to fully concentrate on the surgery was awesome. It was evident that he was a master at performing this operation and performed every step, every cut, every stitch with utmost skill and precision. In the course of five hours, I watched him perform the resection, as well as make connections between the small bowel and the stomach, the pancreas, and the bile ducts. Thereafter, the abdominal incision was closed with the same methodical attention to detail and precision. My first operation with Dr. Wolfe was over, and both the patient and I had made it out alive.

Our second operation—a double bypass—was going to be much easier. The head of the pancreas is located in the center of a C-shaped loop of small bowel called the duodenum. This area is a busy area anatomically, as the food from the stomach, the common bile duct, and the pancreatic duct all empty into the duodenum. Tumors of the head of the pancreas can cause obstruction in any or all three of these physiologic "drainage" systems. A double bypass is a palliative operation for unresectable tumors of the head of the pancreas in which a loop of bowel from the second part of the small bowel (jejunum) is used to re-establish the drainage of the common bile duct and the stomach. As the operation does not involve the resection of the tumor, it is much less complex, and thus less risky to the patient and much shorter in duration.

Dr. Wolfe and I completed this second operation without any major mishap, and before I knew it, my first day operating with Dr. Wolfe was over and it had been much less stressful than I had envisioned. Still on an emotional high, I arranged to meet the interns on the floor and promptly started rounds. It was about six p.m. and after a poor night's sleep and an emotionally draining day, I was very much looking forward to going home to unwind.

We had just arrived on West Wing 10 after rounding on the patients on the other floors when I heard the unmistakable high-pitched voice scream from somewhere around the nurses' station.

"JOE, COME HERE!"

I followed the sound of the voice to a small room adjacent to the nurses' station where Dr. Wolfe was teaching the six medical students who were currently rotating on our service. The loud scream had caught the attention of everyone in the vicinity. I felt all eyes fixed on me as I walked into the room where Dr. Wolfe was standing next to the small table where the medical students sat.

Despite my close proximity to him now, his tone of voice did not change.

"OUR PATIENT IN THE STEP-DOWN UNIT IS NOT PUTTING OUT ANY URINE. HOW COME YOU HAVE NOT DONE ANYTHING ABOUT IT?"

"Sorry Dr. Wolfe, but I was not made aware." I tried to keep my tone of voice low and steady.

"HOW CAN YOU NOT BE AWARE? YOU HAVE TO TELL THE INTERNS TO COMMUNICATE THESE THINGS TO YOU. YOU HAVE TO LEARN TO CONTROL THEM."

Dr. Wolfe was very much aware that he and I had both spent the entire day in the operating room together and that no one had given us any information about Ms. Singleton's poor urine output. He also knew that this was my first day on the service and the first day I had worked with this specific set of interns. Alas, he did not care. All he knew was that our first patient of the day had a low urine output for several hours and nothing had been done about it, and being the senior on the service, it was my responsibility to know about it and address it. I had failed miserably in his eyes.

"I'll go see her." My voice remained intentionally low and steady as I turned to walk out of the room.

"YOU BETTER!"

When healthy patients without kidney disease have low urine output, it is usually due to one of two reasons. One reason is low blood volume in their vessels (low intravascular volume), such as when they are dehydrated from not eating or drinking anything for hours prior to surgery or when they have suffered significant blood loss during surgery. The other reason is "pump failure." This occurs when the heart is not pumping the blood efficiently, such as in instances of heart failure or myocardial infarction (MI), the medical terminology used to denote a heart attack.

The reason why a low urine output after surgery should be managed fairly aggressively is that it is a sign of hypotension (low blood pressure), which if allowed to continue for a prolonged period can lead to cardiac ischemia (low oxygenation of heart muscle) or kidney damage, along with other ominous complications. When a healthy patient has low urine output after surgery, most of the time it is due to low intravascular volume due to blood loss and evaporation of fluid during surgery by having large body cavities such as the chest or abdomen open to ambient air. This fluid needs to be replaced with intravenous fluid infusion during and after the operation. When the blood loss is significant during surgery, sometimes blood transfusions need to be given as well.

Dr. Wolfe had been informed of Ms. Singleton's low urine output when he arrived on the floor after surgery to meet with the students. His initial assessment was that she was "dry" (with low intravascular volume) and he had ordered a fluid bolus (a 500cc intravenous infusion of normal saline). This was the classic way to initially manage hypovolemia (low intravascular fluid volume) leading to low urine output and blood pressure in the immediate post-surgery period. When patients are dehydrated, this fluid bolus is usually followed fairly quickly by a subsequent increase in blood pressure and urine output.

Certain patients require more monitoring than the healthier patients on the regular floor, but not necessarily the intense monitoring of an ICU. For this purpose, some floors in the hospital have a section with greater nursing supervision and more advanced respiratory and heart monitoring equipment and are designated as step-down units. It was here that we had sent Ms. Singleton after her surgery that morning. After examining Ms. Singleton and reviewing her chart for several minutes, I began to suspect the reason for her low urine output was pump failure rather than low volume status. Although she was not complaining of chest pain, she was somewhat disoriented and lethargic, her blood pressure was rather low still, and she had not responded to the fluid bolus with the expected increase in urine output.

Although none of these findings were conclusive, and some of them could also be seen in patients who were severely dehydrated, I thought that the possibility of a heart attack should be ruled out before further fluid boluses were given. Giving too much fluid to a patient with pump failure could lead to a condition called pulmonary edema. This is when the extra fluid given cannot be efficiently circulated by the failing heart and accumulates in the space between the cells in the lungs, thereby causing problems with oxygenation and further compromising the patient.

After I formulated the plan of taking Ms. Singleton to the ICU and ruling her out for an MI (heart attack), I proceeded to walk back into the small room by the nurses' station to inform Dr. Wolfe. Upon hearing my plan of action, he did not seem pleased. "WHAT ARE YOU TALKING ABOUT? SHE IS NOT HAVING A HEART ATTACK—THAT IS CRAZY. SHE JUST HAD A STRESS TEST BEFORE SURGERY. SHE IS NOT PUTTING OUT ANY URINE BECAUSE YOU DID NOT GIVE HER ENOUGH FLUIDS AFTER SURGERY."

It is true that in writing my postoperative orders, I decreased slightly the amount of fluids that I gave her after surgery. This is a prudent strategy for elderly patients and those with weak heart muscles, as giving too much fluid volume to those patients can easily cause fluid overload and pulmonary edema. It was Dr. Wolfe's contention that I had underestimated the amount of fluid she had lost during surgery and that I should have ordered a higher rate of fluid administration post-operatively. I held firm.

"Dr. Wolfe, I will do what you want, but those are my recommendations."

"DO WHATEVER YOU WANT, BUT I TELL YOU, SHE IS DRY!"

As I spoke to Dr. Wolfe, I could see in my peripheral vision all the students' faces turned towards me. I could sense a feeling of empathy emanating from them, perhaps not unlike the way I looked at the senior resident who was operating with Dr. Wolfe on that liver case, during my intern year anesthesia rotation.

The first electrocardiogram (EKG) we obtained on Ms. Singleton was inconclusive, but after transferring her to the ICU and several hours after a thorough work-up, the result of the blood enzyme tests, and the repeat EKGs were conclusive. Ms. Singleton had suffered a heart attack. Exhausted but with an immense sense of redemption, I dialed Dr. Wolfe's home number in order to inform him.

"Wow! You have just saved her life!" His sleepy voice sounded genuinely surprised. The gentleness and contrition in his voice during that conversation was as surprising as much as it was welcomed.

It was four a.m. by the time I left the hospital. My plans were to go home to take a quick shower, change into new clothes, and be back at the hospital to start rounds at six a.m. After rounds, another full day of surgery with Dr. Wolfe awaited me. I had not even had a chance to glance at the charts of the patients for the next day. I carried the two folders full of medical notes, lab, and radiographic results under my arm. I tried to put the events of that day and thoughts of the upcoming two months out of my mind as I walked into the night towards my car.

Ms. Singleton eventually got better and was discharged from the hospital. After a short reprieve on the day after the incidents described above, Dr. Wolfe reverted back to his usual self and I dutifully endured what residents of my program have endured for many years before and since. My views toward Dr. Wolfe during those days can best be described as ambivalent. On the one hand, I could clearly see how great a surgeon he was and how much I was learning from his tutelage. On the other, the amount of stress I was under working with him was close to unbearable. His expectations were borderline unrealistic, and I was running ragged trying to keep up with them.

Several cases come to mind when we initially went into the operating room expecting to do a Whipple but ended up only doing a double bypass instead, after we discovered intraoperatively that the patient's tumor was unresectable. The sudden realization that the surgery was now going to take much less time and be much less stressful for me led to great, momentary joy only to be replaced by extreme guilt upon the subsequent realization that this also meant that the patient's disease was terminal. The feelings of guilt that these types of episodes elicited during my E2 rotation were difficult for me to reconcile and a source of great angst.

In order to feel a certain sense of control, I developed some peculiar defense mechanisms during the rotation. I quickly learned that both apologizing and arguing with Dr. Wolfe were counterproductive as it exacerbated his ire, so I never did. I instead took the stance of not uttering a single word during any of our surgeries unless it was in response to a direct question. It was not long before Dr. Wolfe picked up on this and added a couple of new phrases to his repertoire during surgery.

"WHY WON'T YOU SPEAK?" he would often yell during cases with me. This was the one question to which I would never respond, leading to his utter frustration, adding: "SAY SOMETHING!" Remaining completely quiet and composed during these outbursts gave me a sense of control and helped me cope.

Another habit I picked up was to write down on the small blackboard on the wall of operating room #9 the number of days remaining in my two-month senior-year rotation through E2. This was usually the first thing I did when I walked into the room before the case. I would write the number on the lower right-hand corner of the board. It was not long before Laryssa, the circulating room nurse for Dr. Wolfe, noted what I was doing and asked what the number meant. When I let her in on the secret, she smiled and thereafter would often ask me what the number was that day. She was careful never to ask me that question in Dr. Wolfe's presence. During cases where the level of stress was high, I would often lift my eyes for a few seconds and look at the number. More than once, Laryssa caught me doing this. She would amusingly shake her head and roll her eyes.

I had occasion to see Dr. Wolfe at the Miami Arsht Center Opera House a few years ago. Despite the ensuing years, he looked exactly the same. He was nice and affable and seemed to genuinely care about how things were going for me. I chuckled at myself when I realized that it had been more than fifteen years since I had rotated with him and he had not yet retired. I recently learned that he had finally retired, close to a quarter century after I became aware of him that particular day during my general surgery interview.

This many years later, I still have unreconciled, mixed feelings about that rotation and about the man himself. On the one hand, it was an outstanding educational experience where I got to work closely with a true master surgeon who exhibited great empathy and care for his patients. On the other hand, the education gained was at the cost of significant emotional duress and strain. I have often wondered why Dr. Wolfe behaved towards the residents the way he did. I have asked myself if it was out of frustration at having to put up with poor assistant help by residents who were still new at learning their craft, and have even considered the possibility that there might have been a sadistic streak to his personality. I've then thought perhaps it was because he knew that enduring that time with him would forever change us as human beings, as surgeons, and give us the mental fortitude we would be sure to need in the future as practicing surgeons. As he was a great teacher and mentor, despite my ever-present ambivalence as to my feelings towards him, I have always given him the benefit of the doubt and have come to believe that the reason was the latter.

As a surgeon, I've experienced critical situations in the operating room, sometimes as the senior surgeon in the room, when all have looked to me to save the day. After the initial few seconds of panic, I've instinctively been able to think back to the times when I rotated with Dr. Wolfe and remind myself that I've been in those dire situations before—perhaps even when the surgeries were more complex, and the stakes and the level of pressure were exponentially higher. Thinking of those times has allowed me to regain composure and to better take control in those situations. It is during those times that I genuinely appreciate how much he taught me, not just about surgery but perhaps even more importantly, about what it takes to be a great surgeon. One of those qualities is the ability to maintain composure and be able to perform optimally even under extreme duress.

I also think about him when I do a great job on a case, or at times when I feel that I have mastered a technique or an operation. When humbled during the next case with a difficult situation or a less than perfect execution of technique, I marvel at how he could perform surgery day in and day out with impeccable technique and execution no matter how difficult the case or how tired he was. Nowadays the overwhelming majority of the feelings I have towards Dr. Wolfe are those of awe and gratitude. It has often been said that we most often remember and are most grateful for those teachers who were toughest on us. In the case of Dr. Zach Wolfe, that statement holds true.

Toward the end of my rotation I compiled the notes I had taken on Dr. Wolfe and the E2 rotation. I titled the single-spaced twenty pages "The E2 Manifesto" and penned it under the pseudonym "Anonymous." I passed the manuscript along to the resident that followed me in the hopes that it would make it easier for him to endure the rotation. He continued the tradition, added to the manifesto, and changed its name to the X-Files. I understand that an updated and much larger version circulated for years thereafter.

In our program, there were rotations through the E2 service in our fourth and fifth years. As I was eager to get that service behind me, I chose to start my chief and last year on E2. Thus,

I spent four consecutive months on that service. If I had then whatever wisdom I have now, I would have been well-served in partaking of every opportunity to work with Dr. Wolfe, as he still had many other things to teach me. I, however, was utterly emotionally exhausted by the end of those first two months. It felt like I had been asked to run a marathon at sprint speed and I could simply not take any more. Thus, like many residents before me, I exercised the chief resident's prerogative and assigned the fourth year on the service to work with Dr. Wolfe. My heart rejoiced when I saw Tom Alcalde walk onto the floor the day he was to take over the senior resident responsibilities on the service. I handed him a freshly printed copy of "The E2 Manifesto."

"Starting today," I said to him, "I will be operating with Dr. Wodicka and the other attendings on the service. Over the next two months, you my friend will be communing daily with The Lord."

To Err Is Human

"*Primum non nocere*" is the Latin phrase which means, "First, do no harm." It is the solemn ethos that physicians live by. Many mistakenly believe that this phrase is included in the Hippocratic Oath, a set of ethical rules that historically physicians have been asked to follow and which dates back to ancient times and is traditionally attributed to the Greek physician Hippocrates (470-360 BC). Although not actually included in the Hippocratic Oath, the phrase "First, do no harm" is a bedrock principle that all physicians follow. The thought of doing harm to those whom one is sworn to protect is abhorrent to all physicians. Yet, harm is an unavoidable universal fact of life that sometimes happens to patients at the hands of physicians.

I freely confess that I have done harm. Despite my best efforts and intentions and never on purpose, I have indeed done harm to some of those I've tried to help. That fact and the realization of the probability that it will happen again as long as I remain a surgeon is ever present on my mind, as those instances led to substantial emotional pain and distress for both patient and surgeon. Physicians in general, and surgeons in particular, accept this risk as a reality of their chosen profession. Despite this, however, they persevere in their efforts to help those in need. To me, this speaks to the noble nature of the medical profession and those who engage in it.

Mistakes are familiar to all of us. It is part and parcel of the human experience, especially when acquiring new knowledge or learning a new skill. Most mistakes have negligible or minimal consequences. What makes mistakes different in medicine is that they have the potential of hurting those whom the doctor is trying to help. The consequences of these mistakes for the patients and their families are often self-evident. However, the psychological damage to the doctor making the mistake, although not always clearly evident, can have consequences just as devastating.

Errors in medicine are said to be of two broad categories: omission and commission. Errors of omission occur when the physician fails to do something that would benefit the patient, such as when abnormal labs are not interpreted correctly, or when a constellation of symptoms is not recognized as significant. Errors of commission are characterized by the act of doing something that hurts the patient, as when a certain procedure or operation leads to patient injury (for example, when spinal surgery leads to nerve damage that leaves the patient paralyzed). Surgeons can make both types of errors. Due to the nature of their profession, which involves performing procedures on patients, errors of commission are more common for surgeons than for other medical specialties. Errors of commission at times can be exponentially more catastrophic.

Both types of errors can be psychologically traumatic on the person committing them, but errors of commission can be even more impactful for the physician because they involve the act of doing something that leads to harm. Learning to cope with the realization that one has caused injury to those one is sworn not to harm and is desperately trying to help is one of the most difficult challenges that surgeons confront. While training to learn their craft, residents are prone to making these types of mistakes. At the same time, they have not yet reached a certain level of psychological maturity and professional perspective necessary to allow them to optimally cope with the ramifications of such errors. The combination of these two factors makes this one of the most difficult areas for trainees to deal with on their way to becoming surgeons.

Like all other residents, in the first couple of years of training I had my share of complications. The occasional wound infection, dehiscence, or an unsightly scar from a poor closure spoke of less than optimal performance, but their consequences were not drastic for the patient, and were thus easier to deal with psychologically for the surgeon. While an intern on the trauma service, one of my first attempts at a central line placement resulted in a well-known complication of that procedure, namely a pneumothorax. Dealing with that particular situation and that patient after the fact was not easy on me and it took me several weeks to fully recover from that event. My first memorable major error occurred while a third-year resident in the ICU.

Mr. Collet was a gentleman in his mid-sixties who one week prior had undergone a liver transplant to treat liver failure as a result of a viral infection—hepatitis C. His postoperative course in the ICU had been favorable and he was anticipated to leave the unit in the next couple of days. After the surgery, he had developed bilateral pleural effusions (fluid collections in his chest cavity) for which he had bilateral chest tubes placed in the ICU. This particular morning, however, he was stable, without a fever or major concerns, and was already tolerating feedings by mouth. We had rounded on him about one hour earlier, and all seemed to be going well. I was still on the unit finishing up some notes when Mr. Collet's nurse came running towards me to tell me he was coding. This term usually denotes sudden death as in a heart attack, cerebrovascular event (stroke), etc.

It seems Mr. Collet had suddenly collapsed while drinking a juice. His heart monitor showed that his heart had gone into V-fib, an ominous heart rhythm that often signals impending death. I rushed to the bedside to find a full code in progress. The patient had already been intubated and the respiratory tech was bagging him with the Ambu bag. Meanwhile, the intern was doing chest compression and several nurses were busy around the bed providing support and getting medications ready. The trauma fellow who happened to be in the unit at the time when the patient collapsed was running the code. The patient had been shocked three times with chest paddles as per protocol and the next step was to start giving intravenous medications per the algorithm. Upon seeing me approach the bedside, the trauma fellow put his hand on my shoulder. "His IV is blown and we have no access. Please get me a central line and quick."

A central line is a type of intravenous catheter that is placed in one of the main veins in the body such as the internal jugular veins (neck), subclavian veins (upper thorax), or femoral veins (groin). This catheter is much wider than the catheters we normally place in the smaller veins of the extremities, and it allows for more rapid fluid infusion. More specifically, this is the catheter of choice in trauma cases and in situations where the patient's life hangs in the balance and IV access is poor.

The nurse was opening the kit as I maneuvered myself close to the patient's head. As I gowned and gloved, I glanced toward the side table where the kit had just been opened. I noticed she had taken out a special type of central line called an Introducer Kit. This wide lumen catheter was a good choice for this type of situation as it would allow us to give fluids at a very rapid rate if needed. The catheter is inserted by gaining access to the desired vein with a long needle on a ten-cc syringe. Once it is confirmed that the needle is within the vein's lumen (by the ability to freely draw back dark venous blood), the syringe is disconnected from the needle and a flexible wire is inserted through the lumen of the needle into the vein. At this point the needle is withdrawn, leaving the wire within the vessel, and exiting through the skin. This particular catheter system has a wide lumen, and within it a pointed but soft plastic "introducer," which has enough rigidity that allows for the displacement of the soft tissues around the wire as the catheter/introducer combination is advanced over the wire into the vein. Since the actual catheter is way too flexible, it does not allow for this part of the procedure unless it has the added rigidity of the introducer within it. Once proper position in the vein is confirmed again by the ability to draw back dark venous blood through the catheter, both the wire and the introducer are removed while the catheter is left in place.

The last step is to suture the catheter to the patient's skin at the point where it exits.

By this time in my residency, I had placed dozens of central catheters of different varieties, and even some during codes such as this one. I was not particularly nervous or flustered, as I performed the procedure flawlessly and rapidly. Moreover, I did this while timing my critical movements in between the chest compressions.

"We need a line, now!" It was the trauma fellow again.

"I almost got it." I had gotten venous blood on my first stick to the neck, quickly threaded the wire through the needle, did a small cut in the skin to allow for the wide lumen catheter to pass without resistance, and quickly threaded the introducer/catheter complex over the wire and straight into the vein. My hands were quick and sure, and in one quick motion I buried the catheter/introducer complex all the way in, pulled the introducer and wire out simultaneously after confirming the free return of venous blood, thereby leaving the central line catheter within the lumen of the vein.

"Got it!" I said to no one in particular, and now addressing the nurse: "Give me the line." When she did, I connected it to the catheter and then started to secure the catheter to the skin with a stitch. I silently congratulated myself on a flawless performance in a clutch.

"What's all that blood?" The nurse was looking down when she said this. It had been about thirty seconds after I had placed the central line and we had continued to run the ACLS protocol. The patient had been shocked one more time and medications had been infused while the intern continued CPR. Upon following her gaze, we all noted that the chest tube drainage canister, which was empty several minutes before, was full of dark blood. I had finished doing the central line dressing and was getting ready to relieve the intern with the chest compressions.

"Lisa, easy on the chest compressions." The trauma fellow was addressing the intern. Our initial supposition was that perhaps the chest compressions had broken some ribs leading to some bleeding into the chest.

“That’s way too much blood to be from cracked ribs.” The trauma fellow was now moving to the other side of the bed to check on the other chest tube.

“This side is not bleeding. Joe, what central line did you place?”

“An introducer.” As I said this, I remembered multiple warnings from attendings and senior residents who had supervised me in doing these lines when I was learning that although soft, the plastic introducers were somewhat pointy and had the capacity to cause damage to the thin wall of veins. Thus, they had to be inserted slowly and only part way, never to the hub. Terror struck me as I realized what had just happened. In my rush and after pushing the introducer to the hub, I had most likely torn through the wall of the large vein thereby causing all the bleeding.

“You think that’s what happened?” The liver fellow who had just joined the code was addressing the trauma fellow.

“I think so.” The trauma fellow seemed confident in his answer.

“Should we crack the chest?” It sounded like the liver fellow was making more of a suggestion than asking a question. By this point, the overwhelming guilt I was feeling was making it impossible for me to think straight or be able to make any constructive suggestions. The trauma fellow took charge as he had been leading the code all along.

“No wait. We’ve been here for over thirty minutes, and even if we crack the chest there is no way we will be able to get to the site of injury here without the right instruments and without proper light. Let’s call it.”

Everyone stopped what they were doing and slowly moved away from the bed. The nurse drew the curtain around the patient’s bed in order to allow for some privacy from the other patients and ICU personnel. I stayed behind almost not being able to move. I looked at the chest tube canister again and saw it completely filled with dark-red blood. The capacity of the container was two liters. As the cannister and the drainage tubing was full of blood, this probably meant that there was still a considerable volume of blood backed up in the chest cavity. The container on the left side was completely empty.

I was in a fog for the rest of that day and several days thereafter, continuously perseverating about the episode and reviewing in my mind every single move I made during the procedure. The psychological distress was at times unbearable, as I deeply hoped against all hope that the chest bleeding was the result of the chest compressions and not my central line. The result of the autopsy confirmed my worst fears. The report described a 1.5 cm tear at the junction of the internal jugular and subclavian veins. These are two large veins in the upper thorax that come together in the base of the neck and bring all the blood from the head and the upper extremity back to the heart. The only solace in the report was that the official cause of death was a massive heart attack, from which the chances of survival were nil.

It was several months later during my third year when I was beginning to come to terms with Mr. Collet's death, when I was scheduled to perform a colonoscopy on Mr. Hernandez, a fifty-seven-year-old who had presented to the colorectal surgery clinic with the chief complaint of occasional blood in his stool. A colonoscopy is a diagnostic procedure to evaluate the large intestine (colon) in which, after the patient is sedated, a camera scope in the form of a soft, flexible tube is inserted through the anus and allows for the visualization of the entire lumen of the large bowel (colon) up until it joins the third part of the small bowel (ilium).

I had already performed several of these procedures under the watchful eye of the attending staff and was feeling good and confident as I undertook the procedure on Mr. Hernandez. It was a Friday morning, and I was anticipating a relatively easy clinical day and a free weekend. My plans were to go spend it with Rachel in the Keys. Mr. Hernandez was an affable fellow, and jokingly excused himself for any unsavory language he might use while sedated.

Once the patient was sedated, I started the procedure under the watchful eye of Dr. Thal Johnson, a young colorectal surgeon who had recently joined our staff. The trouble soon began after I quickly traversed the straight end of the colon (rectum) and began to negotiate the S-shaped segment of colon call the sigmoid. Somehow, I was unable to keep the flexible scope on track. I kept my eyes fixed on the TV monitor while both hands worked the controls at the opposite end of the long, flexible colonoscopy tube. I held the flexible scope on my right hand while my left hand worked the control wheel used to manipulate and point the end of the scope. Once I had manipulated the scope into the center of the lumen, I would then use my right hand to gently push and advance the scope further into the colon. These maneuvers are done while the left index finger is used to occasionally press on the button that injects air through the scope in order to keep the colon distended.

I kept having trouble negotiating the curves of the sigmoid colon, and for the life of me, I could not keep the scope centered in the lumen. No matter how hard I tried, the end of the scope would end up abutting the colonic wall to the point that I was no longer able to see the lumen. I repeatedly had to back off the scope in order to find the center of the lumen once again. After several attempts at this maneuver, Dr. Johnson, who seemed to be getting impatient, told me to step aside so that he could take over the controls. As he was saying this and as a last gasp before relinquishing my turn as the operator, which I feared would be relinquished for the rest of the case, I perhaps a bit more aggressively advanced the scope once I managed to find the lumen one last time. Once again it seemed like the scope ended up against the colonic wall; exasperated, I gave Dr. Johnson the controls.

As he pulled back on the scope, we both expected to see the lumen once again on the screen, but what we saw was what looked like a stack of air balloons surrounding the end of the scope. Almost as if on cue, as Dr. Johnson and I looked with curiosity at the screen, Mr. Hernandez began to groan as if in pain. When our gaze went from the screen to Mr. Hernandez, we both saw him grab for his abdomen, which was by this time distended. "I think he is perforated," Dr. Johnson said, almost as if asking a question as he continued to manipulate the controls of the colonoscope.

Mr. Hernandez groaned again as if to answer in the affirmative. I was frozen in place as my mind raced through all the repercussions.

Dr. Johnson put his right hand on Mr. Hernandez's abdomen and pressed on it, eliciting a groan of pain from him. It was obvious by now that all the air which we had inserted into the colon to keep it distended had escaped through the perforation into the abdominal cavity proper, thereby resulting in abdominal distention.

"Yes, he is perforated." The scope was now completely out as Dr. Johnson made this statement. "Let's talk to the family and book him for an emergency exploratory laparotomy." Dr. Johnson was now addressing me, distress notable in his tone of voice.

Speaking with Mr. Hernandez's wife was an exceedingly difficult thing for me to do. As she only spoke Spanish, I took charge of the conversation, although Dr. Johnson stayed by my side the entire time. It was difficult for her to comprehend that we now needed her consent to take her husband to emergency surgery when she had been anticipating an uneventful diagnostic procedure. Rather than getting ready for breakfast with her husband and a drive home, she was now being asked to endure several stressful hours of waiting while her husband underwent emergency surgery for a complication that I had caused. Furthermore, the surgery was to be performed by the same people who were responsible for the complication. She reluctantly gave her consent. I felt sick to my stomach by the end of the conversation.

A couple of hours later, Dr. Johnson and I were on opposite sides of the operating room table while hardly speaking. While mobilizing the left colon low in the pelvis, we easily saw the area of perforation as well as its potential cause. Visible through the perforation and easily palpable about three centimeters above the perforation, there was a large mass that took up about eighty percent of the lumen of the colon. A frozen section biopsy of the mass taken in the operating room revealed that the tumor was cancerous. Dr. Johnson surmised that perhaps the large mass in the colon was tethering it to the posterior abdominal wall, thus making it difficult for me to negotiate the last bend in the sigmoid colon. I was not sure if the explanation was plausible, but it made me feel a little better to know there might have been a reason for the perforation other than my utter incompetence.

I struggled with feelings of guilt and doubt the entire time that Mr. Hernandez was in the hospital recovering from his surgery. Nevertheless, we were able to resect (remove) the segment of colon with the tumor and connect the proximal colon to the skin in the abdominal wall (colostomy) so that his feces could be evacuated. The plan was to wait three to six months and take Mr. Hernandez back to the operating room in order to reconnect the remaining two segments of his colon so that he could defecate normally. I was not meant to participate in that second operation, as my rotation through the service was only for two months. Luckily for Mr. Hernandez, his final pathology report showed that his tumor had not invaded through the wall of the colon and had not spread to any of his lymph nodes. The medical oncology service suggested a short course of chemotherapy, but the feeling among all experts involved was that Mr. Hernandez had a great chance at a cure. I was consoled with the thought that at the very least, his colonoscopy had allowed us to discover his tumor in time.

The psychological wounds of dealing with the aforementioned two mistakes took me the rest of the third year to overcome, though I can say these experiences made me a better doctor. My fourth year of residency started with a more mature perspective of my surgical abilities, as well as a better understanding of how to address less-than-optimal surgical outcomes.

My experiences during the fourth year, however, showed me that there was much learning for me yet to do in regard to this topic. This was especially true when it came time to assert myself if I perceived that the senior residents, fellows, and even attending surgeons had committed or were about to commit a potential mistake.

Residency training is a hierarchical process in which the interns are supposed to be supervised and follow the orders of the more senior residents, who in turn are supposed to follow the orders of the chief residents, who themselves are under the supervision of the fellows and the attending surgeons. This system is meant to protect patients from potential errors that can be committed by those still learning their craft. However, as human beings, physicians at any level of their training can still make mistakes. When a resident perceives or knows that a more senior resident or even an attending is about to make or has made a mistake, the default position agreed to by all is to always do what will protect the patient at all costs. Junior residents, however, often struggle with this as they tend to doubt themselves, their knowledge, and even their ability when making judgments about what is being done by their seniors, who by definition are much more experienced. Thus, residents are often not confident enough to step in and prevent or ameliorate the errors of their seniors.

Once such incident occurred to me when I was the fourth year (senior) resident in trauma working with, and under the supervision of, one of the trauma fellows. This rotation took place toward the latter part of my fourth year. My confidence was extremely high as I anticipated the start of my chief year. It was during a typical weekend night on call that we were alerted by the air transport helicopter that they were bringing in a man in his mid-thirties who had just sustained two gunshot wounds to the abdomen. The patient had stable vital signs but was barely responding to verbal command.

Penetrating trauma such as gunshot wounds (GSW) and stab wounds were always more exciting to the residents rotating through the trauma team, as it meant that most likely the patient would require an operation. The call came in at about ten p.m., and we were full of energy and eager for the opportunity to save a life. I rushed to the trauma bay as soon as I saw the call come through the pager. As I got there, I directed the secretary to make sure the fellow was aware that we had a gunshot wound coming in.

Dr. Katouma Kawamoto was born, raised, and had trained in surgery in Japan. He had come to America to complete his trauma fellowship and anticipated going back to practice in Tokyo once his two-year fellowship was over. I had been rotating with him for over one month now and very much enjoyed his company in and out of the operating room. He had a very thick Japanese accent, which made it difficult for some of us to fully understand what he was saying. I remember his pronunciation of "lap chole" (short for laparoscopic cholecystectomy) to sound something like "rappacoli." In the operating room, however, he was extremely confident, fast, and skilled.

The trauma secretary told me that Kato (his nickname) would soon join me in the operating room for our gunshot wound case as soon as he finished the case he was currently on. Upon entering the trauma bay, I immediately noticed, as the patient's shirt was being removed, a long surgical scar down the middle of his abdomen beginning close to his chest and running down to his pubis. This laparotomy scar was indicative of prior abdominal surgery. On either side of the scar at about the level of the mid-abdomen, I saw two small, round, bleeding wounds indicative of the gunshot wounds he had sustained.

As the patient was still awake, I attempted to inquire as to what other abdominal surgery he had undergone. He was somewhat combative and responded only with unintelligible sounds when he perceived pain. I was not able to get any useful information out of him. Soon thereafter, he was intubated and made ready for the operating room. A thorough inspection of his body revealed no other signs of fresh trauma. Before going to the operating room with our patient and since by now we had his driver's license available, I asked the trauma desk secretary to run his name through the hospital computer to see if his prior surgery had been performed at Jackson. This would have been extremely helpful information, but our search was unsuccessful: Our patient had never been treated at Jackson. I instructed the secretary to track down a next of kin to see if we could find further information as to our patient's medical history and prior surgery.

The patient had been prepped and draped, and I was ready to make my incision when Kato rushed into the operating room already scrubbed and ready to be gowned. "I'm here. What do we have?"

"A guy in his mid-thirties with two gunshot wounds to the abdomen," I responded as I proceeded to make my laparotomy incision right over the previous one. "He has a laparotomy scar." I stated the obvious to make sure we were all of the same mind regarding the potential implications.

"Do we know what from?"

"I tried to ask him, but he was not able to respond."

"Possibly previous trauma?" Kato stated what we all suspected.

"Possibly," I answered.

As Kato approached the table, I had entered into the abdominal (peritoneal) cavity, and a gush of blood rushed out onto the operating room table and floor. Just as we had done multiple times previously during similar circumstances, Kato and I proceeded to start packing laparotomy pads into the patient's abdomen in order to tamponade (compress), and thus slow or stop the bleeding.

After the active bleeding slowed, we allowed some time for anesthesia to infuse blood and fluids to stabilize the patient, and we proceeded to remove the lap pads one by one in order to inspect the damage. We noted several enterotomies (perforations in the bowel), but our attention was directed towards the right side of the abdomen where blood was still seeping from under the pads. The blood was brisk and bright red, indicating an arterial injury. Upon removal of the last pad, the bleeding became profuse and flooded the entire field despite my attempts at suctioning. Further packing did not prove successful as it seems we had unroofed a large hematoma in the posterior aspect of the abdomen.

"His pressure is dropping. You've got to stop that bleeding." The anesthesia team was busy now hanging unit after unit of blood in order to replace the blood that the patient was pouring into his abdomen.

"Give me the scissors." Kato had now taken over the case. He proceeded to cut into the retroperitoneum (posterior lining of the abdominal cavity) and completely unroofed the hematoma. All hell broke loose then, as gushes of blood again poured over the patient's abdomen onto the operating room table and floor.

"Suction. I think I see it. It is coming from the renal hilum. Clamp quick!" His accent made it a bit hard to understand him, but after getting his message across, Kato took the large clamp the nurse had given him and clamped the blood vessels running into and out of the right kidney. This had the effect of ameliorating the bleeding to the point that my suctioning was able to evacuate most of the blood that had pooled in the patient's abdomen.

"I need more room. Scissors." Kato took the scissors in his right hand and began to place it next to and parallel to the previous clamp.

"Wait!" I screamed as I surmised what Kato was about to do. "Remember, he has had previous abdominal surgery. We need to make sure he has the other kidney first."

Kato stopped for a split second but was just as sharp with his answer. "No time. We need to stop this bleeding and I have no access. Besides, his kidney is shot anyway. Look at it." I peered over his hands and now that the field was dryer, I was able to see the right kidney. The bullet had gone right through it and it had made it look like a partially peeled banana, with its outer covering (capsule) torn and displaced circumferentially away from the point of impact. The blast effect of the injury made the kidney look like an unrecognizable lump of tissue.

"Besides, what are the odds his other kidney is gone?" As he said this, Kato closed the scissors, severing in one swoop the renal artery and vein. Shortly thereafter, after clamping and severing the ureter, he handed the severely damaged kidney to the nurse.

I saw this happening almost as if in slow motion, knowing full well that the decision was controversial at the very least and potentially a monumental mistake. Furthermore, I was well aware of the potential negative consequences of this action and yet, had not been strong enough to stop it. As the senior person in the room at that time, this life and death decision was Kato's to make, but I could not help thinking that we might have had a couple of minutes to discuss it first, as the bleeding by this time was partially controlled and the patient was not necessarily crashing.

After much difficulty, we sutured the bleeding vessels and were closing the multiple enterotomies (intestinal tears) when the attending walked into the room. Dr. Scott Conner, the attending on call that night, had just finished another case next door and walked into our room to get a status report. We proceeded to tell him the sequence of events as he joined us after scrubbing up. I thought I noticed him pause for a split second as Kato related to him that we had removed the damaged right kidney in order to stop the bleeding. I remained quiet throughout the exchange. Dr. Conner turned to the scrub nurse. "Please make sure to put that kidney on ice." The nurse had already done so, anticipating the potential need to repair the discarded kidney.

After the repair of the last two enterotomies, with great anticipation and under the watchful eyes of our attending, Kato and I started dissecting on the left side of the posterior abdomen looking for the left kidney. I silently prayed that we would find it. As we dissected deeper and deeper into the posterior abdomen, our sense of dread increased until finally our worst fears were realized as we discovered that the left kidney was not there. Undoubtedly, it had been removed during the previous operation.

The kidney transplant team was called in. The kidney was meticulously sutured together on the back table and replanted back into the patient. The transplanted kidney looked like a Frankenstein creation, a poor replica of its former self, now with multiple missing pieces and covered with multiple sutures. Kato and I mostly stood by and watched as the transplant team did their work, which took several hours. Both of us were afraid and perhaps too ashamed to walk out of the room. It was past ten o'clock the next morning when the patient was finally wheeled out of the operating room. I walked out dripping in sweat, self-doubt, and guilt.

The transplanted kidney never put out any urine and had to be removed one week later. This case became widely discussed among the trauma residents and attendings alike. It was the consensus that the only way to salvage the kidney was if somehow we had been able to arrest the bleeding and figured out a way to repair the renal vessels and then reconstruct the kidney while still in situ (in place) in the patient's abdomen and still connected to its blood supply, a tall order indeed. In retrospect, it is hard to ascertain if the decision made by Kato was the right one. Perhaps his decision, despite causing the patient to lose his only remaining kidney, was the right one because it had saved the patient's life.

Although it had not been my decision per se, I felt greatly responsible in that I had failed to exert myself and stop Kato. I felt a great sense of embarrassment and guilt for the rest of that rotation and beyond. As a matter of fact, I still think of this case often even today. I will always feel terrible for whatever my role was in condemning my patient to lifelong dialysis or, if lucky, a future kidney transplant. I will never know if there was a possibility of saving that kidney, but I do know that the actions we took during that operation most likely eliminated whatever possibilities there were. I chose to console myself by believing that the decision to sacrifice the kidney had saved the patient's life.

Looking back now and taking into account all the mistakes that I've made during my residency years and ever since then, which in one way or another have caused my patients some form of harm, it is easy to see how for some surgeons those types of mistakes cause significant psychological difficulty in dealing with their aftermath. For those surgeons who persevere with enthusiasm despite this painful reality, finding a way to cope with these mistakes is paramount.

After much introspection, I've made a commitment to myself to do everything in my power when it comes to didactic study, mental preparation, and technical development to minimize these mistakes. When mistakes inevitably occur, I've committed to promptly accepting the due responsibility and learning from them so as to never repeat the same mistake again. It is this personal and professional ethos that has allowed me the psychological fortitude to persevere through these exquisitely painful episodes and times of distress, which come from unwittingly harming those we are sworn to protect.

The perforated colon during my third year E3 (Elective 3) colorectal service rotation was not prominent on my mind when four years later as a chief resident in plastic surgery I went to meet one of the patients who was scheduled to undergo surgery that day. As was customary then, all the patients who were to undergo surgery at the Jackson Memorial main operating rooms were kept in a large waiting room on the second floor of the center building. One by one they were taken by the residents into one of several private examination rooms which were set up to allow the residents to do their physical exams on the patients prior to surgery, as well as to have the patients sign preoperative paperwork, including surgical consents.

As I walked toward my first patient for the day, I heard a man's voice coming from my right calling out my name. I turned in the direction of the voice and saw a man getting up from his chair and walking towards me. I did not recognize his face and presented him with a blank stare as I shook his extended hand. "Dr. Garri, you don't remember me? I'm Mr. Hernandez. You perforated my colon a couple of years ago."

This statement was made loud enough to be heard by almost every person in the large waiting area, which contained at least twenty people. My heart sank as I perceived all eyes in that room, including those of the patient on whom I was about to operate, fixate on me. The embarrassment made it difficult for me to react as Mr. Hernandez shook my hand enthusiastically and with a broad smile on his face. "Boy, I'm glad I finally got to see you. I never got a chance to thank you. Because of that perforation, you guys found that tumor and saved my life. I had to have chemotherapy, but now the doctors say I am cancer-free and cured. All that I have left now is a hernia from the surgery and I am getting that fixed today. I am sure glad I saw you again so that I can thank you in person."

I thanked him as I exhaled in relief. I knew Mr. Hernandez was assigning credit where none was due, but I was overwhelmingly grateful for the way he had chosen to interpret my mistake. All is indeed well that ends well.

M&M

Seeing Kato in the cafeteria was odd, as I had never seen him there before. Come to think of it, despite rotating with him for close to two months on the trauma team, I had never seen Kato eat. However, it seemed that on this occasion eating was not on his mind. As soon as Kato spotted me sitting at one of the center tables with a few of the medical students, he made a beeline for me. "Sorry, Joe. Our kidney case got picked to be presented at M&M (Morbidity & Mortality Conference) for next week, but I have to make an unexpected trip. I need you to present the case."

I knew immediately what he was doing, and I empathized with him...really, but there was no way I was going to take the hit for this one. "Then either delay your trip or tell them to postpone the case presentation. It was your decision, Kato. You have to take responsibility for it."

I felt completely comfortable taking such a rigid and perhaps confrontational stance with my senior—even if Kato actually did have an emergency of some sort that prevented him from presenting the case. I already felt guilty enough as it was for having participated in that case, and for not being assertive enough to stop Kato from resecting the kidney. I thought the patient was stable enough at the time to allow the decision to be made after a bit more consideration. I felt having me present the case was unjust because for better or worse, the decision to sacrifice the kidney was his. At the same time, I understood his reluctance and felt sorry for him. Presenting at M&M is not for the weak of heart.

The Morbidity and Mortality Conference is the most dreaded event for all residents. The goal behind it is lofty, and perhaps even noble. Mistakes that are made are discussed in excruciating detail so as to learn from them and ensure that they never happen again. The conference is meant to be an educational exercise with the goal of protecting patients from mistakes by educating doctors as to how mistakes occur, and what steps can be taken to prevent them. In practice, however, these conferences are more akin to gladiator games, a spectacle where the condemned (residents) are thrown to the lions (the surgical attendings) and devoured without mercy while the spectators (the entire audience of medical professionals in attendance) watch in amazement and are thoroughly entertained.

The particular resident who made the mistake has to stand up in front of the entire attending surgical staff, the residents and fellows on the program, and the medical students rotating through the surgical services (in all usually between 50-100 participants packed into a conference room), and describe his/her mistake in painful detail. This is followed by a barrage of questions and sometimes even insults, when the attendings feel the appropriate punishment must be handed out for egregious mistakes. Three case presentations are made at each conference, which usually lasts anywhere from one to two hours.

As complications are recognized during the week, there is a self-reporting format where residents and involved attendings are expected to enter such complications into a master database from which the most interesting and educational cases are chosen for presentation. Thus, the first step in ensuring that one is not picked for M&M is to be less than diligent in reporting one's complications. As these complications usually became common knowledge quickly, however, this tactic hardly ever worked. If a particular resident failed to enter the complication in the database, it was usually entered by either a more senior resident, a fellow, or the attending involved. Dr. Hamil Socas, who ran the M&M conference and was responsible for picking the cases, was at times referred to by some of us as "Big Brother," as he always seemed to know about every single mistake made in the hospital. An unexpected call from him during the week was a bad omen, as it often meant that you were one of the three lucky ones chosen to present the following week.

As a medical student and junior resident, attending an M&M conference was entertaining. There was always something to be learned, but even more rewarding was the guilty pleasure one gained from watching senior and chief residents, who at times seemed to be one's personal tormentors, squirm under the onslaught of highly suspicious questioning, which at times seemed to be carefully coordinated and downright cruel. There was always the underlying message that, "There is a price to be paid for each and every one of your mistakes, and this is the place where the bill comes due." However, what seems like sport during the junior residency years takes an ominous turn for the more senior residents, as they find themselves alone in front of that room describing professional shortcomings and failures that they would rather keep secret.

This overwhelmingly negative experience was handled in as many different ways as there were senior residents. I personally watched in a mixture of bewilderment, amusement, and shock as some residents bent the bright light of truth beyond recognition, while others succumbed to the experience with near emotional meltdowns, which at times were plainly revealed by the uncontrollable shaking, cracking voice, or the profuse shedding of tears. Sitting through multiple M&M conferences during my junior years taught me that the greatest sin a surgical resident can make is that of laziness. If a complication or negative outcome resulted from the failure of a resident to come check a patient or follow up on a patient because they were too tired or lazy to bother, then there was no reprieve from the oncoming punishment, which was handed out in large portions and without mercy during the conference and beyond. The attending staff at times reacted downright cruelly, as if to let the residents know that this particular sin was never to be committed or tolerated. Once I learned this, I made a resolution that laziness would not be my downfall. I made a personal pledge to make sure never to refuse to come in to see a patient whenever there was the slightest doubt regarding anything that might require my personal attention. This was easier said than done, as it meant I came in many times to the hospital for naught, often when I was so tired and sleepy that neither driving nor taking care of patients was advisable.

Having resolved to banish laziness from my repertoire, I also paid attention and tried to learn from my predecessors in as many ways as possible to ameliorate the pain of presenting at M&M. I learned that lying and covering up for mistakes was counterproductive, and the sooner and more freely one admitted to mistakes, the better. Thus, I freely sprinkled my presentations with phrases such as: "The mistake I made...", "Mistakenly I assumed...", "My error in judgment was..."

Then there were the props. While on my fourth-year trauma rotation, the new chief of the trauma surgery service had provided each of the senior residents and fellows of the trauma teams with digital cameras. He encouraged us to take pictures of anything we felt was educational so that they could enhance the learning experience during the following day's morning report. I had found this innovation extremely helpful in enhancing the educational value of these conferences. It was one thing to listen to the description of a particular stab wound or laceration of the liver, and yet another, richer experience to see that description coupled with an actual image to match it. I noticed during these conferences how such images had the effect of getting everyone focused on the topic being discussed and away from any strenuous side issues, such as assigning blame for potential errors committed. It occurred to me that these types of images might have the same effect during M&M conferences.

Thus, after watching the overwhelmingly positive reception a senior resident received for putting up a slide of a pathology specimen during an M&M presentation one day, I resolved to give this technique a try. I purchased a small digital camera and carried it with me always in the hospital. If any of my cases got picked for M&M, I would take pictures of anything that I thought might add value to the presentation. While keeping patient confidentiality, I would take any clinical pictures I thought relevant such as infected incisions, wounds, pathology specimens, etc. Moreover, I would take pictures of X-rays, diagnostic studies, and even chart entries that I thought pertinent to the issue at hand. I would then include these images in a short PowerPoint presentation, which I started using routinely to present my cases in the form of a visual story with relevant images. I could not claim to be the first resident to use props at M&M conference, but I can safely say that I was the first resident to do so routinely.

The result of this technique was miraculous, in that everyone seemed to be engrossed by these presentations, and along with my frequent, self-deprecating admissions of failure, the end result was that I seemed to draw far fewer personal attacks and negative comments than the other presenters. I was determined to either dazzle the audience with eloquence and brilliance or baffle them with mea culpas and props. The positive effects of this technique lasted well into my chief year, by which time it had become routine for most residents to present utilizing the same format.

By the middle of my chief year, I felt that I had things well under control, including the dreaded M&M conference presentations. I had mastered techniques that mitigated any personal damage and strangely enough, I was beginning to actually enjoy presenting my complications. That is, until one particular day when I innocently and unknowingly walked right into the middle of an unexpected ambush, which came from an even more unexpected source.

"I've been performing this operation for over thirty years and have never had this particular complication. Over the past month since I've started operating with Joe Garri, I've had two in a row." This statement, made by one of the most senior attending surgeons in the program, left me stunned and speechless.

"Really? Joe?" Dr. Willoughby, the chairman of the surgery department stared at me with an inquisitive look on his face. I felt the same gaze from every single face of the more than fifty people sitting in conference that day. I was utterly surprised and could only muster a half-smile and a shoulder shrug. Perplexed, I really did not know what to say.

What Dr. Holland had said was technically true, however, the implication of the statement was not. It is true that I had been present in both cases and I took it at face value that he had not had such complications before. However, there were two people in that room who knew that my participation during the two cases being discussed was minimal, and other than perhaps bringing bad luck, I had not been responsible for the complications. One of those two people was me; the other was the person who had made such an off-base comment. Regardless of Dr. Holland's intention for making that comment, the damage had been done. For every other person in that room, I was now somehow the responsible party, and that was that.

Dr. William (Billy) Holland hailed from the Carolinas, an alumnus of our program, who had decided to stay in Miami after finishing his training. His subspecialty was endocrine surgery, which involved the surgical treatment of the endocrine (hormone-producing) organs such as the thyroid and parathyroid glands. He had a strong Southern accent, an easy-going demeanor, and was always very courteous to residents and hospital staff alike. I always thought of him as the perfect Southern gentleman. From the time I was an intern, there had been rumors that he was thinking about retirement. This news was heard with universal sadness as all chief residents genuinely enjoyed rotating with him. Now here I was in my chief and final year and he was going as strong as ever while already in his late sixties. As residents, we only rotated with him during our chief year. We all very much looked forward to the experience and I was no exception.

Dr. Holland's passion and academic interest focused on the parathyroid glands. There are four of these pea-sized glands, two on either side of the thyroid in the neck, and they secrete a hormone that mobilizes calcium stores in the bones and thereby regulate the circulating calcium levels in the blood. When one or more of these small glands is diseased and secretes excess amounts of the hormone, the increased amount of circulating blood calcium can reach such a high level as to cause severe metabolic derangement and potentially even death.

With great enthusiasm and expectations, I started my rotation with Dr. Holland. Not only was he a most respected attending surgeon, but he had an elective practice mostly devoted to endocrine surgery, a fascinating field to most residents. His practice was slow-paced, and he spent ample time teaching the chief residents in and out of the operating room. On our first day operating together, Dr. Holland and I had two cases. The first was the removal of half of the thyroid on a lady who had a very indolent form of thyroid cancer. This case was highly enjoyable and uneventful.

The second case involved a middle-aged female who had presented to her primary care physician with generalized aches and pains. Her work-up had revealed multiple brown tumors, a bony lytic (destructive) lesion that occurs when bone is demineralized by excessive loss of calcium. Further tests revealed a blood calcium level that was through the roof, accompanied by an extremely high level of parathyroid hormone, indicating that the problem was with at least one, several, or all of the parathyroid glands.

Dr. Holland explained that this increase in serum calcium was either the result of a benign tumor (adenoma) of one of the four parathyroid glands, or the result of hyper-function of multiple of these glands. If the cause was the former, our job was to surgically explore, find the adenoma, and remove the affected parathyroid gland. If it turned out that all of the glands were involved, our task was to rule out an adenoma surgically and then remove three or maybe even three and a half of these glands in order to ameliorate the condition. He explained that the parathyroid glands were small, and that we did not really have good quality diagnostic imaging studies that could tell us ahead of time which of the glands was involved. Thus, this was a disease that required true surgical exploration for diagnosis and treatment. He further explained that this was easier said than done, as the glands were quite small and could be found in atypical locations.

Sometimes identifying and finding the four glands is a challenge. Furthermore, it is important to be able to confirm that removal of a particular gland or a group of these glands would have the desired result of reducing the circulating levels of parathyroid hormone. To that end, Dr. Holland had developed a blood assay that within a few minutes could check for circulating levels of parathyroid hormone. After the removal of one or more of the glands, a concomitant drop in the circulating parathyroid hormone level would confirm that the surgery was a success.

Dr. Holland went on to explain the potential complications associated with this operation. The recurrent laryngeal nerves are responsible for innervating the vocal cords. There is one on each side of the neck, and they run posterior and lateral to the thyroid gland, right in the area and in close proximity to where the parathyroid glands are located. Damaging these nerves during the surgical exploration could lead to severe hoarseness if unilateral (only on one side) as the affected vocal cord would lose function during speech. However, in the unlikely event that it happened bilaterally (both sides), both vocal cords could be affected, causing them both to move toward the midline. This situation would leave a narrow slit through which little air could pass, thereby potentially preventing the patient from being able to move sufficient air in and out of the lungs while breathing. He explained that this particular complication was extremely rare, but it was a theoretical possibility and a great concern if it were to happen.

The neck is an area of the body where quite a bit of anatomy is packed into a small space. Operating in the neck requires thorough knowledge of the anatomy involved, and an exceptionally fine touch, which is a bit different than the one needed for surgery that involves larger organs, like abdominal surgery for example. Dr. Holland had told me that he would do the first side himself in order to show me what to do, and then he would let me perform the contralateral dissection under his watchful eye. I was impressed by Dr. Holland's knowledge of the involved anatomy and did not perceive any significant problems during our first parathyroid surgery, other than having some difficulty in finding the parathyroid glands. The patient had an unusually large thyroid gland, and mobilizing it to the right and left through the small incision on her neck was challenging to say the least.

After a smooth start to the case, we stalled when, after mobilizing the thyroid gland, we could not find the parathyroids. After much manipulation, dissection, and suctioning, Dr. Holland finally found the two parathyroids on the patient's right side. I was not used to seeing these glands on a live patient, but they both were the same size and looked normal in appearance. It was unlikely that either of these two small glands housed an adenoma.

After allowing me to do minimal dissection on the left side without success, Dr. Holland lost his patience and took over the case on my side. After a similar struggle, we eventually visualized the two other glands, which looked normal as well. We then proceeded to remove three of the glands and after confirming a significant drop in circulating parathyroid hormone levels with the blood assay, we irrigated and closed. As we turned over the case to anesthesia for extubation, I remained in the room while Dr. Holland walked out to dictate the surgery and speak to the patient's family.

While I was sitting in the room writing my notes, the patient was extubated routinely enough, but shortly thereafter seemed to be struggling to breathe. After using a mask and bag to help the patient breathe, the anesthesiologist informed me that he thought the patient was yet too groggy to safely be allowed to breathe on her own. He then proceeded to re-intubate the patient and informed me that she would be extubated again later when she was fully awake and able to maintain a patent airway. I did not think much of it at the time and went to perform my other scheduled surgeries for the day after transporting the patient to the recovery room.

After finishing my scheduled cases, I went to do rounds with the interns on the service and found our patient still in the recovery room and still intubated. I inquired from the attending anesthesiologist on duty in the recovery room and was advised that the patient was still too groggy and could not keep a patent airway. I was told that Dr. Holland was made aware of the situation, and that it had been decided to keep the patient intubated overnight as it was not safe to attempt extubation late in the afternoon when all hands might not be on deck. I agreed with this plan of action and went home fully expecting our patient to be extubated by the time I did rounds the next morning. However, she was not.

"We tried it again early this morning and she failed." The anesthesiologist who had given the anesthesia for the operation was again involved with the case and seemed concerned.

"Do you think it is swelling in the neck? She looks pretty swollen. Maybe she has a hematoma." I proposed potential reasons, without mentioning the potential cause we both by now dreaded. I had considered the possibility but discarded it because, despite our difficulty finding the glands, we had not been particularly aggressive during the dissection and we had not used any sharp instruments that might have caused inadvertent transection (cutting) of the recurrent laryngeal nerve.

"Joe, I looked in her trachea with a scope and both her vocal cords are medialized (displaced towards the midline). I think her nerves might be down."

"Down? Really? Are you sure?"

The anesthesia attending shrugged his shoulders. "We might need to give her a couple of days to see if her nerves recover. Maybe get some advice from ENT."

"Okay, I will call Dr. Holland and let him know." Speaking to Dr. Holland and describing the situation was uncomfortable to say the least. He sounded deeply disappointed and unhappy when I relayed the anesthesiologist's fears.

"It has to be the swelling. Tell anesthesia to try again this afternoon." I relayed the message.

Three days later the patient was still intubated after failing extubation several times. The ENT service was now on the case and EMG studies were ordered to check nerve function. The consensus seemed to be that both her recurrent laryngeal nerves had been injured during the procedure. Our expectation was that it was an injury due to blunt trauma (neuropraxia), rather than the nerves being severed, which was highly unlikely as most of the dissection we had done in the neck was blunt. We never used sharp instruments other than when we removed the small glands under direct vision while away from the nerve. We were comforted by the knowledge that most neuropraxias resolve in time, the only problem being that it was impossible to determine how much time this recovery would take. If the patient was to require airway support with intubation for a prolonged period of time she would then be required to undergo a tracheostomy, a procedure in which a small, curved tube is placed in the trachea, through an incision in the lower neck, at a level below and which bypasses the vocal cords. A tracheostomy would allow our patient to leave the ICU and eventually the hospital, as with proper care, patients can function with tracheostomies for extended periods of time.

We were still dealing with this particular patient and her complication when the following Monday, Dr. Holland had a similar case scheduled for surgery. The patient was a lady in her mid-fifties who on a routine physical exam by her primary care physician had been found to have increased serum calcium levels. Further work-up revealed increased levels of circulating parathyroid hormone. She was otherwise healthy and without symptoms. A bone scan had revealed no evidence of lytic bony lesions.

I entered the room that morning with a sense of dread. Dr. Holland seemed his normal self, except that he did not seem inclined to let me operate. This was one of the few times during my residency that I really did not want to. I had been dealing with the patient from the previous week nonstop over the prior few days, and I did not want to do the slightest thing that might lead to a repeat of that experience. I figured letting someone operate with the most experience in this delicate dissection was the proper course to follow. Entering the neck was a breeze, and I held the retractors gingerly as Dr. Holland manipulated the thyroid while searching for the parathyroid glands. I remember thinking that I wished he would be gentler with the tissues as by this time I was petrified of reliving the experience of the prior week. Does he not remember the patient from last week? I thought. However, I trusted his better judgment and held my tongue.

I was much relieved when the case was done. Dr. Holland had not invited me to operate and I secretly thanked him for it. This patient's thyroid gland was not as large as the one from the previous week, and although not easy, we had managed to find all four parathyroid glands and the last one we found on the lower left was much larger than the other three. Dr. Holland thought this was a clear case of an adenoma, and after removal of this particular gland the serum assay showed the expected drop in circulating hormone levels. We washed the wound and closed the neck in layers. Dr. Holland did the entire closure himself while I watched with relief and cut the sutures.

After the surgery was finished, I was sitting down writing the postoperative orders while Dr. Holland was still in the room dictating the surgery on the phone by the door. Very quietly at first, but progressively increasing in volume over time, I heard a high-pitched sound emanating from the patient as she was being extubated. The sound immediately caused in me a great sense of dread. Stridor, as this sound is called, occurs when there is some sort of airway obstruction. The rapid flow of air through a narrowly constricted airway causes this unmistakable high-pitched, whistling sound. I stopped writing and sat there watching the anesthesiologist attending and resident struggle trying to ventilate the patient. For several seconds I froze as if watching a surreal scene like a plane crash or a train derailment.

Eventually, I mustered the courage to stand and walk over to Dr. Holland who continued to speak into the phone. I grabbed him by the arm so as to have him turn towards me.

"Dr. Holland, hear that? She has stridor."

I was close enough to him to see his eyes widen and his pupils dilate momentarily as he internalized what I was saying. "No. It can't be!" He put the phone on the hook and we both walked towards the patient's bedside.

The following two weeks were dreadful, and they culminated in the statement Dr. Holland made at the M&M conference after I presented the two cases. I remember thinking how unfair it was that attendings were never expected to present at M&M, the task being assigned to the most senior resident on the case, no matter his/her involvement in actually performing the surgery. If there was ever a case to break that protocol, it was this one as my participation in both surgeries had been nil.

Both patients were found to have bilateral damage to their recurrent laryngeal nerves. Both required prolonged intubation, eventually tracheostomies, and were discharged home after respiratory rehab with indwelling tracheostomy tubes. Throughout the entire time Dr. Holland and I worked together before and after those two cases, he always was a gentleman and kind to me. I sensed after the two incidents that he was not as jovial and seemed more tired than usual. However, I never noticed any hostility towards me. He was clear in his praise of the way I handled the patient's postoperative course and arranged for all the subsequent required treatment and follow-up. It was, therefore, a great surprise to me to hear Dr. Holland utter the statement he made during my M&M presentation. He had to have known that he left the impression that the complications were directly attributable to me. I felt betrayed and angry. After all, I had presented the two cases in a very neutral and nonjudgmental way and in no way assigning blame. After the conference, he never brought up the matter to me and I always remained too afraid to bring it up to him. Besides, the damage had already been done.

For months and even years after the incident I would occasionally ponder as to why Dr. Holland had done what he did. The thought always brought the same feelings of anger and betrayal, the same way I felt the day the comments were made. As time passed, these feelings ameliorated somewhat. Eventually I was able to think of the incident from a more objective perspective. Since he was always the kindest of mentors and an obvious great surgeon and teacher, I took time to consider what could have possibly caused him to make that comment. I will never know for sure, but with the passage of time, I have begun to look at that incident through a different lens and from a much more empathetic perspective.

Now that I've been in practice for several years, I am more able to put myself in Dr. Holland's shoes. I have considered how I would feel and react if I had two such devastating and rare complications back to back in an operation that I specialized at, and for which I was considered an expert. Even more concerning would be if these complications occurred at a time when I was reaching the end of my career and rumors swirled among my colleagues and associates that perhaps the time was getting close to when I should be considering retirement.

By this time in my career, I've had the occasion to experience some of my senior colleagues and mentors wrestle with operative complications, particularly if they are unanticipated and occur as the surgeons get on in years and others wonder or make comments about the surgeon's retirement. I've come to learn that this process is not easy. Most surgeons are extremely motivated and focused on their work. For some, the job becomes their life. Facing the realization that one has to turn away from the only life one has known for many years can be heart-wrenching and downright scary.

Even more difficult is trying to make an objective judgment of one's own abilities, and whether one can still perform at a level proficient enough not to put patients in undue danger. And all this while friends and colleagues continuously ask you when you will retire. Their question at times must seem like they carry the implication that you have reached an age where you can no longer perform surgery at a level to ensure that you are not a danger to your patients. I will freely admit that I have no way of knowing if this is what was behind Dr. Holland's actions in attempting to refuse or at least divert to a certain degree the responsibility for what happened. Short of any other likely explanation, I've to come to believe that this might have been the reason why, although I freely admit that this is conjecture on my part.

I can only imagine how painful it must have been for Dr. Holland to face back-to-back dreadful complications in an operation that he had been performing flawlessly for years. I can only imagine how the incidents might have brought to the fore questions that he might have harbored about his ability to still perform surgery at a high-enough level and with a certain measure of safety. I only knew him for a short time, but I still think him incapable of doing anything to purposely hurt another human being, myself included. I think the statement he made during my M&M presentation was not meant to hurt me, and came out of a sense of self-preservation or perhaps utter frustration—not necessarily with me, but just at the fact that such complications occur. I have since forgiven him in every way and will forever be thankful for all he taught me in the short time we worked together.

At no time while operating with Dr. Holland did I ever feel that he was unsafe or had in any way put any of the patients we operated on at risk. His intellectual prowess was obvious, his knowledge of anatomy extensive, and his surgical skills were sound and true. It is hard for me even now to ascertain what could have happened in those two consecutive cases to cause such dreaded, rare complications. Perhaps it was a matter of getting too comfortable and complacent with procedures one feels have been mastered, or perhaps it was just bad luck related to scheduling two anatomically difficult cases back to back. The true cause was just as hard to ascertain then as it is now looking at the situation in retrospect.

Dealing with mistakes despite our best efforts is something that all physicians face at one level or another. These incidents can happen at any point in a surgeon's career starting from the first day of residency all the way to the day the surgeon retires. Often it is a private reckoning that takes place only in the mind of those involved. Presenting at M&M conference is one of the most difficult undertakings that physicians are asked to do. It is a place to confess your errors and make them public for the whole world to see. It is a place where one is asked to stand up in front of colleagues to face and confront one's demons. That particular Thursday afternoon when I presented back-to-back cases of bilateral recurrent laryngeal nerve injuries, I stood up and confronted my demons. I am now convinced that somewhere in that room, sitting in the audience, Dr. Billy Holland was confronting his, as well.

Kato eventually did present our kidney case about a month after it happened. It turned out that he did have an emergency trip and asked Dr. Socas to postpone his presentation until after he got back. I was sitting in the audience during his presentation and saw him stand and take responsibility for his decision to remove the kidney with humility and contrition. He took well the questioning and punishment that followed. It was, however, the consensus of all those present that it was his decision to make on the spot as to whether leaving the kidney in situ could have cost the patient his life. If his judgment as an experienced surgeon was in the affirmative, it was the consensus of every senior surgeon in the room that he had done the right thing in sacrificing the kidney. In dire situations such as this, life trumps all. I was proud of the way he handled himself and began to feel more at-ease with my involvement in that case.

Dr. Tom Alcalde was a fourth year when I was chief resident. He followed me as the senior on the E2 service and has since, like me, become a plastic surgeon who practices in South Florida. Several years ago, I received an email from him with the subject heading "FYI." In it, he told me about a patient he had recently met in consultation. The patient was a woman in her late sixties who had recently been diagnosed with breast cancer and he was being consulted to do her breast reconstruction after her planned mastectomy. During the consultation, he noticed a scar on her neck and asked her about prior surgeries. She then proceeded to tell him a story of how years prior, she had undergone a neck surgery at University of Miami Hospital to remove an adenoma of one of her parathyroid glands. There had been complications during the surgery and the nerves innervating her vocal cords had been damaged, leaving her temporarily unable to breathe on her own. She needed to remain intubated after the surgery and several days later underwent a tracheostomy so that her damaged vocal cords could be bypassed. She remained with the short tube protruding through her lower neck for nearly a year. Repeat testing eventually determined that her nerves had regained function. Her tracheostomy tube was removed shortly thereafter, and she went on to a complete recovery, except for some mild residual hoarseness in her voice.

Dr. Tom Alcalde had been in the audience that day. Even years later, he remembered my presentation and what transpired during that particular conference. I had never discussed the incident with him nor tried to set the record straight after the email. I chose to let bygones be bygones. I thanked him for remembering my presentation and affording me some closure by letting me know that in the end, all had ended well with my patient. It is my ardent hope the other patient had a satisfactory recovery as well.

THE FIFTH YEAR:

CHIEF RESIDENT

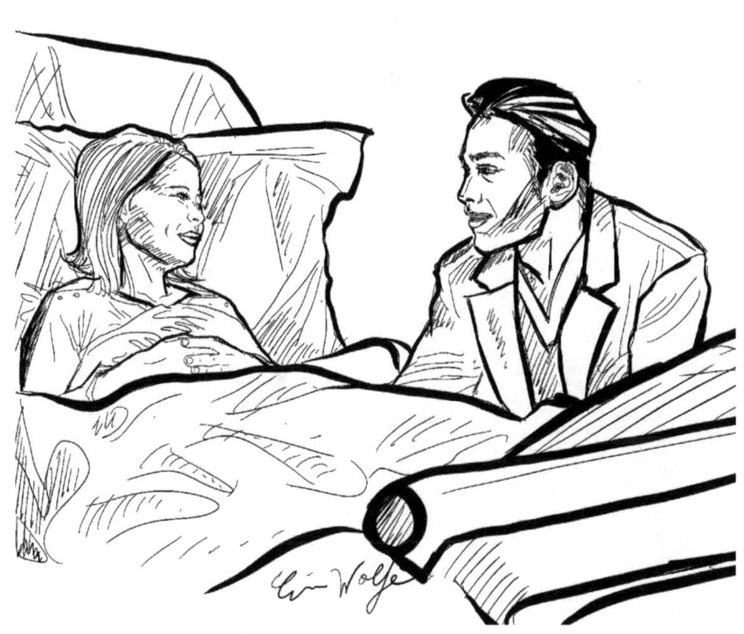

YELLOW PEOPLE

Finally, my chief and last year had arrived. As a group, our resident class had decided that the two chiefs who were destined to stay at Jackson Memorial for fellowships, namely Tony Cicilio and myself, were to have the two worst rotations of the year last, the VA hospital and trauma, respectively. The rest of the residents were to have the more elective rotations, such as to leave Miami to their next destination, be it private practice or fellowships elsewhere, two weeks before the official end of the academic year on June thirtieth. I used this bargaining chip to secure that I could remain in E2 and have it as my first rotation of my chief year. I was determined to get this rotation over and done with as soon as possible.

It was with great anticipation that I waited for the fourth-year (senior) resident to arrive on the service. Tom Alcalde was one of my favorite residents. Like me, he had started medical school and general surgery a bit older than the rest of the class, as he had spent some years in business—Wall Street, specifically—before deciding that his true calling was to become a surgeon. He was mature, organized, and had a great work ethic. I felt that he would do well in the rotation.

As for myself, I was ecstatic not only to have started my chief and final year, but also because I was going to get to work with Dr. Gerald Wodicka, one of my favorite attendings in the entire program. Not only was Dr. Wodicka a great surgeon, but he was also extremely easy-going and very much a resident advocate. He always appreciated the residents' efforts on his patients' behalf and was acutely aware of how hard the residents worked. His occasional words of encouragement did not necessarily lead to less work on one's plate, but they did make the burden easier to bear. However, the best aspect of working with him was that he treated the residents more like junior colleagues than as residents or mere personal assistants, as some of the other attendings did. Perhaps this was because he usually worked with chief residents, who naturally had more knowledge and experience, and were thus much more capable than their more junior cohorts. No matter the reason, his demeanor and behavior toward the residents in general and me in particular was always greatly appreciated.

After a couple of weeks, I found myself energized and enjoying the rotation immensely. I was in a great mood one Tuesday afternoon rounding on the floor after having finished a case with Dr. Wodicka, when one of the interns broke away from hurriedly following Dr. Wolfe and Tom for afternoon rounds to hand me a consult sheet.

"There is a 'yellow people' consult for the service in the medicine floor. I've already seen the patient and all pertinent info is already on the consult." As I took the consult from him, he rolled his eyes and quickly turned to resume rounds but stopped in mid-stride and turned towards me again. "Trust me, Joe. You want to go see this consult right away."

"Is it an emergency?" I asked, given that painless jaundice consults never were.

"No," he said, as a smile briefly flashed across his face before he hurried back to join the others.

Service consults were generated by residents and handled by residents. These were usually patients who came through the clinic or were admitted through the emergency room to a medical service and who did not have a "private" attending of record. The patients were usually managed in all services by senior or chief residents under the supervision of a rotating attending physician. When service consults were requested, the senior or chief resident who was consulted had some leeway as to which attending to get involved in the care of that particular patient. The attending chosen was usually someone the resident liked and trusted, and from whom the resident felt he/she could learn the most. For me, there was no doubt as to the attending I was going to direct the consults to, that being Dr. Gerald Wodicka.

Jaundice is a condition in which the skin takes on a yellow hue. It occurs due to an increased level of bilirubin in the blood, a pigment formed as a result of red blood cell breakdown. This pigment is conjugated (processed) in the liver. When there is liver failure for whatever reason, for example in hepatitis or inflammation of the liver caused by noxious stimuli or infection, this pigment is not properly processed by the liver and accumulates in the bloodstream, causing jaundice. Usually the urine and sclera (the white portion of the eyes) turns bright yellow first, followed over the course of the next few days by the skin. Besides the skin turning yellow, another common symptom of jaundice is uncontrollable itching, the result of bilirubin deposits in the skin. In cases of hepatitis, the jaundice is usually accompanied by nausea, vomiting, and abdominal pain in the right upper quadrant from the inflamed liver. Blood tests reveal increased levels of total and unconjugated (unprocessed) bilirubin and the pathological (disease) process occurs within the liver itself, resulting in this organ not being able to function properly.

However, when the jaundice appears without any other associated symptom except for itching and when blood studies reveal that the bilirubin has been processed by the liver (conjugated), the issue is usually one of a blockage of the biliary tree, by which the liver releases digestive hormones and metabolic byproducts such as conjugated bilirubin into the intestinal tract so they can be discarded through the feces. The presentation of painless jaundice can potentially be an ominous sign as it can indicate blockage of the common bile duct by a mass or tumor either of the common bile duct or on the head of the pancreas, which sits just behind it. On the hepatobiliary oncology service (Elective 2 or E2), we were used to seeing and treating patients who had presented with painless jaundice and had gone on to be diagnosed with pancreatic cancer, a terrible and most often fatal diagnosis. Some of us residents used to refer to those patients colloquially as "yellow people," due to the bright yellow hue of their skin.

I put the completed consult sheet the intern had given me in my lab coat pocket, and promptly forgot all about it as I went on to complete the many tasks on my list for that day. It was not until early evening when I was contemplating the possibility of going home that I was reminded about the pending consult. Although I knew it was not an emergency, I thought it best to go ahead and see the patient that night, so I could discuss the case with Dr. Wodicka the following morning. Tired as I was, I headed toward the adjacent building, which housed the medical wards, to see the patient.

I found the patient's room easily enough. It was the usual two-patient room that was common at the time on the medical and surgical floors. The first bed was empty, and the partition curtain was pulled halfway, not allowing me to see the second bed by the window. I knocked on the door in order to announce my presence while simultaneously looking down at the consult sheet so that I could call out the patient's name. "Terri Neely?" I called out as I walked around the curtain, gently pulling it back.

In the bed lay a young woman of twenty-five years of age who seemed to be in deep thought. Her appearance was most striking in that along with her blonde hair, her skin and the sclera of her eyes were bright yellow like an orange, and yet, she was stunningly beautiful. This was my third month on the hepatobiliary oncology service where most of my patients had been at the youngest in their sixties and ranging up into the high eighties. Not only her age, but the striking bright yellow appearance of the hair, skin, and eyes in such a beautiful young woman was uncanny. The smile on the intern's face as he handed me the consult made complete sense now.

As I struggled to introduce myself, she managed a smile and sat up in bed as if to hear her fate. She expressed some frustration at having been in the hospital for several days now without anyone clearly finding a solution to her peculiar problem of turning yellow. I explained to her that I had been consulted by her medical team to help them diagnose and offer recommendations as to how to manage her condition, but I was new to the case and was not ready to reach any conclusions or make any recommendations yet.

As I knew the potential dreadful diagnosis that the medical team was considering and requesting our help for, I first needed to know how much she had been told, which turned out to be not much. She explained that she had been totally healthy all her life and, just two weeks prior, had moved to Miami with a friend who worked at the coast guard base on Miami Beach. Terri was interested in pursuing a career in the coast guard like her friend or perhaps law enforcement. As her family was in Maryland, the only person she knew in Miami was her roommate, and she was becoming very concerned that this illness was going to interfere with her plans to start looking for a job and help her roommate pay the monthly expenses. She emphasized that other than her skin turning yellow, she felt perfectly fine.

I explained to her that jaundice in young patients was almost always due to some form of liver inflammation (hepatitis) and that we needed to get to the bottom of why she was jaundiced before we could formulate a treatment plan. I told her I needed to perform a thorough medical history and physical exam and review all her labs and studies so that we could figure out what was going on before making appropriate recommendations. I inquired about potential causes of hepatitis such as certain contaminated seafoods like oysters, blood transfusions, etc., all of which she denied having been exposed to. I further mentioned that alcohol and/or drugs were sometimes the culprits and managed a smile as I inquired if perhaps, she had been partying too much after her arrival in Miami. She denied drug use and stated that besides having had a couple of beers the first day she arrived, over the past two weeks she had been so busy settling in that she had not had time to go out. Besides, she added, her funds were getting low from the move and she had not yet secured a job and did not have extra money to spend on such things.

Next up in the process was the physical exam. Somehow, I found myself saying this almost apologetically. I thought it best to make sure I had a nurse as a chaperone for the exam, a customary practice per protocol, but which residents sometimes ignored due to impatience and time constraints. With the nurse present, I performed a cursory exam everywhere else other than the abdomen, where I pressed somewhat firmly in the area above the belly button, particularly on the right side, secretly hoping that she would experience pain, indicating an inflammatory process. She did not react at all. Her belly was soft, her liver did not seem enlarged on physical exam, and she did not complain of tenderness no matter how firm the pressure.

I told Terri that this part of the process was done. I was going to review her labs and studies and would then discuss her case with my attending, Dr. Wodicka. I promised her that I would visit the following day with some answers. "Please do," she replied. "I really need to get out of here and find a job."

As I walked out of the room, I was struck by how blessed she was that she did not yet know the potential gravity of the situation, and that her biggest worry in the world seemed to be finding a job. I dreaded the prospect of having the conversation with her that I'd had several times with patients over the past couple of months.

As I sat down in front of the computer to review her labs and her radiology studies, I hoped against all hope that her studies did not show what I feared they might. Then I proceeded to read the results of her abdominal CT scan: "There is a large mass encompassing the head of the pancreas." Moreover, her labs showed increased levels of serum total and conjugated bilirubin, indicative of an obstructive process of the biliary tree from a mass in the head of the pancreas. I was sick to my stomach all the way home and found it awfully hard to sleep that night.

Dr. Wodicka and I discussed the case in the morning. He and I were in agreement that a tumor was unlikely. As our patient was way too young for a tumor, he felt that the lesion was most likely a non-cancerous inflammatory process. However, neither of us could explain why our patient was not experiencing any pain at all. He postulated that the mass in the head of the pancreas could be from an atypical case of pancreatitis, or inflammation of the pancreas. Pancreatitis is a profoundly serious condition usually associated with a great amount of abdominal or back pain, nausea, and vomiting, where patients deteriorate very rapidly and become severely ill, often necessitating ICU care. Terri was in no way ill, and she had absolutely no pain, abdominal or otherwise. Dr. Wodicka wisely suggested that we discuss Terri's puzzling clinical presentation with a much more experienced surgeon, Dr. Zach Wolfe—The Lord.

Here I now was, without a definitive answer to give her, but was compelled to fulfill my promise to Terri and go see her that day. As I walked into the room, I found Terri and her roommate sitting in bed looking at a magazine and giggling. The scene seemed somewhat strange given the potential gravity of the situation. If not for one of the women being completely bright yellow, the scene resembled any college dorm room where two female friends get together to relax and talk. They both seemed startled when I walked into the room but eager to hear what I had to say.

I felt uncomfortable having any serious medical conversation with Terri while her friend was in the room, so I told her that unfortunately we would need a bit more time before deciding on what our recommendations would be. I again promised to come see her as soon as possible with something concrete to report. I sensed her growing frustration at having to sit in the hospital for days without a definitive answer to her predicament, but told her at this time she needed to concentrate on getting well and that we needed to take our time to make sure we studied her condition. I told her that her case was not typical, and we would need to discuss with experts so as to make sure we arrived at the right diagnosis. I assured her that we were working hard on her behalf and that I would come back as soon as we had some answers. Her face reflected a sense of gratitude as I spoke. As I walked out of the room, the two women went back to their magazine, conversing and giggling as if nothing at all was amiss.

Dr. Wolfe suggested, rather than an impromptu case discussion with Dr. Wodicka and myself, that I should present the case at our weekly E2 conference. There in attendance were usually not only the surgeons on the service, but also associated services such as radiology, pathology, nutrition, et al, where I could get the best recommendations to this interesting case. Dr. Wodicka relayed the message and I promptly complied. After I carefully went over the case history, the physical exam, and lab findings, I put up the pertinent ultrasound and abdominal CT scan of the mass on the viewing board located in the front of the room. After my best attempt at reading the films, the head radiologist opined that he agreed with me that the mass did show peripheral "stranding" around the head of the pancreas, a radiological term which is consistent with inflammation. He further stated, however, that this did not necessarily mean the process was entirely inflammatory, but rather it could have started as a neoplastic process (tumor) that had eroded through the pancreatic tissue, thereby releasing pancreatic hormones that led to the peripheral inflammation. Someone inquired from the radiologist as to whether there was any way to get a tissue diagnosis with a CT scan guided needle biopsy.

"No, we can't. Even if we could biopsy some of the tissue involved in all that inflammation, there is no way we can be sure we are taking a representative sample of the original lesion, as the entire head of the pancreas is involved with this inflammatory process."

Next, the pathologist chimed in that although pancreatic malignancies were unusual in someone in their twenties, there certainly existed case reports, particularly of some of the pancreatic endocrine (hormonal tissue) malignancies, in patients who were younger, some even in their late teens. She agreed with the radiologist that the only way to tell for sure if this was strictly an inflammatory process or one associated with a neoplastic process (tumor), was to take out the whole specimen and study it.

With bated breath, all in the room, but particularly Dr. Wodicka and I, waited for Dr. Wolfe to speak. "It is indeed an unusual case, but if it is a malignancy, we only have one chance at saving this patient's life, and that is to excise it. We will not do right by this patient if we sit around hoping and wishing for this to be an atypical case of pancreatitis, because if we are wrong, she will surely die sooner rather than later."

Thus, as if the words had been uttered directly by God, there was unanimous agreement in the room. Terri Neely at twenty-five years of age was to undergo a pancreaticoduodenectomy (Whipple) and it was my job to break the news to her. Dr. Wodicka directed me to fit her in the surgery schedule for the following week.

I knew talking to Terri was going to be difficult. As she was not scheduled for surgery until the following week, I decided to talk to her on Saturday morning after rounds. This way I would not be rushed and could spend enough time with her and answer all her questions and try to allay any concerns and fears. I still went to see her every day that week but stalled her by telling her we were still reviewing her case. On Saturday morning after rounds I headed to the medical floor to see her. I was happy to see the bed next to Terri's was still unoccupied and that her friend was not around. She was just walking out of the bathroom after taking a shower as I entered the room. With her hair wet, she appeared to me more beautiful and yellow than ever. As usual, she greeted me with a beaming smile.

I asked her to sit on the bed and I pulled a chair and sat in front of her. "Terri, we've had ample time to study your case and have taken in the input of very experienced clinicians and surgeons and are ready to make a recommendation. As I've told you, your case is very unusual because it appears you have an inflammatory process in the head of the pancreas called pancreatitis. Usually, however, this is accompanied by a lot of other symptoms like pain, vomiting, and nausea, and it leads to the patient becoming terribly ill. You are not experiencing any of that." Attempting to break the news easily, I continued, "It is probably a case of atypical pancreatitis. However, there is a small possibility that it is not inflammation but a mass...."

"A mass...you mean cancer?"

"A mass does not necessarily mean cancer, and I can tell you that pancreatic cancer is almost unheard of in someone your age, but the problem is that there is no way to tell unless we take the mass out. And that is what we are recommending...an operation to take the mass out."

"If it is cancer, you can take it all out, right?" Her face was more inquisitive than fearful.

"Terri, we are going to take it all out. Whatever it is, it is coming out. We won't talk cancer until we are sure that is what it is. Again, that would be highly unusual."

"When is the operation? How long will I have to be in the hospital?" Her words and expression seemed very matter of fact to me, and I remember thinking that she was either extremely brave or was not completely comprehending what I was trying to tell her. I tried to put myself in her shoes and wondered how I would take such news. I realized it was not a fair comparison as she and I had a totally different set of facts and information. This was in part my fault, as I had not divulged the entirety of the situation or the potential dreadful possibilities. I had discussed these issues previously in great detail with many patients on the service, but somehow could not bring myself to do so with Terri. I felt somewhat oddly protective of her. I made a mental note that I should check my emotions and not to get too personally attached to this patient.

I shifted to doctor mode and made an attempt to explain to her in layman's terms the Whipple operation and what would be involved, how long it would take, the need for her to go to the ICU, and the average total hospital stay of one to two weeks after the surgery, as we had to make sure her intestinal plumbing was working properly. During the middle of the explanation I noticed that her eyes were glazed over, and I realized that by then she was not taking in much of what I was saying.

"Will I be able to have children?" The question came out of the blue and startled me. "Not that I am planning any right now you know, but maybe in the future…possibly. Yes, I would like to have children."

I tried to be as positive and sensitive as I could muster. "This operation should not prevent you in any way from having children. When you are ready, you should be able to have as many children as you want."

She smiled briefly and then lapsed back into thought. Then she abruptly asked, "Hey, would you mind talking to my mom on the phone? I am sure she is going to have a million questions for me after you leave."

I agreed. Terri got her mom on the phone and I conveyed a short version of the conversation I'd just had with her daughter, who was all the while staring at me without much emotion on her face. Her mom told me that if we recommended surgery, that is what Terri should do. She further stated that she was in the process of making plans to travel to Florida to be with her daughter and would be there the following week for her surgery.

I continued to round on Terri daily until her surgery date. Her mood always seemed to be cheerful to a degree, and somewhat detached from the matter at hand. I marveled at this and wondered if it was due to sheer bravery, lack of knowledge of the potential dreadful outcome (of which I was responsible in part by withholding some of this information from her), or some inexplicable psychological defense mechanism yet unknown to me. A couple of times the following week, Dr. Wodicka came to round on Terri with me. Her innocent, trusting nature and demeanor brought out my masculine, protective nature, and I suspected also in him. It somehow felt as if I were walking hand-in-hand with a child through a dark forest, in which untold dangers lurked. I sensed that Dr. Wodicka too, like myself, was developing a special affinity toward her.

Finally, the surgery day arrived. As per routine, Dr. Wodicka and I came to see Terri in the preoperative holding area, but after our business was done, he left to go get ready. I lingered and then walked beside her stretcher as it was wheeled into the operating room. As she was being put to sleep, she seemed to search for me with her eyes and reached out her hand to grab mine. I stood there, feeling somewhat uncomfortable, holding her hand until she slipped into a deep sleep.

Next I knew, all was set and I was standing, knife in hand, in front of Dr. Wodicka across the operating room table. Terri was prepped and draped, with her abdomen exposed, ready for us to begin. I dreaded the thought of what I feared we would discover within our patient's abdomen, a malignant pancreatic tumor. I hesitated…

"Joe, let's go." Dr. Wodicka's distinctive voice was calm but firm. I reminded myself that the best thing I could do for Terri was to stay detached. I put the knife to skin and made the cut.

Three hours later we were all business. Dr. Wodicka and I were working synergistically and harmoniously. The mood was serious but pleasant. I felt that both Dr. Wodicka and myself were of the same mindset—i.e., acutely aware that Terri would somehow be a special patient in both of our careers. Perhaps it was due to the uniqueness of her case, perhaps because of her age or demeanor. We both felt that she was somehow special, and we were bound to do the best we could on her behalf.

Terri was fit and thin, and it did not take us long to dissect down to her duodenum and pancreas. From there, however, things changed as her abdomen was very "hostile," as we surgeons often refer to tissue that is matted down and difficult to dissect due to a pathologic process such as inflammation or tumor. Dissection around the mass was terribly slow and bloody. We took turns doing the surgery with Dr. Wodicka letting me do the portions he felt comfortable I could handle.

As we began to mobilize the duodenum and pancreas from the attachments posteriorly in the abdomen with Dr. Wodicka dissecting, he plunged his instrument into some loose inflamed tissue and a gush of blood poured out. The blood was significant and overpowered my suction's ability to retrieve it and thus began to flood our surgical field. Dr. Wodicka attempted to visualize where the bleeding was coming from by dissecting further. This move in turn caused the bleeding to increase significantly. Within seconds, there was lots of blood pouring out and we soon realized we were in trouble.

"Oh, Jooooeeeeee…" Dr. Wodicka's voice was always peculiar, but this time I thought I sensed a certain component of fear, an emotion I had never associated with him.

"Let's pack." I reflexively grabbed a stack of lap pads sitting on the scrub tech's table and handed half to Dr. Wodicka. As we would have done in any trauma case with significant intra-abdominal bleeding, Dr. Wodicka and I started packing lap pads into the surgical field and applied pressure to arrest the bleeding. After packing, Dr. Wodicka and I continued to apply pressure and stood still in silence waiting for the bleeding to stop. After some very tense moments, eventually it did. As the minutes passed, the blood coming out in the suction was less and less. As the situation stabilized, our hands still in Terri's belly applying pressure, we took a couple of minutes to take a breath and relax.

My thoughts went back to the fear I thought I heard in Dr. Wodicka's voice. Was it possible that such an accomplished and experienced surgeon had momentarily shown signs of panic, and I had not? Was this even conceivable? As the possibility seemed at least plausible, I mentally congratulated myself on my composure as a surgeon under duress. I did not experience any fear that day in the operating room, but have experienced it many times since, even in situations of much less gravity.

I have come to understand that there is a huge difference between being a resident or an assistant surgeon on a case and assuming the responsibilities of the surgeon of record. With this designation comes all the responsibility of all decisions and the outcomes, good or bad, that occur during any particular operation. This is a solemn responsibility indeed, particularly when things do not go well. I still do not know if it was fear that I heard and saw in Dr. Wodicka that day, but if it was, I am very understanding and empathetic of it now. I have myself experienced panic in the operating room many times since and can personally attest to how uncomfortable and incapacitating it is when things suddenly and drastically turn for the worse in the middle of an operation. It is during these times when the mettle of surgeons is tested. It is during these dire situations when elite surgeons shine by being able, against all instincts, to suppress their fear and perform at optimal levels.

Eventually the field became dry enough for us to remove the lap pads one by one and search for the source of the bleeding. We suture-ligated the large retroperitoneal veins, which were the culprits. This process was tedious and slow as we took every precaution not to get into significant bleeding again. Eventually we were able to fully mobilize and remove the specimen. It took us another three hours to make all the intestinal, pancreatic, and bile duct connections that are part of the operation.

Finally, seven hours after beginning the case, we finished closing the midline incision on Terri's abdomen. We were finally done. Both Dr. Wodicka and I were utterly exhausted from the physical exertion and mental strain of the operation. Before stepping out of the room, he reached out from across the table and grabbed my forearm. "Great job, Joe. Please keep me updated as to how she does."

I watched him walk out of the room and could not help feeling that something special had happened in that room between Dr. Wodicka and myself. We had bonded in a special way that day. I felt that during the operation he truly began to see me more as a junior colleague than as a resident.

To this day, whenever I see Dr. Wodicka at a conference or just around town, right after the usual pleasantries, he never fails to inquire about Terri. Seeing him always reminds me of that one particular case we shared and of that particular patient that the two of us will never forget. In one of our recent conversations about Terri, Dr. Wodicka mentioned that certain blood assays have been developed that can tell whether a pancreatic mass like Terri's is due to tumor or inflammation only. He summed it up by saying: "It is a shame she became ill in a different time."

It is a shame that Terri ever became ill at all.

I was too exhausted to help move Terri from the operating room bed to her stretcher. I stepped back and watched the nursing staff move her. As they shifted her body in order to do so, I noticed a small tattoo of the sun that Terri had in the small of her back. I chuckled at the thought that I had not noticed it before. Surely my professors in medical school would have been more than disappointed at my less than thorough initial physical exam on my patient. I pondered their reaction as I walked out of the room to go talk to Terri's family.

Youth definitely has its advantages and Terri sailed through her recovery as expected. She was out of the ICU in two days and walking and eating normally in less than a week. I saw her religiously two times per day and followed her progress closely, keeping Dr. Wodicka informed all the while. In order to allay her worries and prevent her from getting anxious, I told her that the pathology report on the mass would not be out for at least a week. I checked the computer multiple times daily and was ecstatic to finally read that the mass was all inflammatory tissue—no trace of tumor, let alone malignancy, was ever found. I immediately stopped everything I was doing and rushed to tell her personally. Her smile upon hearing the news was dazzling. She was no longer yellow and was feeling much better. She now had a future full of possibilities.

About a week and a half after her surgery, Terri was discharged home, leaving an empty place in my daily schedule, my thoughts, and my heart. I saw her for two to three visits in the clinic while I was still in the rotation. During the last visit with her, I told her that I was moving on to another rotation, but that I was happy to see she was doing great and progressing right along. I then did something that I had never done up to this point in my residency. I offered her my personal cell phone number and told her I would be happy to hear how she got along from her surgery and with her future plans of getting a job and eventually becoming a police officer.

Over the next several months as I moved on through my chief year, Terri and I did keep in touch, as she would text occasionally. She eventually moved down to Key Largo and started working at Hobo's Café, a popular local restaurant, as she concentrated on her recovery and planned for the next phase of her life. I often vacation in Key West and have been doing so for years now. Every time I drive past that restaurant on my way down and back, I am reminded of her.

I had not heard from Terri for a while, when one evening approximately ten months after her surgery I received a text from her. She had been feeling terribly ill for several days with nausea and vomiting and it was getting worse to the point that she could not keep anything down and was feeling awful. She wanted to know if her symptoms had anything to do with her pancreatitis or her surgery. After hearing the story, I immediately inquired as to whether she was passing any gas.

"Excuse me?" She seemed genuinely surprised and a bit irritated at my question.

"I mean, have you gone to the bathroom to pass stool or are you passing any gas?"

"I don't know about gas, but I have not passed any stools for several days."

Her answer was concerning. I explained to her that there was a possibility that she had developed some adhesions on her bowel from the surgery and had what we call a small-bowel obstruction. I explained to her that this was one of the potential complications of abdominal surgery and that we needed to rule it out right away, because if we delayed treatment too long it could potentially lead to bowel perforation. When she asked what she should do next, I told her to sit tight and I would call her right back.

At the time of this conversation, I was at the end of my chief year and had just started my final rotation in trauma. I was taking call every third day, and this was my night off. Normally emergency surgery consults went to the trauma team on call; however, I felt compelled to deal with this case personally, as I felt a responsibility to her as a prior patient. I thought it best to bypass the normal emergency surgery channels and reach out to Dr. Wodicka directly. He said it was okay for me to see her out of sequence with him as the attending. He volunteered to operate on her with me if she needed it. I immediately called Terri back and told her I would meet her in the emergency room. We both arrived within an hour.

The trauma staff was surprised to see me at the hospital on my day off, but I explained to them the situation and made preparations to take care of Terri the moment she arrived. Her work-up did confirm a small-bowel obstruction. I admitted her to my service, kept her NPO (without eating or drinking anything), and started her on intravenous fluids. Lastly, I inserted a nasogastric (NG) tube down her nose into her stomach to suction out her stomach/intestinal contents, a procedure she did not particularly appreciate and had some trouble tolerating. I explained to her that sometimes, with the actions we had taken, these small-bowel obstructions resolved on their own, but that if she did not get better within twelve hours, Dr. Wodicka and I would have to operate to release the scar band causing the obstruction. "Do what you have to do," she said. It was easy to tell she was not feeling well.

The following day, she was not much better so once again, Dr. Wodicka and I found ourselves across the operating room table with Terri as our patient. Right before she was taken to the room, I came to see her in the preoperative area. She pulled her gown high enough to show me her belly. "Please be careful with my scar and do a nice closure. As you can tell, I've taken care of it and kept it out of the sun like you said. You can hardly see it now."

I promised her I would.

As soon as we opened Terri's abdomen, we saw the scar band causing the kink in her small bowel. We promptly released it and "ran her bowels," examining the entire span of her small and large bowel to make sure there were no other obstructions. There were none. Her bowel looked otherwise healthy without any signs of ischemia (poor blood supply) or gangrene. We washed her abdomen with saline solution and proceeded to close. Dr. Wodicka noticed me taking longer than usual with the closure.

"Come on, Joe. I have other cases and you are not in plastic surgery yet." Five days later, Terri was discharged from the hospital yet again.

Several weeks later, I received a call from Terri who said she had made a decision about her future and wanted to share it. She had come to Miami thinking she wanted to get into law enforcement or perhaps the coast guard. However, after the experience she had with her illness and surgery, and after being exposed to so many kind people who diligently worked on her behalf and took great care of her, she realized that her true passion was helping others heal and she had decided to go to nursing school instead. I was extremely happy to hear this and was as encouraging as I could be. We ended our conversation very amicably and she promised to let me know how she was getting along. I did not hear from Terri again for three and a half years.

After completing my plastic surgery two-year residency, I went to UCLA to complete a one-year fellowship in craniofacial surgery. After completing my fellowship, I decided to fulfill a lifelong dream of taking six months off and driving the periphery of the country and into Canada, camping along the way. I used the idle time to work on my notes and the original outline for this book. I was in the last month of my journey making my way through Maine traveling south when out of the blue, I received a call from Terri. She was very cheerful and said that she had been thinking about me and figured I had just completed my plastic surgery training and wanted to congratulate me. I told her she was one year late but that I appreciated the thought nonetheless.

She confessed that she had other news to share: She had just graduated from nursing school and had gotten a job at Johns Hopkins University Hospital so that she could be closer to her mother, who lived in Baltimore. Moreover, she also wanted me to know that she was engaged and would soon be married. I was very joyful to hear this and promptly congratulated her. I mentioned to her what I was doing, taking the six months off to travel, and was making my way down the East Coast. Upon hearing this, she insisted that I stop by her mother's house on my way down. She said both she and her mother wanted to see me and that she wanted to introduce me to her future husband. I begrudgingly agreed, not realizing it would lead to one of the most uncomfortable moments of my life.

I called her a couple of days before I was to pass by Baltimore. She told me where to exit off I-95 and where to wait for her. She said her mother's house was not far from the interstate and that she would come fetch me. I arrived at the particular exit in the early afternoon and waited at the gas station she mentioned. It was a balmy, sunny day and I had been driving since morning in my Jeep and was wearing shorts, a T-shirt, and sandals. She came alone to get me and stepped out of the car in jeans and a T-shirt. She looked as beautiful as I remembered. I was extremely happy to see her. We hugged and she asked me to follow her to her mother's house.

There were several cars parked in front of her mother's house, which did not register at first, but for which the reason became apparent soon thereafter. After walking through the front door, I was confronted with a room full of about twenty nicely dressed people who seemed present for some sort of an event. Seeing the perplexed look on my face, Terri explained that afternoon was to be her formal engagement party at her mother's house. Her extended family and the future groom's family were present, and other guests would be arriving within the hour. She further said that she had been getting things ready all morning and when I called, was just about to take a shower and get dressed.

At my obvious distress, she was quick to tell me not to worry, as she had explained to the entire family the whole situation and that they had all encouraged her to invite me, as they were all eager to meet me. Most of her family and her fiancé's family were familiar with her prior medical issue and her surgery story. She said they all were aware and understood that I had been driving all day and would not be dressed for the occasion. She further added that her entire family was eager to meet me. She confessed that she had not told me about the party as she feared that if she had, I would have refused her invitation to come. How correct she was about that assumption, she will never know.

I met the groom-to-be, both families, and several other guests that began arriving shortly thereafter. They all could not have been nicer people, but I could not have felt more uncomfortable, especially when Terri went off to take her shower and dress, thereby leaving me alone with them. Despite my stomach being in knots, I forced myself to eat the food they kindly offered, all along praying I could keep it down. As happy as I was to see Terri, I could not wait to get out of that house as the entire time I felt utterly uncomfortable being there, especially dressed the way I was. I finally made my escape, leaving a heartwarming family scene behind—a scene in which I did not belong. I rejoiced at Terri's happiness as I happily resumed my trip relaxed, carefree, and with my Jeep top down.

As I reflected how thrilled Terri was regarding her upcoming plans, I realized that I too was starting a new phase in my life. After completing a long educational journey, which included many years of school and training, I was weeks away from starting my new plastic surgery private practice in Miami Beach. Driving south on that warm, sunny day, I experienced a deep sense of optimism and excitement about her future and mine.

Terri did get married, went on to have three children, and worked several years as an emergency room nurse at Johns

Hopkins University Hospital, the mecca of hepatobiliary (liver and bile system) surgery. She delighted in telling the general surgery residents she came into contact with at her job, that she'd had a "Whipple" at age twenty-five, leaving most of them in utter disbelief. She eventually followed her husband to Massachusetts, where she currently lives and is extremely happy by all accounts.

Not long ago, Terri contacted me yet again to let me know that after many years of working emergency room duty, she had decided to go on and get her nurse practitioner's certification, as she had developed a great interest in aesthetic (cosmetic) medicine. Upon finishing her advanced degree, she was hoping to work with a plastic surgeon. I told her that I had no doubt she would be great at it, thinking all the while that it was a shame she no longer lived in Miami.

In The Chairman's Oncology Service

Throughout the course of my career as a surgeon, both while training and since being in private practice, I've come in contact with many surgeons, perhaps over one hundred, with whom I've worked with very closely. Of those, I would say about a dozen belong to a group I consider outstanding, and a handful of those I consider elite surgeons, several of whom I've been lucky to have had as mentors. Dr. Henry Willoughby definitely qualifies as an elite surgeon, and although I officially trained under him while he served as the chairman of the surgery department at Jackson Memorial Hospital, he and I spent too little (and yet precious) time directly working together for me to consider him a mentor, per se. Nonetheless, in the short time we spent together, I did manage to learn much from him about what elevates surgeons to the elite category.

Dr. Willoughby was born in Canada and trained at the University of Miami before returning home. He eventually made his way back to Miami and served as the chief of the surgical oncology (E1) service before assuming the position of chairman of the department of surgery during my second year of training. I don't remember meeting him during my residency interview, and only became aware of him after arriving in Miami.

My first encounter with Dr. Willoughby was during my intern year while rotating on his service, in which he took me through my first hernia repair, right after jokingly berating me for shaving half the patient's pubic hair off. He threatened to make me explain the unusual haircut on our patient to the patient's wife, but thankfully he never followed through. Other than that embarrassing moment during what was a landmark case for me, our interactions during the month of my rotation were what was expected between an intern and the chief of the service, i.e., nil. Dr. Willoughby was always courteous and jovial, and he commanded a certain unspoken respect among residents and attendings alike.

The rest of my interactions with Dr. Willoughby over the next four years were few and far between, limited to conferences such as grand rounds and M&M conferences. On more than one occasion, I was the victim of his sharp, insightful questioning, and even, at times, his criticism when he felt I had done something wrong. For most of my residency, I pretty much convinced myself that he did not know who I was. He proved me wrong when I decided to call him out of the blue to intervene on Rachel's behalf regarding a categorical spot in the surgery program. He was chairman of the department by then and was keenly aware of each and every resident and fellow in his program, no matter their level of training.

During grand rounds and teaching conferences, he was outspoken, extremely intelligent, and demonstrated great breadth and depth of knowledge of all things related to surgery, including some of the subspecialties. I once overheard a chief resident say that Dr. Willoughby had "a very fast computer processor," referring to his brain. His mental prowess was enhanced by the fact that he was very articulate and had great command of the English language. He had an immense vocabulary and a very particular way of putting his words together, which was accentuated by his peculiar, high-pitched, crisp tone of voice. Listening to him speak, it was easy to be convinced that Dr. Willoughby could easily pass for an expert on any topic human.

In my time, I've known brilliant surgeons who fall disappointingly short when it comes time to exhibit their surgical skills. In this area, however, Dr. Willoughby excelled; he is what

I commonly refer to now as a "master samurai." He was not as methodical and detailed as Dr. Zach Wolfe (another elite surgeon for sure), but he operated with great purpose and always at a surprisingly fast pace. He operated at a rapid clip as if to make his hands keep pace with his mind. In the operating room he was very impatient and operated as if he had other things and meetings to go to (perhaps because he did), but at the same time was exquisitely focused and never lapsed in concentration. He stressed efficiency and focus, qualities I've come to realize are essential in getting complicated tasks, such as difficult cancer resections, accomplished efficiently. As if his considerable mental and manual abilities were not enough, there was something else about him that put him in a different echelon altogether. I sensed it in him from the beginning, but it took working with him several weeks before I could identify it. The quality that made him special is a double-edged sword, however, and one I struggle with to this day: He was supremely confident and self-assured.

My interactions while chief resident with our department chairman started way before I had the opportunity to rotate on his service. He held weekly conferences with the chief residents, which took place Wednesday mornings from seven to eight in the small conference room at the administrative department of surgery offices. I did not know if this was a tradition with all prior surgery department chairmen, or if it was something that Dr. Willoughby had instituted, but I found them very enjoyable. For one thing, it gave us chief residents a respite from running rounds (the senior residents were very aware that they had to take up the slack) but it also gave us a chance to get together with our cohorts on a weekly basis (many of us had never actually worked together despite being in the same year). Most importantly, it gave us a taste of what I call business-related administrative responsibilities, to which many of us had never been exposed; they are an integral part of running any business, including a surgery practice.

During those meetings, Dr. Willoughby discussed issues pertaining to the department and his future plans to make it better. He sat back in his chair and spoke eloquently, his words enhanced by a habit of making a loose fist with his right hand and suddenly flexing his wrist and extending the fingers all at once toward us to drive his point home. After he was finished, he asked each of us in turn for our opinion and invited us to discuss any particular issues we were having with our services or junior residents. He inquired as to our thoughts on improving the training program and seemed to value our opinion and recommendations. He brought up residents who were falling behind their peers in performance or were having difficulties for whatever reason and asked our opinion on how to handle the situation. Finally, he seemed interested in our future plans and freely offered suggestions on how to achieve them.

I always found these meetings quite enjoyable and helpful in many ways. Some of the administrative and management qualities I learned from our chairman I use to this day in dealing with the business aspects of running our practice. In my life, I have come across many physicians who think that because they are good clinicians or surgeons, it automatically means that they are good businessmen or women. I have come to understand that this is not necessarily true, but in Dr. Willoughby's case I saw what was possible. When the same qualities that make someone a good surgeon are applied to other areas of human endeavor, such as business, one can indeed excel in those areas as well. This is yet another lesson out of many that I learned from Dr. Willoughby.

By the time I rotated on his service as a chief resident, I thought I had a rather good feeling for Dr. Willoughby and the way he was as a surgeon and a person. For the most part that was true, however, I did not fully appreciate his sense of humor and his never-ending supply of energy. Walking with him to conference was an exercise in physical endurance, even for us residents who were younger. The pace at which he walked was dazzlingly fast and he talked all the while, never appearing to be short of breath. He took the stairs rather than elevators and offered dissertations on all pertinent topics; residents and fellows followed him around the hospital as if attracted by some sort of magnetic force.

Working on his service gave me a glimpse of how the health-care system should ideally work. Almost as if everyone in the hospital was in on the master plan, Dr. Willoughby's patients received first-rate treatment by anyone they came in contact with at the hospital. The patients who required consults by other services were seen right away and usually by the senior attendings on the other services. The patients who required lab tests and radiographic studies somehow got them done right away, no matter how busy the respective departments were. Even the nurses and hospital ancillary staff such as secretaries, transporters, etc., seemed to snap to attention and get matters taken care of when it came to Dr. Willoughby's patients.

By this time, I had been used to certain attendings getting special treatment by the hospital services and personnel, but I always got the impression that those providing that special treatment did it either out of fear or found it easier to perform the task being requested than to deal later with the wrath of that particular attending. With Dr. Willoughby, however, I got the impression that hospital personnel complied out of respect rather than fear. Thus, all ancillary staff seemed happy to perform the tasks required of them, making it very pleasurable for residents to work under those circumstances, a rather surprising and pleasant experience for me.

Spending time with him in clinic was yet another education in optimal people skills. Because of his position as chairman and his unique surgical expertise, he was much in demand. He saw and treated those considered to be the pillars of the community, but no matter who the patient was, whether they were wealthy businessmen or common laborers, he treated everyone the same. He had a way of walking into a room and making some jovial remark as a way of breaking the ice—while rotating with him, I was the target of some of those jokes—and he made it a point to give everyone in the room one of his business cards. This had the effect of making everyone relax and feel included in the conversation, which often revolved around some very distressing diagnoses.

Dr. Willoughby was an oncological (cancer) surgeon with a special area of expertise dealing with cancer of the intestinal tract, particularly the distal esophagus (a cylindrical structure through which food travels from the mouth to the stomach). This type of cancer is profoundly serious, as it is often diagnosed late, after it has had a chance to metastasize (spread), and thus carries with it a very dire prognosis. Even in those patients in which the cancer is discovered early and there is a chance for a cure, the position of the esophagus in the back of the thorax (chest cavity) behind the heart makes it very difficult to access, and renders the operation to resect it extremely difficult technically and fraught with a multitude of potential complications. Very few surgeons dare tread in that territory. Dr. Willoughby was one of those rare few who happened to be the absolute best at it.

When a cancer develops in the mid portion or distal (far end) of the esophagus, if it has not yet had a chance to spread, the surgical treatment of choice is to resect it and reconstruct the esophagus. The esophagus is a two-foot-long structure that connects the oral cavity and pharynx (throat) to the stomach. As it travels inferiorly to the stomach, the esophagus takes a position behind the trachea and the mediastinum, an anatomical zone that contains the heart and the great vessels. It then perforates the diaphragm, the fibrous membrane that separates the chest from the abdominal cavity, posteriorly and slightly to the left, and close to the spinal column before it connects to the stomach in a muscular tissue band called the gastroesophageal sphincter.

The operation to resect a cancerous esophagus was developed in the 1940s by a surgeon named Dr. Ivor Lewis, involving incisions in the abdomen and the right thorax. A newer technique that Dr. Willoughby preferred involved incisions both in the neck (usually left side) and the abdomen in order to sever the esophagus in the neck and the stomach, so as to resect most of the esophagus including a portion of the proximal (top end) of the stomach, so as to include the entire cancerous tumor with the surgical specimen.

The remaining portion of the stomach is fashioned into a tube-like structure that is then mobilized into position in the chest and sutured to the esophageal stump above, thereby reconstructing the esophagus and restoring the continuity of the gastrointestinal tract. In theory this operation is logical; it makes perfect sense. In practice it is technically exceedingly difficult, mostly due to anatomical considerations. Once the surgery is done, it is a matter of waiting for the surgical connections to heal to allow the patient to resume eating and eventually embark on the way to full recovery. As often happens with these big, intricate operations, however, the path to recovery is not always a smooth one.

Mr. Adam Harris was a man in his early sixties who had developed what he originally thought was chronic indigestion. Being a remarkably busy businessman, he found it hard to make it to the doctor on a regular basis, so his diagnosis was slightly delayed. His symptoms progressed to the point where he could no longer wait and eventually, he made it to a gastroenterologist, who upon performing an upper endoscopy noted and biopsied a lesion on Mr. Harris's distal esophagus. The pathology report revealed adenocarcinoma of the esophagus. By the time he made it to Dr. Willoughby's office, where he and I first met him, our patient had undergone a full work-up that revealed he did not have any spread of his cancer, thus making him an ideal candidate for a curative resection. Being in excellent shape for his age, he had an otherwise clean bill of health and was deemed to be an ideal surgical candidate from that standpoint as well. Even better, he was lean and had a flat abdomen, giving us the hope that his surgery would not be particularly challenging from a technical standpoint.

Mr. Harris came to his visit with Dr. Willoughby with his wife and teenage daughter. In typical fashion, Dr. Willoughby walked into the room with a very jovial attitude and after giving everyone in the room his business card, he made the usual introductory funny, cursory remarks and got to the issue at hand. After allowing the patient to start by explaining the reason for the visit, Dr. Willoughby eventually jumped in, letting the patient know he was fully aware of his situation after having had discussions with both his referring gastroenterologist and primary care physician. He reviewed the findings of the diagnostic work-up that had been completed so far. He did all this out of memory without referring to the chart or asking the patient for any information. This had the effect of making the patient feel that Dr. Willoughby was very immersed in the particulars of his case. I could sense the patient's confidence in Dr. Willoughby increasing by leaps and bounds as he spoke.

"I agree with both of your physicians that we seemed to have caught this lesion early and we should be able to completely take care of it with surgery." Dr. Willoughby's professorial explanation and demeanor seemed to be very soothing to the patient and his family and above all, inspired a great confidence in them. I sat back and watched the whole scene, alternating my attention among Dr. Willoughby, the patient, and the two family members, learning all the while.

"I am ready." The patient's statement was brief, determined, and calm, what you would expect from someone used to being in charge and making firm decisions. Mr. Harris's expression did not show the grave concern that was apparent in his wife and daughter. He seemed to mirror the same jovial mood that Dr. Willoughby was displaying, which I found somewhat strange in view of the dire subject being discussed. I was further struck by the lack of questions I often encountered from patients when discussing surgeries, such as what the surgery entailed, hospital stay, recovery time, etc. Those questions eventually did come, but they came from the wife and not from the patient, who just seemed eager to get the surgery done. Dr. Willoughby eventually did touch on all those issues, but did so in a roundabout, optimistic way—almost as if a great outcome to the surgery were already preordained.

Another benefit of working in Dr. Willoughby's service was that most of the patients we took care of were from his private practice, which meant that all of the logistics of getting the case into the operating room were handled by his secretarial staff without any assistance or input from me. All I had to do was show up for the case and then make sure to handle the medical aspects of the patient's postoperative care. The administrative logistics were completely taken off my plate, and I welcomed that change.

Approximately a week and a half after our visit with Mr. Harris in Dr. Willoughby's office, he was on the operating room table, ready for us. Dr. Willoughby allowed me to make the incision and begin the dissection through the abdominal wall. It did not take long before he became impatient. "Faster, Joe. We don't want to kill this patient with kindness."

I was in the process of using the electrocautery to stop all small bleeders in the field of my dissection. True to fashion, Dr. Willoughby was getting impatient with my progress.

"Come on, faster. Don't worry with the bleeding. Remember, all bleeding eventually stops."

Dr. Willoughby was a true believer in this old-fashioned surgical dictum. He practiced it as if it were a religion. Incidental bleeding to him seemed inconsequential. He endured my slow progress through the abdominal wall and allowed me to dissect a bit around the stomach. When he could no longer stand it, he took over the case and never relented. As this was his private patient, I had anticipated this and did not take it personally. I was happy to be able to assist a true master on this intricate case, which promised to be a great learning opportunity.

One of the images I will forever hold in my mind is of Dr. Willoughby, elbow-deep in our patient's abdomen while his hands reached through the diaphragm around the esophagus in order to completely free it up from the adjacent tissues. His body twisted over the patient in this uncomfortable position took great effort and concentration—as the dissection was completely blind. Finally, he pulled his hands out, and as a gush of blood followed from where his hands were withdrawn, he triumphantly announced that the dissection was complete. Eventually we stapled off and severed the esophagus in the neck and the lower aspect of the stomach and, having freed the entire surgical specimen, were able to remove it. Dr. Willoughby carried the specimen with both hands and deposited it at a back table that had been set up for that purpose. Dr. Willoughby then used surgical scissors and longitudinally opened the esophagus and stomach so as to be able to look within its lumen.

"There is the culprit." Dr. Willoughby pointed the cancer out to me as I stood by his side studying the specimen carefully. We were happy to note that it looked like the tumor had not completely perforated through the esophageal wall—indicating, we hoped, that the cancer was caught in its early stages and that the surgery was potentially curative. We would have to wait for a pathological evaluation of the specimen to be sure that no cancer was detected in any of the associated lymph nodes. Ultimately, we would need to wait for five years and no return of the malignancy before we could designate our patient as officially cured.

Upon completion of the teaching session, Dr. Willoughby put the "dirty" (soiled) instruments on the back table, changed gloves, and walked back to the operating room table. We then proceeded to properly mobilize the remaining stomach and pass it through the opening in the diaphragm up into the chest and neck where we completed the anastomosis (connection) to the remaining esophageal stump. A couple of hours later we were done with what seemed like a close to perfect operation. Upon finishing, the patient was taken to the ICU where he received outstanding postoperative care.

The ICU, including some of the more senior fellows and attendings, devoted a great amount of time and effort to Mr. Harris. I visited him twice per day, usually in the mornings with

Dr. Willoughby in tow. Jovial as usual, Dr. Willoughby would make funny statements in the patient's presence to which Mr. Harris was usually oblivious.

Things developed according to plan in the first couple of days. Mr. Harris was extubated the first postoperative day after we made sure his lungs were inflating properly and that there was no air trapped inside the chest (pneumothorax) from inadvertent lung injury during the surgery. His vital signs were stable, and we were all anticipating a potential discharge to the regular floor when, on the third postoperative day, Mr. Harris began to develop high fevers—up to 102.5 degrees. As per protocol, all potential sources (lungs, urine, surgical wound, etc.) were considered and studied and all potential etiologies (causes) were entertained and addressed. All the patient's lines and tubes were changed, and the tips submitted to the lab for culture. Blood, sputum, and urine cultures were also submitted to ascertain the potential responsible organisms. In that way, antibiotic therapy, which at this point was broad-spectrum, could be chosen to specifically target the responsible organisms.

While waiting for the results of the studies and for Mr. Harris's condition to improve, the ICU care team began to ponder the possibility that the cause of the fever might be related to a failure (leak) of the surgical anastomosis (surgical connection) or perhaps inadvertent bowel injury while the stomach was being mobilized to be transposed into the chest. They also theorized that perhaps the stomach was ischemic (poor blood supply) and potentially gangrenous from being manipulated and mobilized. Anastomotic leaks as the source of the infections, particularly when the patient is still not being fed, are rare at two to three days postoperatively. However, the ICU team expressed that they wanted to be as thorough as possible and intended to entertain and potentially study any possible cause.

To rule out the possibility of an anastomotic leak, we needed a CT scan of the abdomen and chest in order to look for potential fluid collections indicating an abscess, and/or dye studies to see if we could find the dye outside the gastrointestinal lumen, confirming the leak. Checking for gangrene of the stomach would require direct visualization of the gastrointestinal mucosa by inserting a scope through the mouth into the stomach lumen, a potentially dangerous maneuver in lieu of the recent suture line from the anastomosis.

From the moment that the possibility of an anastomotic leak or ischemia was brought up, Dr. Willoughby was insistent that this was not the case, and that the etiology of the fever had to be due to another cause, which the ICU team had failed to find. While discussing the issue with me and with the ICU team, Dr. Willoughby reiterated that it was too soon for the fever to be related to a leak, which usually presented one week out from surgery. Besides, he stressed, so soon after surgery, there was bound to be fluid and air seen on a CT scan of the abdomen, but this did not prove anything, as it could be due to the results of the surgery itself and not related to an infection or other complication.

Moreover, Dr. Willoughby objected to moving the patient from the ICU to the CT scanner to obtain a test that he felt had an overwhelmingly low probability of being diagnostically useful, and could potentially damage the patient's kidneys by exposing them to the iodine dye that was necessary to perform the study. Moreover, an endoscopic study to evaluate the stomach lumen carried the obvious risks of disrupting the anastomosis. Up to this point, his reasoning was very sound and made perfect sense. Thus, the ICU team would bring up these issues as potential sources but would immediately relent when faced with Dr. Willoughby's firm objections. For most of those back-and-forth discussions, I was the designated intermediary.

As the days passed, Mr. Harris's condition worsened and he developed frank sepsis, an overwhelming systemic infection associated with organ failure. He soon developed respiratory failure leading to reintubation and prolonged ventilator use. His blood pressure progressively dropped—another common feature of sepsis—and his vital signs became unstable, requiring vasopressor support—medications that raise and stabilize blood pressure—and compromising his kidney function, as kidneys need a certain blood pressure threshold to function properly.

As our patient's condition deteriorated, the ICU team became more and more insistent that we needed to rule out an anastomotic leak and gangrene as potential sources of the infection. In dealing with this patient, I was reminded of a similar incident I experienced with a difficult case in the ICU during my third-year rotation. In that case, I had been on the ICU side of the equation and was continuously prodding the liver transplant surgery team to perform an exploration. In that particular case, the patient eventually expired, and I desperately hoped this current situation would turn out differently.

After repeatedly talking to the ICU residents, fellows, and even attendings, it became clear that they were convinced that the cause of the sepsis was related to our operation. Dr. Willoughby was just as convinced of the opposite. "Joe, our surgery was textbook and there is no way we have a leak or dead bowel. The clinical course does not support that diagnosis. The cause of the sepsis is something else. Tell them to find it." Dr. Willoughby was insistent to the point of being irrational. I understood his concerns that moving an intubated and unstable patient to the radiology suite for a CT scan of the abdomen was fraught with risk and so was an endoscopic study, but if we were wrong and did nothing, the longer we waited, the less the chance we would be able to act and save the patient from a very dire outcome.

Since I was the conduit of communications between the ICU team and Dr. Willoughby, they put more and more pressure on me to talk some sense into him. I must admit that as days went by without any improvement in our patient, I began to think the ICU team's suspicions were right. After all, so far the chest X-rays had not shown any signs of lung infection (pneumonia), all the urine, blood, and central line culture tips kept coming back negative, and we could not figure out where his sepsis was coming from. Eventually I suggested to the ICU team that it was up to their attending to get Dr. Willoughby to agree to the studies. I told the ICU fellow that although I agreed with their assessment, my efforts to convince Dr. Willoughby had not borne fruit. I suggested that the ICU team attending should contact Dr. Willoughby directly to make the case. By this point, I had become fully convinced that the studies the ICU team wanted were warranted and the right thing to do.

Finally, more out of frustration than anything else, Dr. Willoughby relented and in short order preparations were made to obtain a contrast CT scan of chest, as well as an upper endoscopy, in order to rule out ischemia or frank gangrene. Although not technically my responsibility, as these tasks were usually assigned to the ICU rotating resident, I accompanied Mr. Harris down to the CT scan unit alongside the ICU nurse, respiratory therapist, and resident. Later, I stood by his bedside as the gastroenterology attending and fellow brought up their endoscope and inserted it into the patient's mouth, past our anastomosis, and down towards the abdomen, visualizing the lining of the bowel, all along looking for anything amiss. Thankfully, Mr. Harris made it through the studies no worse for wear and once I safely had tucked him in and made sure the ICU team was hovering, I made my way to inquire as to the final readings and results of the tests.

It turned out that there were no collections in either the abdomen or chest consistent with an abscess from an anastomotic leak. The upper endoscopy showed an intact anastomosis and viable mucosa throughout the entire length of the bowel they were able to study. I immediately called Dr. Willoughby to tell him the news. He seemed as jovial as ever and no less resolute than before. "Told you, Joe. Our surgery was perfect. I'm glad they did not kill the patient with all these studies. Now tell the ICU team to figure out why the patient is septic."

I had mixed feelings when I talked to the ICU fellow again the following morning, and rather than finding him despondent, he seemed somewhat encouraged when discussing Mr. Harris. "We think it is pneumonia and are setting up for a bronchoscopy at bedside."

I interjected that this was unlikely since none of the daily chest X-rays we had on our patient had any findings consistent with pneumonia, and he had no sputum (pus coming from respiratory tree) to indicate such a diagnosis, which we had been looking out for all along. The fellow explained that the ICU attending, upon further study of the chest CT scan with the radiologist, had noted an area of consolidation in one of the posterior lobes of the left lung, which was very suspicious for pneumonia. The reason we had not seen it on routine bedside chest X-rays is that it had been obscured by the mediastinum (heart shadow) and the surgical fluid and blood accumulated in the posterior thorax as a result of our surgical dissections.

I skipped clinic that morning and waited for the ICU fellow, with the attending by his side, to perform a bronchoscopy. He inserted the flexible scope down the endotracheal (breathing) tube and went into the left lung as far down as he could in the posterior lobe and triumphantly announced that he had found pus, which he promptly aspirated through the suction encased within the scope tube. After taking a sample from suction reservoir, I personally took it to the lab for immediate gram stain and for culture and sensitivity studies. When I called Dr. Willoughby with the good news, his response was predictable: "Glad they finally found out what was going on. It took them long enough."

We had a gram stain within the next half hour and within forty-eight hours we had the culprit organism that conveniently and belatedly began to grow in our blood cultures. Once the necessary adjustments were made on the antibiotics, along with aggressive respiratory therapy and almost daily bronchoscopies to wash out the pus from the lungs, our patient made a slow but eventually a complete recovery. I happily monitored Mr. Harris's progress as he was discharged from the ICU to the floor, and eventually home.

Dr. Willoughby and I continued to visit Mr. Harris daily together in the mornings prior to going to surgery or clinic. One particular morning after the crisis had passed and Mr.

Harris was being prepped for discharge to the floor, we were joined at bedside by the ICU fellow who, proud of his efforts, had come over in search of some recognition and accolades. "I'm glad we got him through this," the fellow uttered with a confident smile as he joined us.

"What do you mean?" retorted Willoughby. "I do a beautiful operation and you guys let my patient get sick. I should have known to keep him away from the ICU."

At first the fellow seemed perplexed and did not know how to react to Dr. Willoughby's statement, much like I had felt about Dr. Willoughby's threat pertaining to the pubic hair shaving incident during my first hernia surgery with him. The fact that he said it with a big smile on his face bespoke that the comment had been made in half-jest, however, with a certain admonition contained therein.

"What a jerk!" the fellow whispered in my ear as Dr. Willoughby walked off. I, not knowing what to say, trailed off behind the chairman.

It was later, while pondering on this particular interaction with the fellow in the ICU and Dr. Willoughby's statement, that I was finally able to put my finger on the quality that made Dr. Willoughby so uniquely special. It was his remarkable self-confidence. At no point during our care of this particular patient, even as his condition deteriorated dangerously, did I sense any doubt in Dr. Willoughby as to what his opinion and medical assessment of the situation was. I always felt his reasoning was sound, logical, and left little room for doubt. Yet I also sensed that his position was never based on ego or emotion, but rather a result of his sound clinical judgment and experience.

There are several qualities common to great surgeons such as intelligence, dexterity, and clinical judgment, to name a few. Another intangible quality, as mentioned previously, is confidence. Insecurity in surgeons is dangerous and can even be deadly, but just as dangerous is false bravado or unfounded overconfidence, as it makes surgeons take on cases and do things that are beyond their abilities. The optimal amount of confidence, when tempered by good judgment, is indispensable in making a surgeon elite, as he/she must be able to persevere for the sake of their patients in dire circumstances where less confident surgeons would desist or throw in the towel. That self-assuredness is vital when surgeons must persevere, hold the course, or take certain actions that raise doubt in the minds of others.

Great surgeons tend to be extremely confident in their intelligence and abilities, and they have an almost irrational level of optimism—an expectation that operations will turn out as planned. In the rare instances when they don't, these surgeons trust their abilities and skills to get them out of any situation they might encounter in and out of the operating room. I'm convinced that unshakable confidence, when tempered by great clinical judgment, is that one intangible ingredient that above all else makes a surgeon elite.

The critical issue when it comes to surgeon confidence is to decide what is the ideal level that allows for optimal performance but also makes room for human fallibility—the possibility of being wrong, no matter how good or experienced the surgeon is at his/her job. After many years in practice, I've come to understand that elite surgeons walk that fine line between extreme self-confidence and arrogance. By the time I rotated with him as a chief resident in the chairman's oncology service, Dr. Willoughby had found his sweet spot along that line. After many years of training and private practice, I find myself still searching for mine. When things in surgery don't go exactly as planned and, God forbid, complications ensue, insecurities and self-doubts plague me to this day.

You Can't Win Them All

"Stab wound to the chest. ETA seven minutes."

It was a typical Saturday night gun-and-knife club, so the trauma alert on my pager was not unexpected. I had finished a case and was in the process of writing postoperative orders. The walk to the trauma bay took me no more than thirty seconds. There, the whole team was present and getting ready for the incoming patient. Each team member represented my personal journey through my training program. The intern getting ready to do the three sticks, the second year holding "the bricks" getting ready to run the code, the fourth-year resident ready to be my wingman, and then there was I, after five long years, finally in the position of "top dog"—chief resident on the trauma service.

All members of the team had put on their booties, surgical gowns, and masks, and were ready to go when the doors at the end of the hallway swung open, allowing us to see the ambulance crew bringing in the patient. "This is gonna be a big nothing," I murmured to my fourth year, Chris Castrellon, as I surveyed the scene.

For years in trauma we had discussed the musings of one of our long-time attendings who believed that if the patient came into the trauma bay with his/her legs crossed, arms leisurely resting on the stretcher side-rails, and casually chatting with the ambulance personnel, there was almost a 100 percent chance that the patient was okay. To his original description our attending had added "and smoking a cigarette" but this was done to drive home the point that the picture was not consistent with someone who had sustained a serious injury. I almost considered taking all my protective gear off and letting the more junior personnel deal with the "code," but thought the better of it, as it was important for me to set the tone and never appear to let my guard down. However, I did stay back and let Chris and the second-year resident lead.

As the patient was being transferred to the trauma stretcher, with the entire code team swarming, the paramedic explained that the patient had been involved in a fight with a friend and had undergone a stab wound with a screwdriver to his chest. While he said this, he pointed to the patient's anterior chest where just a few millimeters to the left of the midline of his chest we noted a small dark circle more consistent with a pen marking than a serious injury. From its location, I surmised that even if the stabbing had been deep enough to perforate through the skin and deeper tissues, it was sure to have bounced off the sternum (breastbone).

As the patient was totally stable, reasonable, cooperative, and conversing pleasantly with the staff, there was not much hurry in undertaking the necessary trauma steps of cutting all his clothes off, turning him to look for other injuries, doing the three sticks (I told the intern to hold off on the femoral stick and the rectal exam), and necessary X-rays. These steps were performed as per protocol by the assigned staff but at a leisurely pace. Once the chest X-ray was read as negative for pneumothorax, foreign bodies, or any abnormal findings, we allowed the patient to sit up on the stretcher as we were making final arrangements to get him admitted for overnight observation.

The team began to wander off to their respective duties as the nurses were making arrangements to send the patient upstairs. I was contemplating a midnight food run with the fourth-year resident and, while waiting for him to finish his notes, I stepped up to the foot of the stretcher and engaged our patient in conversation. The patient still had all the monitors on, and I could see and hear the heart monitor, which was on the back wall right above the patient's head. He began to describe how the fight happened. He had already explained to us that it was not much of a fight, but rather a verbal argument, after which his friend took offense and used a nearby screwdriver to stab him once in the chest and then took off running. After that single act, there had been no other blows, injuries, etc.

I was interested in knowing how the patient had been taken by surprise to allow such an injury in the middle of his chest; the patient was telling me how the stabbing had been completely unexpected. All of a sudden, in mid-sentence, the patient's head slumped to one side and he went limp. At first, I thought the patient was playing some sort of a sick joke, especially since I noted the heart wave was still clearly visible on the monitor. It then took me less than two seconds to recognize the possibility of a condition that I had never personally seen, but had reviewed countless times in classes, rounds, exams, and mock trauma discussions. I confirmed it by placing my fingers on the patient's neck and finding no pulse.

"Chris, we have to crack his chest. He is in PEA." The senior resident was just outside the room, but I yelled loud enough that everyone around took notice and came rushing in. As the room became hectic with activity in order to intubate the patient and get everything ready, Chris and I once again confirmed my diagnosis by making sure that the patient had no pulse, but did have an electrical heart rhythm wave on the monitor.

Pulseless Electrical Activity (PEA) is a condition in which the heart's electrical impulse is still intact and can be detected with heart monitors such as EKG equipment, however, there is no pulse, which indicates that the heart is not mechanically contracting and therefore not pumping blood. There are several medical or metabolic situations that can make this happen, but in our particular patient, the cause was clear. There was a compressive force on the heart from outside preventing it from being able to expand and contract. In lieu of a normal chest

X-ray ruling out any lung injury possibly causing air to be this compressive force (tension pneumothorax), there was only one other possible cause, that being blood accumulation in the pericardium, the fibrous membrane that encases and surrounds the heart. This condition is called pericardial tamponade and if not treated emergently, it inevitably results in death.

I immediately took a scalpel with a number ten blade and cut the patient's chest just under the fifth rib from just left of the midline all the way down the side of his chest until my blade could go no further due to the stretcher. Although the cut was deep, I still was not full thickness through his chest wall, and it took one swipe with large, curved scissors from the back towards the front to get this done expeditiously. Next, I placed the rib retractor and rapidly turned the knob so as to cause the ribs to spread. I was able to clearly see the patient's pericardium and left lung. There had been no rush of blood when I entered the patient's chest, thereby confirming my diagnosis that the blood was not within the chest cavity proper but contained within the pericardium. The left lung appeared intact but as expected, the pericardium was distended, tense, and bulging, like a balloon.

As I performed each step with an acceptable level of proficiency that confirmed my original diagnosis, I became aware of a certain confidence swelling up in me. From now on, my task was clear: Open the pericardium as I had been taught, parallel to the phrenic nerve, find the hole that was sure to be in the heart or one of the great vessels, and plug it by sewing it shut. Right before incising the pericardium I consciously told myself that I could do this. I had not exactly done this before under similar circumstances but had practiced for it many times. I had learned the theory, studied the steps, even performed the steps in animals (pig trauma-lab at the zoo) and cadavers. I had entered the chest multiple times during my rotations and had previously entered the pericardium during my cardiothoracic rotations. I had even previously sewn on a beating heart. Yes, I was sure I could do this.

The rush of blood that came in my direction as I started cutting into the pericardium startled me. It had been under pressure and came pouring out onto the stretcher, all over my gown and the floor. Chris used the suction as best he could to enable me to see the heart. Sure enough, in the middle of the left ventricle (one of the chambers of the heart) there was a pencil-wide hole pouring out blood from what now was a fibrillating heart. Again, without hesitation I called out for a 2-0 silk suture. With it, I placed a figure-8 stitch over the hole, immediately stopping the leak from the ventricle.

"What's going on, Joe?" I recognized the voice immediately as that of the trauma attending who had rushed into the room still putting on his protective gear. As I explained to him what had happened as I finished tying up and cutting my stitch, he directed me to quickly look for any other holes. I flipped the heart as much as I could quickly and told him I did not see any.

"Great job! Start compressions." I was already doing compressions with my right hand on the heart, which was shaking (fibrillating) rather than beating. As I did this for several seconds, the nursing staff was busy getting the internal heart paddles ready.

For those few seconds while I waited, my thoughts flashed on the situation, which I had not been in since I was an intern, in this same trauma center working with Jack Rio. Every step I had just performed I had watched Rio do five years prior with one huge difference. He had been given a situation that was almost certainly going to end in a bad outcome, as his patient had multiple injuries and had expired minutes before arriving at the trauma center.

My chance at an emergency thoracotomy was as optimal and as textbook as they come. A young and otherwise healthy patient, one single injury, who had arrived totally stable and had collapsed right in front of my eyes. Furthermore, the procedure had been executed expeditiously and the injury had been addressed favorably. The rest was academic. All that was left to do was to shock the heart back to life, an almost guaranteed outcome when a young, healthy heart had been in fibrillation for less than two to three minutes. I had seen this take place time and time again during my cardiothoracic rotation as we reactivated the heart and took patients off the heart-lung bypass machine at the completion of open-heart surgery.

In the process of dying, the heart does not go from normal, synchronous contractions to asystole or complete cessation of activity. There is usually an intermediate stage called fibrillation, a period of unsynchronized, irregular muscular activity more consistent with shaking than contractions. Heart fibrillation does not allow the heart to properly pump blood, its main function, and within minutes leads to asystole and death unless this rhythm is reversed. The best way to convert fibrillation to a functional heart rhythm is through the application of electrical current. This can be done with external paddles where two large defibrillator paddles are applied to the patient's chest in order to deliver the electric current. However, in rare situations where the heart is exposed, much smaller internal paddles are used and a much smaller electrical current is delivered, as the two paddles are placed in direct contact with the heart. When the chest is open as in this case or during open-heart surgery, air enters the chest cavity and surrounds the heart. This air does not allow for the conduction of electricity and thus makes external paddles ineffective as a way to defibrillate a patient whose chest is open. In these situations, which usually occur due to trauma or surgery, internal paddles are the best way to deliver the current.

Now with the attending by my side congratulating me all the while, I grabbed the internal paddles, applied them to the patient's heart, and got ready to press the buttons that deliver the shock.

"Ready?" I asked, looking at the nurse.

"Ready," was her prompt reply, indicating that she had finished setting up the defibrillator.

"Clear!" I gave the signal to have everyone step away from the patient so as not to get shocked. A second later, I pressed the buttons on the paddle handles to deliver the shock.

For a split second, I pondered how great I was about to feel after saving this patient's life. This was the kind of case that we surgeons dream about and few have a chance to perform, let alone have the positive outcome of saving the patient's life. Even more impressive, I had performed the entire procedure by myself as the attending did not make it down to the trauma bay until the whole thing was done. The exhilaration I felt was intense. This was to be the crowning achievement of my general surgery residency and it was happening at the perfect time, during my last month of training. This was going to be a perfect ending to my residency story.

After I pressed the blue buttons on each paddle simultaneously, I could almost visualize the heart beginning to beat in rhythm. Everyone in the room expected that to happen as in a young heart, after such a short time of PEA, it was almost a sure thing that we should be able to convert the fibrillation to a normal rhythm. I saw the heart contract for one to two seconds as the current was delivered, but once the initial contraction passed, the heart continued its irregular fibrillation. As per the protocol of three consecutive shocks, I repeated two more shocks with increasing energy settings, but the heart rhythm did not change.

"Let's continue with ACLS protocol." I was still fully composed.

ACLS protocol calls for three consecutive shocks followed by intravenous medications that stabilize the heart muscle membrane and optimize such muscles to break the rhythm with the subsequent shocks. I continued compressions of the heart within my hands so as to allow the medication to circulate.

"Make sure to place the paddles correctly." This uttered from the attending in a calm, commanding voice.

"Clear!" Again, I pressed the buttons and saw the heart contract for one to two seconds and then promptly revert back to fibrillation.

"What's going on? This is not working." I was still composed and in control.

Someone suggested we try the external paddles, but the attending stated that the open chest would not allow for the electrical energy to reach the heart.

"Get another machine, and a new set of paddles." The attending's voice was still calm.

I resumed my compressions as the nurses scrambled to get everything ready. Blood was hanging by now along with the intravenous fluid and I could feel the fibrillating heart fill up with blood in my hands and then empty as I squeezed it out with my compressions. I would then release my fist and repeat the process.

While waiting for all to get ready, which took mere seconds, as the other machine and paddles were merely steps away, I once again had a flash come into my mind of how lucky I truly was to be able to experience saving this patient's life in such a dramatic fashion. I would be the only resident in my class to have done this. This procedure had a positive outcome in approximately one out of a thousand times tried. Who knows how long it had been since a resident had performed a successful emergency thoracotomy at Jackson Memorial Hospital. I knew Rio never got the chance. I mused as to how all residents and attendings in the department of surgery would somehow hear about what I had done. I was to be a hero.

"Clear!" Now we had a new machine, new paddles, and all was again ready. The nurse had made sure all the buttons were turned on and everything was connected. We were by now at the maximum recommended current for internal defibrillation. We had gotten a new machine and paddles to rule out any technical issues and thus I fully expected the heart to convert after the next shock. Inexplicably, the heart did not convert.

"Oh, come on!" Now I was no longer in control and everyone else was beginning to panic.

"Joe, you sure you are pressing the buttons?" The attending's voice showed great exasperation by this time as well.

"Of course, you see the heart contracting after I shock it," I replied in the affirmative with some irritation as the nursing staff kept trying to troubleshoot the issue. I continued my heart compressions with the heart's fibrillation now appearing visibly weaker. The attending asked for one of the defibrillators from the second floor to be brought down.

A couple of minutes later, one of the defibrillators from the trauma ICU, which looked just like the others, was brought down. Yet another new set of paddles was made ready and the situation repeated itself first with me holding the paddles, and then with the attending performing the task. At this point, with the heart fibrillation continuing to get weaker and weaker, we were all at a loss as to what to do; the situation seemed more surreal by the second. In between shocks, I continued to perform heart compressions all the while. We continued repeatedly to follow the ACLS protocol while desperately trying to figure out why we could not get the heart to convert.

Out of desperation, we decided to try still another machine. The attending approved the suggestion and also called for one from the hospital emergency room, which was not as far. Those two units were older and of different vintage and model, but they should do the trick. They both arrived simultaneously. By that time, however, the heart lay motionless in my hand with absolutely no contractions of any kind. We immediately deployed the internal paddles and shocked the heart several times but despite our efforts, it again failed to start.

Physicians choose their profession mainly due to a desire to help people. Surgeons choose their profession for similar reasons but also because with surgery, the help you can offer is often dramatic in scope and timing. In surgery, with your intellect and your hands, there is truly the possibility, in a matter of seconds, of saving someone's life. But even if not that dramatic, the positive outcomes of surgery can have an amazing, exhilarating, and rewarding effect on the surgeon. However, complications, the ultimate being death, can result in exquisite pain and have untold negative sequelae on the surgeon's psyche. In no other case in my career have I experienced such extremes of emotion as in this one case during my chief year trauma rotation. I went from the sheer exhilaration and self-validation of accomplishing something truly special to the depths of anguish, despondency, and self-doubt at not being able to see it through to the end.

I walked out of that room drained emotionally and in utter disbelief. We all felt the same and were walking around like zombies in an altered reality, not being able to fully comprehend what had just happened. While sitting at the trauma desk not knowing what to do next, Chris, with an empathetic look on his face, approached and put his hand on my shoulder. "Sorry, Joe! You tried your best. You can't win them all!"

To this day, I struggle with finding an explanation as to why our patient's heart did not convert to a normal rhythm. The patient and situation were ideal for it to happen, the execution was fast and flawless, the ACLS protocol was followed to the letter, and we even tried multiple defibrillator machines and paddles to rule out that as a potential issue. Despite our best efforts and no matter how hard we tried, our patient's heart would not start again when by all indications and probabilities, it should have. I've even considered the possibility that my hubris at celebrating the anticipated positive outcome before it happened might in some way have had something to do with the ultimate negative outcome.

I felt guilty for counting my chickens before they hatched. More importantly, however, I learned a most important lesson that day. Surgery is a science, but it has a component of art as well. Despite having the ideal situation and doing everything right, it does not necessarily mean that all will be well at the end. Sometimes for inexplicable reasons, and despite your best efforts to the contrary, things do not go as they should. When involved in these situations and particularly when the negative outcome results in a fatality, the emotional swing for the surgeon can be extreme and psychologically devastating.

Minutes later, I was called to go see the patient's family who had just arrived. Looking into the mother's crying eyes, I told her that her son had been stabbed in the heart with a screwdriver and despite our best efforts, we had not been able to save him. What was left unsaid that day has haunted me for years ever since. Sometimes I think that my failure to relate the full story was the ultimate act of mercy in not telling a grieving mother about how close we had been to saving her son and the inexplicable reason we had not been able to. At other times, I think it was the ultimate act of cowardice for not owning up to my epic failure. As time passes, I have come to the painful conclusion that the reason was most likely the latter. I will live with that realization and burden for the rest of my life.

A life was lost that for all accounts should have been saved. I will forever feel guilty for the thoughts of personal glory that flashed through my mind while in the act of attempting to save my patient's life. I can't help but think that I might have performed that much better if my mind was clear of everything else except for the tasks I was performing on my patient's behalf. For all I know, that might have made the difference that could have led to saving his life. At the end of the day and no matter the reason, I was solely responsible for the negative outcome, and will live forever with my memory of the resulting mental anguish.

THE LAST MAN STANDING

Finally, the last rotation of my chief year arrived. The trauma two-month rotation had not changed much since my previous exposure to that service. Due to the new rules implemented by the CIR negotiated contract, call was now every third day, but the clinical responsibilities were still the same. These responsibilities included taking care of all emergency patients coming to the hospital, both in the surgical emergency room and those injured patients who came through the trauma center. The only difference now was that I was rotating as a chief resident and in charge of one of the teams. Although I very much looked forward to these last two months of my residency, the rotation started off on a rough note with my failure to save the patient with the stab wound to the heart. That episode took the wind out of my sails for several days. However, in time, I was able to recover and genuinely enjoy what was left of the rotation and appreciate what it portended for my future as a surgeon.

From the first day I took over the service, I noted I was being treated differently to the way I had been treated during my past rotations on that service. Everyone, including medical students, interns, junior residents, and even the attending staff showed me a certain extra level of deference that I had not experienced before, including in my other rotations during my chief year. It was as if everyone suddenly simultaneously recognized that I was about to go through a metamorphosis and reach a different stratum in my professional development. I was very much aware and was anxiously anticipating the impending completion of my training, but to me that was a mere formality. I was going through a metamorphosis for sure, but while to me it was five years in the making, the way people treated me during my last rotation seemed as if they perceived it to be of a more drastic nature, like I had all of a sudden arrived at my destination. It was as if they all in unison suddenly realized that I was about to undergo a long-standing rite of passage—going from resident to attending surgeon.

The first month on the service, the changes in the way I was being treated were apparent but subtle. During the last month, however, the change became progressively starker. I noted this in all hospital personnel I came into contact with, but most profoundly in the way the attending staff dealt with me. During the last month on the service, the attendings did not feel the need to be in the room with me for every case, whether scrubbed or hovering. As my tenure got towards the end, it was not unusual for the attending to retire to his/her on-call room with instructions for me to call in case I needed help. The attending instructions went from "Call me when you are in the operating room," which universally meant that they would come participate in the case, to "Call me if you need me," which meant they would not show up in the operating room unless I requested their presence. I got the sense that allowing the chief resident to fly solo during the last couple of weeks of the residency was an integral part of the surgical training. After all, many of my coresidents were already functioning as general surgeons in the community.

This would put the onus on me to call whenever I thought I needed it, but at the same time allowed me the freedom to perform most of the cases by myself, with Chris Castrellon, the fourth-year resident from the US Air Force as my assistant. I loved working with him, as we had similar personalities and worked synergistically in the operating room. In our free time in between cases, Chris and I would often retire to the cafeteria or the sandwich shop in front of the trauma center and sneak a few minutes of conversation to discuss issues related to the service, but also other issues of mutual interest like boating, fishing, etc.

The last month of my residency, I was walking on air and having the time of my life. I had successfully surgically treated Terri Neely for a bout of intestinal obstruction, and had seen her go home several days later, fully recovered. Furthermore, I was working with a great team, made that much better when Ramiro Beguiristain, the medical student whom I recruited in the elevator to help me in the vascular rotation, decided to come and rotate with us for one of his electives during his senior year. It turned out that the previous year he had to deal with a family health emergency that necessitated taking a year off from medical school. I was extremely happy to welcome him to the trauma service as I always loved working with him.

The cases I got to do those last two months offered great variety and an optimal level of complexity for my level of training. Moreover, I was allowed to do a fair number of them by myself without the direct supervision of an attending, enabling me to develop a great feeling of confidence and the assurance that I could walk out the day after my training was over and perform proficiently as a general surgery attending in any setting. My plan, however, was to stay at Jackson Memorial Hospital and continue on to a two-year residency in plastic surgery. However, knowing that I felt comfortable and competent to perform as a general surgeon was exhilarating. After all, I had devoted by now five years of my life to reach that plateau.

As I drove in for my last day of the rotation and in fact, my residency, I was in a very jovial, energized mood and felt an underlying current of something pivotal happening in my life. It was a bittersweet feeling of being about to accomplish a great life goal, yet at the same time knowing that life as I had known it for the past five years was about to change drastically and forever. I was about to live my last day as a general surgery resident.

Fully realizing that the following week I was to transition to a plastic surgery residency, I was very much aware that I was no longer going to get to do cases that were routine for me in general surgery. Thus, this was my last day to get my fill. Very much like a starving man in front of an all-you-can-eat buffet, I was determined to make my last day count. I was keen to do as many good cases as I could get in. Not only to get my fill, but also to prove to myself once and for all that I had indeed accomplished my goal of becoming a competent, self-sufficient general surgeon. The day could not have started any better. During the trauma service change-over rounds, I learned that there were several cases on the docket lined up for me to tackle.

Mr. Gimenez was a gentleman in his mid-fifties who had experienced two prior episodes of diverticulitis. He had presented to the emergency room the previous evening with left lower quadrant abdominal pain, signaling his third episode. He had been evaluated and diagnosed with acute diverticulitis and had been admitted to the medical service for routine medical treatment of his condition. However, over the previous night, his pain had worsened, and he developed peritoneal signs. The trauma fellow had evaluated the patient right before rounds and had diagnosed a surgical abdomen. The case had been booked for me to do first thing in the morning.

Diverticula are small out-pouchings that sometimes occur in the bowel wall. Although they can happen anywhere in the intestinal tract, the most common anatomical location is the large bowel toward the end in a region called the sigmoid colon, which topographically is located in the left lower quadrant of the abdomen. Pain in this area, particularly in patients already diagnosed with diverticulosis, can indicate an inflammatory process of these out-pouchings. This condition is called acute diverticulitis and is normally treated with bowel rest (nothing by mouth) and intravenous antibiotics. Peritoneal signs in the setting of acute diverticulitis can mean potential bowel perforation and thus surgical exploration is indicated.

Just as trauma rounds finished, Dr. Scott Conner, the attending who was to be on call with me for that last day, approached me and told me to call him once I entered the abdomen so that he could see what was going on. I took this as a very good sign, as I surmised that he was going to give me plenty of leeway to run my own show that day, something that I very much wanted to do, if only to prove to myself that I could. Chris and I immediately headed for the preoperative holding area so that we could meet our patient and examine him.

It was easy to see that Mr. Gimenez was sick. He did not seem comfortable, had an NG tube connected to wall suction, IV fluids were running, and he was lying in bed quietly in obvious distress, with his wife by his side. After introducing myself and getting the best history I could out of him, I proceeded to examine him so as to prove to myself he had surgical indications. His abdomen was distended, and he exhibited significant guarding and rebound tenderness, particularly in the left lower quadrant. I went over his diagnosis again with him and his wife and explained the likely outcome of the surgery: a colostomy. When I explained that a colostomy is a procedure in which we bring a loop of bowel through the skin and that he would need to wear a stool bag for several months until the colostomy was reversed, he and his wife became somewhat alarmed.

"Why not treat him like the other two times with fluids and antibiotics?" The wife seemed even more distressed than our patient.

"Because his physical findings are telling us that this time the infection is a lot more severe and to the point that we are worried that he might have a bowel perforation. If that were to happen and we are late in intervening, he can get extremely sick and even die." I assured them that this was the right thing to do. There was really no other option and the sooner we operated the better.

With my explanation, both Mr. Gimenez and his wife relented and promptly agreed to proceed with the surgery. As this case was already scheduled and ready to go, it did not take long for us to be in the operating room with my first case of my last day. In my mind, I pretended that I was already a general surgeon, finished with my residency, and out working in the community. It was not to be so for me, but it was to be the typical scenario for three of the six of us chief residents in our class. Tony Cicilio and I had decided to stay at Jackson Memorial to complete our fellowships and Tracy Trott had decided to pursue her fellowship in colorectal surgery at another institution. The other three residents in my class had decided not to pursue further training and had already gone off two weeks prior to fill private practice jobs. Some of them, even that same day or at least shortly thereafter, were to be in this same scenario as I was, taking care of their own patients, although no longer as residents, but as attending surgeons. I mentally put myself in their shoes to see how I would fare.

By this last day of my rotation, Chris and I had gelled beautifully and were having lots of fun working together. Having Ramiro now rotating with us was like icing on the cake. Thus, it was with great zest and zeal that the three of us undertook this case. I apologized to Chris in advance for doing most, if not all of this case, as I explained to him what I wanted to accomplish. He completely understood and told me that he was happy to play my assistant all day long if I wanted to. I told him not to worry, I would let him take the lead on some of the other cases already on the docket for that day.

After entering the abdomen through a lower midline incision, we found the left lower quadrant to be a huge inflammatory mess. It took us a significant amount of time and considerable difficulty to dissect the inflamed, matted sigmoid colon free of all adjacent tissues. Thankfully, we did not find any frank perforations of the bowel wall. However, the affected segment of bowel was grossly inflamed, and I thought it best to resect it so as to avoid potential future rupture. I thought this was the appropriate time to invite Dr. Conner into the room as he requested so that I could tell him what I was about to do.

Dr. Conner walked in but did not scrub. He was holding his untied mask to his face when he peered over Chris's shoulder on the other side of the table from me. I showed him the released inflamed sigmoid colon and explained to him where I was planning on doing my resection. I told him of my plan to leave the far (distal) end stapled off in the lower abdomen (mucous fistula) and bring out the proximal (near) end through the left lower quadrant abdominal wall as a colostomy.

"Proceed." This was all he said as he promptly turned around and walked out of the room. Watching him do this felt really good as it meant he had enough confidence in me to allow me to proceed without scrubbing and staying in the room to watch my every step.

After releasing the mesenteric (root) attachments of the sigmoid colon, we stapled off both ends in adjacent healthy colon and delivered the specimen off to the back table. After washing out the abdomen, we chose the correct spot for the colostomy and made a perforation on the abdominal wall, through which we brought out the now released loop of bowel. We finished suturing the colostomy and closing the abdomen without any issues. Chris and Ramiro both seemed genuinely happy with my performance on the case and told me so. Their comments were well-received indeed.

Having this case under my belt, I felt satisfied enough to take a back seat and help Chris do two laparoscopic gall bladder removals (laparoscopic cholecystectomies) and even walked our grateful intern through an appendectomy (removal of an inflamed appendix). By late afternoon, our team had done several cases and, it being a weekend night, I anticipated some great trauma cases for the evening fare. I was not to wait long.

At around nine o'clock that evening, a patient was brought to the trauma center with a slash wound with knife to the abdominal area. The patient was stable the entire time and at first the wound seemed superficial and would not require a trip to the operating room. However, a peritoneal lavage, the procedure that is done to assess the possibility of intra-abdominal injury, turned out to be positive, indicating that he would need surgical exploration of the abdomen.

Once again, Chris, Ramiro, and I were in the operating room together, this time working on a real trauma case. The patient being thin, it did not take us long to enter his abdomen. Upon entering, I immediately noted blood inside the abdomen, which indicated the knife had perforated the abdominal wall. It did not take us long to find an injury in the small bowel and the adjacent mesentery. We temporarily placed a clamp in the hole so as to prevent further spillage of intestinal contents and proceeded to run the bowels and search for other injuries. We found none. We went back to the injured bowel and made the assessment that the injury of small bowel and mesentery could be repaired and did not require a resection. After cleaning the area, I securely sutured both of the bowel holes, washed the abdomen, and closed. Another great case finished for the day. This one in particular I managed all by myself, this time just with a courtesy call to the attending, who never came into the room.

It was close to midnight by the time we finished this case and had the patient tucked in. I suggested to Chris and Ramiro that we take a food break. We got some sandwiches and drinks and decided to go eat at the trauma resident library, located on the second floor of the trauma center. We found ourselves all alone in the library and had a great time eating and talking as we anticipated a great night of operating together. Sitting in the large, comfortable library recliners, soon our conversation shifted to talking about the future. Chris and Ramiro were both finishing their rotations the following day as well. Chris was traveling back to his base at Biloxi, Mississippi, to start his chief resident year. Ramiro had a week off before starting another elective rotation. They were both extremely interested in what it felt like to be finished with residency. I tried my best to put my feelings into words for them, as they tried to picture themselves in my shoes. Within one year, they would both be going through similar experiences. Chris, like me, would be finishing his general surgery training and Ramiro, medical school. As we talked about accomplishments, personal pride, and future plans, I felt myself drifting off to sleep.

At 5:30 a.m. my watch alarm went off and I woke up still in the chair, but now all alone in the room. I surmised that Chris and Ramiro had already started doing rounds on the floor, so I decided to go to the on-call room to freshen up and brush my teeth before doing my rounds in the ICU and preparing for trauma morning report. As I walked out of the library, I happened to see Ramiro coming down the hallway on his way to the elevator.

"Isn't that unbelievable, not one trauma alert the entire night." While saying this, I tried to remember the last time I had slept undisturbed through a trauma call night and realized that this had never happened to me before. It was as if the whole world knew it was my last night and decided to take a rest.

"I don't know what you are talking about, Skippy. Chris and I have been operating all night." Ramiro uttered the words with a huge smile on his face. He had recently started calling me Skippy on occasion. Ramiro called everyone he liked Skippy, so it made me happy to hear him call me that. I immediately and instinctively reached for my beeper and noted it was off.

"Crap! Sorry, bro. My battery must have died."

Again, with a smile on his face: "I turned your beeper off after you fell asleep, Skippy. Chris and I thought the best we could do for you on your last day was to let you sleep undisturbed. But don't you worry, the attending knows. We had his blessings."

That day, trauma morning report was uniquely pleasant. I came into the room to receive many heartfelt good wishes and warm handshakes and sat in the back of the room as Chris insisted on taking the podium to present all the patients from the previous day and night. I felt extremely satisfied that we were leaving the incoming team with a well-managed service. All operated patients were on their way to a full recovery and most importantly, we were not leaving any disasters or sick patients behind that would need to be cared for by the new team. I felt satisfied and proud of a job well done by a great team.

As Chris was about to start his presentation, Dr. Conner got up and stopped him. "I want to take this opportunity to thank and congratulate Joe on completing his general surgery residency as of today, and also for performing brilliantly for the last two months and his last day on call. As most of his fellow chief residents already left two weeks ago, I want to specially note that he worked until the last day. Out of his class, he is the last man standing."

As everyone in the room looked at me, smiled, and clapped, Dr. Conner ended his remarks:

"Joe, as of this moment, you are no longer a resident. Chris can take it from here. You are officially dismissed."

Once again, everyone smiled and applauded as if on cue. I stood up, took a bow, and exited the room.

Walking towards the parking garage I felt a great sense of personal satisfaction and immense pride. It was one of the few times in my life when I literally felt as if I were walking on air. The mood I was in can best be described as sublime. While pondering the words of Dr. Conner, for which I was most grateful, I then thought of Tony Cicilio. He was the other resident in my year who, like me, was to stay at Jackson Memorial Hospital to complete a fellowship. I had chosen plastic surgery and he had decided on transplant surgery, like his father. Because we were to continue on at Jackson, we had been "volunteered" by our fellow chief residents to end our year with the two rotations that would require us to work until the last day. I was to do trauma and Tony was scheduled for the VA hospital rotation.

Without a doubt and by a long shot, Tony Cicilio was the hardest working and most dedicated resident in our class. As sure as I was walking toward the garage at that moment, I knew he would be rounding at the VA hospital and would stay there as long as necessary to make sure his replacement was well-versed on all the patients on his service and fully up to speed with all pending matters on those patients. It was he, much more than I, who was truly deserving of the grand title of "the last man standing."

Reflections On Becoming A Surgeon

The first of July 2001 happened to be a Sunday. As I drove home that morning after being excused from trauma change-over rounds, I pondered how for the first time in a long time, I was literally unemployed and free of any job responsibilities. I would remain thus for a full twenty-four hours until I was to report for my first day of plastic surgery training the following day at seven a.m. Sure, I had taken multiple vacations during my general surgery residency, but no matter how far away I traveled, I never could completely clear my mind of my ongoing responsibilities, pending surgeries, upcoming rotations, etc. This time and for the next twenty-four hours, it was to be different. I was about to start training in an altogether different specialty and even if I wanted to, legally I was not able to step foot at Jackson Memorial Hospital, as for that day I no longer worked there.

Driving the short distance from the hospital to my apartment in Miami Beach, after having slept a full night, I found myself full of nervous energy with a multitude of thoughts and feelings. I was to have a celebratory dinner with my family that Sunday evening but until then, I was completely free of anything to do. In a very introspective and emotional mood due to the many profound changes happening in my life at that time, I thought it best instead of going home, to drive some place where I could take some time to collect my thoughts and clear my mind. Thus, I searched for the gym bag I kept in my car trunk, and after changing from my scrubs into my shorts, I drove directly to South Beach.

It promised to be a warm, typically sunny Florida summer day, and as I got to the beach early in the morning, I had it all pretty much to myself. I walked into the warm water and dove into it headfirst. I then floated on my back in the waves for what seemed like hours as many thoughts simultaneously rushed to my head. I attempted to quiet my mind and ponder what the last five years of becoming a surgeon really meant, just as today, almost twenty years after that day and a full twenty-five years since I started my residency, I once again quiet my thoughts to ponder what the last twenty years of being a surgeon has truly meant to me, not only professionally but also intellectually and emotionally as a human being.

Being a good student, college was always in the cards for me. However, as I entered college, I was not yet fully focused and wrestled with what to do with my life. My mother, who was born into a family of a long line of physicians, lovingly always tried to nudge me toward medicine and often encouraged me to become a "professional man" like my father. He, having come from a much more modest family of salesmen and clerks, never tried to push me toward any particular career, let alone medicine or surgery. His advice was always that I should try to find something to do that was worthwhile, but which I could be passionate about. He further encouraged me to try to explore as many potential careers and fields of endeavor as possible, to be able to make an educated decision. Toward that end, at the University of Florida I joined a club called PSO (Preprofessional Service Organization), which was devoted to offering exposure to the health fields of medicine and dentistry to interested college students.

PSO also sponsored meetings, where speakers representing different specialties exposed us to what it was like to practice their chosen profession. During one of those meetings, a gentleman came to speak to us about what it was like to be a general surgeon. I will never forget his opening words when he said, "I am a surgeon by trade"—words that appeared contradictory at face value. Of course, all of the students in the audience knew that surgery was a profession and not a trade. It turns out that we were all wrong; it is actually both.

My father, like me, was also a surgeon by trade. As a matter of fact, for many years he was the only surgeon in our town of about fifty thousand people on the southern coast of Cuba. From as early as I can remember, I recollect more times that I can count, my father being called away from the dinner table, family gatherings, and awakened from his bed to go care for a sick patient in need. Not once did I ever hear him complain or in any way begrudge or fail to fulfill his personal responsibility and oath as a doctor. By the time we emigrated to the United States, my father was already too old and, with a family and two small children, had too many responsibilities to embark on another general surgery residency. For many years, he worked in a state hospital near Jacksonville, Florida, where with a limited license he was allowed to practice minor surgery. Eventually he was promoted to an administrative position at the same institution, one that he felt compelled to accept so he could bring more prosperity to his family, but that at the same time took him away from direct patient care.

Several years later, now of advancing age, my father started picking up shifts at a local VA hospital covering their surgical ICU overnight. At the time, I did not quite understand why he was doing this and assumed it was for financial reasons. We were never a wealthy family, but we did not have any concerns about regular living expenses as a typical middle-class family, so his decision to take call at the VA hospital did not make sense to me. When I asked my father why he felt compelled to take this extra work at his age, his unexpected answer spoke volumes of his love for his vocation.

"Son…" he said, "…that is the only way I can go back to taking care of patients again, something that I miss terribly. A surgeon is not just something that I do, it is what I am."

At that time, I did not fully appreciate the full meaning of his words, nor the passion he felt for his chosen profession.

Sometime during my late twenties, I came to my own personal fork in the road. I was finishing my four years of training in oral surgery after having completed four years of dental school and one year of a general practice hospital dental residency. It was then that I became painfully aware that the career path I was on would not take me to the place where I wanted to be professionally. I hoped to acquire the advanced expertise and ability to care for the soft and hard tissue of the face in order to treat children and adults with complex and severe craniofacial deformities and injuries. This realization was profound, for if I were able to reach what had by that time become my true passion and dream, it would mean that I would have to go back and complete medical school, then general surgery, followed by plastic surgery, and finally a year of craniofacial fellowship. Altogether, this was an investment of another twelve years of education and training, in addition to the nine years I had already invested after college.

It took me a while to fully come to terms with the reality of the situation and the consequences of the decision I was pondering. When I finally did, as I always did on important matters, I reached out to my father for his opinion. He did not take long before giving me the sagest advice: "No question you should pursue your dream no matter how long it takes, and the sacrifice involved. I will always be here to help you in any way I can." He further opined: "Son, if you are lucky like me, you will live a long life. I can't think of a greater tragedy for any person than to endeavor for years in a job or profession that they do not enjoy or for which they do not have any passion."

Surgery is a profession because it requires formal advanced education to learn certain concepts and theory, but it is also a trade, because the way surgeons learn their craft is more akin to an apprenticeship, where the skills learned are taught by experienced surgeons and mentors who teach by doing. As a profession, surgery provides a certain level of respect, prestige, and standard of living. But the process of becoming a surgeon is so grueling, both physically and mentally, that those who enter it seeking these superficial rewards usually desist and drop out either during residency or soon thereafter. They find that the price they are asked to pay for the privilege is way too dear.

However, it has been my experience after having worked and interacted with multiple surgeons at all levels of training and abilities, that for those who endure and practice surgery with zest and zeal, those financial and superficial benefits are not what appeals to them at the core. There are other intangibles that are much more personal and offer a much deeper and profound level of motivation and satisfaction. If one is lucky, our mentors and surgeons whom we learn the trade from will impart some of those values in us as part of the process of teaching us to become surgeons.

Surgery is up-close, intimate, and violates all personal boundaries. Moreover, it offers a particular mix of both intellectual and physical challenges and gratifications. Surgeons are doers, men and women not afraid to get their gloves dirty with blood, bodily fluids, and tissues in order to fight a deeply personal, hand-to-hand battle with disease and injury, so as to benefit their patients. When things do not go well in surgery, resulting in bad outcomes, complications, and God forbid, loss of life, surgeons experience deeply personal, gut-wrenching, and severe emotional pain and self-doubt, which can be hard to imagine or describe. However, when surgeries go right and lead to cures, amelioration of symptoms or pain, or lives saved, surgeons can experience deep and even spiritual, emotional exhilaration and self-validation rarely experienced by those in other human endeavors or professions. These emotions are satisfying beyond measure and deeply cherished by all surgeons alike. The ability to help others, particularly those who entrust us with their most valued possession—their health, and their lives or that of their loved ones—is indeed a very noble and lofty endeavor to dedicate one's life to. This is the essence of what it means to be a surgeon. It is the lofty, higher calling that surgeons are extremely grateful to be able to participate in and dedicate their lives to.

My father was diagnosed with Alzheimer's disease shortly before I started my general surgery residency. Over the ensuing years, his condition progressively deteriorated to the point that by the time I finished my five-year residency, his mental faculties had left him and he was not able to fully comprehend what I was saying when I triumphantly told him that I had finished my training, in no small part thanks to his advice. Had he been able to understand my remarks, I know he would have been very proud, not only because I had achieved something special and had followed in his footsteps, but especially because his son had taken his advice and somehow found the drive, motivation, and endurance to pursue his dream no matter the sacrifice. Of that, we could both be proud. I finished my general surgery residency the morning of July 1, 2001. My father passed away nine days later, the evening of July tenth.

Due to an early acceptance to dental school, I do not have a college degree. However, I do have two professional degrees, dentistry and medicine, and proudly hold three surgical boards: general surgery, oral surgery, and plastic surgery. For all three, I eagerly undertook the challenge of the written and oral exams required to achieve the original board certification, and later, the written exams required for the ten-year recertification. For oral surgery and plastic surgery, this sacrifice made sense because I currently practice those two professions. However, for general surgery, board certification for me was not necessary as it was never to be part of my practice. Regardless, I did it as a validation of what I consider to be my life's most important academic and professional accomplishment, as becoming a general surgeon required the most personal effort and sacrifice by far.

I proudly display my board certificates in my office. Although I value all three of them, it is the general surgery certificate that I contemplate and reflect on when my spirits falter due to the challenges of being in the practice of surgery. When disheartened, discouraged, or feeling "less than," I look at that certificate with pride. It reminds me of the time when I felt that with the knowledge gained, the skills acquired, and a number ten surgical blade in my hands, I could, all by myself, save the world.

GRADUATION SPEECH

Not wanting to get too emotional, I will reserve my comments for my family for a more private setting. I do, however, want to say a few words. The last five years, without a doubt, have been the best five years of my life. As was mentioned earlier in the introduction, my journey here has been a long one. However, it was here at Jackson for the first time along that road that I felt at home and that I truly belonged. The surgery program at Jackson Memorial Hospital is truly top notch and only getting better. No matter where my professional path takes me, I will always mention with pride that I trained here in general surgery. That is something we can all be proud of.

I would like to thank Dr. Willoughby and the attending staff for teaching me and my fellow residents the art and science of surgery. One of the greatest strengths of this program is the people that make it up. They provide for an excellent working environment where education and learning are paramount. I would also like to thank the nursing and ancillary staff who through their efforts helped us take care of the sick and injured.

Finally, and specially, I would like to thank my fellow residents. First, I would like to thank those residents that came before us who, by example, taught us what to do and not to do. My fellow chief residents for their friendship and support, and particularly the junior residents, who through their efforts and hard work, allowed my fellow chief residents and I the time and freedom to concentrate on learning surgery. I hope they had as much fun working with me, as I had working with them. For me it was also a solemn honor to have had the opportunity to work and serve with them. Thank you, one and all, very much.

Joe Garri
June 2001

EPILOGUE

The final editing process of this book took place in the midst of the 2020 coronavirus pandemic, nearly twenty-five years after I first started documenting the events depicted in it and twenty years after the completion of my general surgery residency. During this process, I had the chance to read multiple times each and every chapter, some of which I had not read for quite some time as they had been completed years prior. As I relived the stories and experiences recounted in this book, I was struck by no matter how unique these particular experiences and people involved have been to me, the themes that these stories represent are universal, timeless, and apropos today in the middle of this terrible worldwide plague.

As the numbers of those afflicted grow each day and the stories in the press tell of the experience of those sick and dying, and their families, I can't help but be reminded of the people and events that this book recounts. As unique as this pandemic is to most of us living it, the health, ethical, and even humanitarian issues that it raises are not unfamiliar to those in the healthcare fields. From dealing with the insurmountable amount of work required to care for the sick, to the ethical implications of having to decide how to allocate limited resources, to the real-life danger of healthcare workers falling victim to communicable diseases, these are all universal themes that each and every healthcare provider comes face-to-face with during the course of their careers, surgeons particularly so.

Most striking of these themes is the nobility of the healing professions and those who devote their life to them. When humanity is stricken by sickness and suffering, there are those who out of a deep calling, respond to that need. Even when facing the possibility of personal harm or even death, they put on their uniforms, lab coats, and scrubs, and quietly but resolutely march toward the front lines to do their part in providing care for those afflicted. We see them do this whether personally or on television; we read about them and we listen to their stories. We witness their nobility and are inspired by it. I am proud to be the son of one of them, glad to have gotten to know a lot of them, and thankful to have the opportunity to proudly serve alongside many of them. Indeed, I am proud to humbly count myself as one of them. Most of all, however, I am grateful to have had the opportunity to answer my calling and fulfill my dream of becoming a surgeon.

Joe Garri
April 2020

APPENDIX A

THE EVOLUTION OF SURGICAL TRAINING IN THE UNITED STATES

by
Elena Sheppard

Courage, ingenuity, dexterity, resourcefulness, are such prominent characteristics of our countrymen that it would have been surprising if from the labors or her many earnest and devoted teachers and practitioners there had not resulted contributions to the science and art of surgery which have carried the fame of American surgery throughout the civilized world.

— William S. Halsted, Yale University, June 27, 1904

The word *surgery* is derived from the Greek *cheirourgos,* meaning "working by hand." Surgery has existed in some form or another throughout the history of man. During the Roman Empire, both Galen and Celsus—renowned physicians of their time—preached the importance of surgery; trepanation—making a hole through the skull to treat a variety of diseases—was practiced as long ago as the Neolithic period and can be placed to such far off corners of the world as Ancient Greece, the Far East, Africa, and North and South America. As for surgery in the United States, the practice dates to colonial times, and was formalized via the 1766 formation of The Medical Society of New Jersey, the first organization of medical professionals in the colonies. Even so, The Medical Society of New Jersey was not a place to train surgeons; it was designed as a place to regulate and license practitioners. The actual formalization of a training process was not introduced until much later.

Until roughly the mid-nineteenth century, the most common method of training surgeons was through apprenticeships, during which students learned how to perform surgery through observation and imitation. Apprenticeships were variable and not standardized, but as the country creeped toward the twentieth century all that began to change—much of that thanks to a surgeon named Dr. William S. Halsted.

The nineteenth century was a highly prolific era for surgical history, during which roughly 100 new surgeries and surgical techniques were created. Dr. Halsted led the change in America toward formalizing and structuring the training process. At the turn of the nineteenth century, Dr. Halsted was the chairman of the Department of Surgery at Johns Hopkins University. In 1897, he introduced the idea of a surgical residency, based on the German model of training surgeons that he had observed while studying in Europe. There were a few core principles to his training model:

- The resident must have intense and repetitive opportunities to take care of surgical patients under the supervision of a skilled surgical teacher.
- The resident must acquire an understanding of the scientific basis of the surgical disease.
- The resident must acquire skills in patient management and technical operations of increasing complexity with graded enhanced responsibility and independence.

In a famous address given at his thirtieth college reunion at Yale, Dr. Halsted described the surgical resident training program he had devised: Interns served for six years as assistants to a resident surgeon and two years as a house physician before they could take on the position of resident surgeon themselves. He also mandated surgical training that involved original research. His training model quickly began to spread across the country.

While Dr. Halsted's training model yielded countless beneficial attributes with respect to surgical training and patient care, there was one aspect of his model that proved detrimental: the relentless work schedule it instituted. Dr. Halsted promoted a highly restrictive lifestyle, which had residents living and working in the hospital, and essentially being on call every hour of every day all year long. In hindsight, Dr. Halsted himself may have been able to keep this pace due to his reported addiction to cocaine. In 1884, he read a report about the potential anesthetic qualities of cocaine, and he began to experiment on himself. Those experiments eventually contributed to the creation of local and regional anesthesia. They also led to Dr. Halsted's lifelong cocaine addiction, which he tried to treat various times to no avail.

The formalization of the surgical training process also led to the establishment of important professional organizations, which became the bedrock for surgical education from that time forward. In 1913, the American College of Surgeons (ACS) was founded as an organization dedicated to the ethical practice and standardization of care. It was also founded to improve training opportunities for surgeons. Relatedly, the Council on Medical Education and the American Medical Association (AMA) were among the first organizations to standardize graduate medical education. In 1927, the ACS published a set of surgical education standards, the *Fundamental Requirements for Graduate Training in Surgery,* which became a cornerstone of surgical education moving forward.

In 1937, the American Board of Surgery (ABS) was founded to establish a comprehensive certification process as a means of protecting the public and improving the specialty. By 1940, the AMA, ACS, and ABS had joined forces to create the ACS's *Manual of Graduate Training in Surgery,* which lays forth the minimum standard for graduate training in surgery. The ACS also produced a list of 200 US and Canadian hospitals that met their standards. In 1950, the Residency Review Committee in Surgery (RRCS) was established and the surgical certification and accreditation process was split between the ABS and RRCS.

To ensure that all these guidelines were standardized and coordinated, the Coordinating Council of Medical Education was established in 1972, ultimately leading to the Accreditation Council for Graduate Medical Education (ACGME) in 1982. The ACGME has made several landmark changes to graduate education, including shifting focus onto evaluation of outcomes, as well as establishing guidelines under which residents work. The ACGME also introduced six core competencies that residents must achieve:

- Medical knowledge
- Patient care
- Interpersonal and communication skills
- Professionalism
- Practice-based learning and improvement
- Systems-based practice

Surgical training, historically speaking, included a broad curriculum where residents received exposure and training in multiple areas of the body and in disciplines that are now considered subspecialties. The term "general surgery" was not a category in the ACS directory until 1965. Today, general surgery is mostly confined to surgery of the abdominal cavity as the field of surgery has greatly diversified. The current trends in surgical education lean towards specialization. Currently more than eighty percent of surgical residents go on to pursue fellowships in subspecialties. The trajectory now is that after completing medical school, a general surgeon goes into a five-year residency program. After that, a subspecialty fellowship can be completed, the lengths of which vary depending on the particular discipline. For instance, colorectal surgery or laparoscopic surgery requires one additional year of training, while subspecialties such as trauma/critical care and cardiothoracic surgery require fellowships that are two years long. Plastic surgery is currently a three-year fellowship. Through the years, these trends toward specialization have allowed surgeons to develop and perfect techniques for the area of the body or pathologic conditions on which they concentrate.

In 2002, the ACS, RRCS, ABS, and American Surgical Association (ASA) joined forces to appoint a Blue Ribbon Committee on Surgical Education, which in 2004 put forth a slew of recommendations for those studying medicine and interested in specializing in surgery. One of the changes was that fourth-year medical students who wanted to study surgery would be focused on preparing for surgical training. The Blue Ribbon Committee also suggested executing a nationwide standardized curriculum for surgical residency. This resulted in the formation of the Surgical Council on Resident Education (SCORE), which is a voluntary consortium focused on the improvement of surgical education through standardization. Under current ABS and RRCS standards, surgical residency is now sixty months of training at an accredited program, with fifty-four of those months devoted to clinical training. Forty-two of those months are considered essential and, in order to graduate, residents must log a minimum of 750 major operative cases.

Surgeon scientists are an integral part of academic surgery and contribute to the understanding of diseases and the innovation of new therapies, procedures, and treatments. In addition to the five years of surgical training, surgery residents interested in research or academic careers can opt to spend one or two extra research years during their residency participating in either clinical or basic science research. One exemplar of the surgeon-scientist is Dr. Joseph E. Murray who in 1954 performed the first successful organ transplant, when he transplanted a healthy kidney from one identical twin into the body of the other. In 1990, Dr. Murray was awarded the Nobel Prize in Physiology and Medicine. He is the most recent of four surgeons to receive that honor.

An inflection point in medical (and surgical) residency training occurred in 1984, when an eighteen-year-old college student in New York City named Libby Zion died in a hospital under circumstances that many deemed unnecessary. She was admitted to the hospital with a high fever and jerking movements and went on to expire the following morning. After her death, the patient's parents sought an investigation into the particulars of their daughter's medical treatment. They learned that the only doctors who participated in Libby's care were residents, and that those residents worked thirty-six-hour shifts on a regular basis. These findings led some to believe that errors made by overworked and tired residents might have resulted in Libby's demise.

The case eventually went to trial and the legacy of it was a change in resident training, particularly as it related to the number of hours that residents were expected to work. Residents were thereafter to work no more than eighty hours per week, and no more than twenty-four hours in a row. More direct supervision was also implemented. The Committee of Interns and Residents union (CIR) was integral in the codification of these changes. The CIR was established in NYC in 1957 and was the first union in the United States to represent interns and residents. CIR has played a significant role in negotiating contracts between residents and training institutions through the years and has grown to the point that it now represents thousands of residents in multiple states throughout the nation.

Over the last few decades, the biggest change in surgery has been the development of minimally invasive techniques such as laparoscopy and endovascular surgery. While these techniques often lead to better outcomes and faster recovery for patients, they also require more advanced technological training for surgeons. More recent, and perhaps more dramatic, changes are due to the impact of robotics on the field. Robots have revolutionized surgery in situations like thoracic or pelvic surgery where exposure and access are an issue due to anatomical considerations. With respect to surgical education, simulators have been developed that offer a great advantage in terms of acquisition of new skills, and assessment of young surgeons. National efforts are currently underway to standardize simulation-based surgical skills.

The number of those who go into the field make it as competitive as ever. In 2019, there were 1,432 (categorical) general surgery residency positions available throughout the United States and every one of those positions was filled. Surgery, which has long been a field dominated by men, remains that way but changes are slowly occurring. According to 2017 numbers amassed by the Association of American Medical Colleges (AAMC), the percentage of active surgeons who are male is 79.4 percent, meaning women make up 20.6 percent, a number that is progressively increasing as more female medical students opt to become surgeons.

Much of what Dr. Halsted imposed during the early days of formalized surgical education in terms of concentrated, focused training has withstood the test of time and remains the same to this day. Nonetheless, medicine and the specialty of general surgery are forever evolving. Advancements in gene therapy, individualized antibody therapy for solid tumors, and new technologies may very well herald the day when certain operations, such as large cancer resections, will become a thing of the past.

However, there will always be a vital need for the specialty of general surgery. The specialty's evolution will most likely lead to more targeted, less-invasive procedures resulting in better patient outcomes with decreased morbidity and faster recovery. Besides advances in clinical modalities, efforts are also underway to discover new, better, and more efficient ways to approach surgical education, as well as the assessment of resident surgeons as they progress through their years of training. It seems safe to say that the twenty-first century will see enormous advancements in the field of surgery, including the way it is taught, learned, and practiced.

REFERENCES

Halsted, William S. "The Training of the Surgeon." Yale University, June 27, 1904. https://ia600407.us.archive.org/12/items/b2246413x/b2246413x.pdf

Wallack, Mark W., Chao, Lynn. "Resident Work Hours: The Evolution of a Revolution." *JAMA.* https://jamanetwork.com/journals/jamasurgery/fullarticle/392566

Hobert, Leah, Binello, Emanuela. "Trepanation in Ancient China." *World Neurosurgery.* https://www.sciencedirect.com/science/article/abs/pii/S1878875016310397

"Doctor of Medicine Profession." *Medline Plus,* US National Library of Medicine. https://medlineplus.gov/ency/article/001936.htm

Polavarapu, Harsha V., Hamed, Osama. "100 Years of Surgical Education: The past, present, and future." *Bulletin.* https://bulletin.facs.org/2013/07/100-years-of-surgical-education/

"Dr. William Halstead: The Cokehead Who Fathered Modern Medicine." *History Daily.* https://historydaily.org/cocaine-and-modern-medicine-a-twist-you-didnt-see-coming

Abboud, Carolina. "William Stewart Halsted (1852-1922)." *The Embryo Project.* Arizona State University. https://embryo.asu.edu/pages/william-stewart-halsted-1852-1922

Grant, Scott B., Dixon, Jennifer L., Glass, Nina E., Sakran, Joseph V. "Early surgical sub specialization: A new paradigm? Part 1." *Bulletin.* https://bulletin.facs.org/2013/08/a-new-paradigm/

Valentine, R. James, Jones, Andrew, Biester, Thomas W., Cogbill, Thomas H., Borman, Karen R., Rhodes, Robert S. "General surgery workloads and practice patterns in the United States, 2007 to 2009: a 10-year update from the American Board of Surgery." National Library of Medicine. https://pubmed.ncbi.nlm.nih.gov/21865949/

Goldstein, Allan M., Blair, Alex B., Keswani, Sundeep G., Gosain, Ankush, Morowitz, Michael, Kuo, John, Levine, Matthew, Ahuja, Nita, Hackman, David J. "A Roadmap for Aspiring Surgeon-Scientists in Today's Healthcare Environment." US National Library of Medicine. https://www.ncbi.nlm.nih.gov/pmc/articles/PMC6298819/

Dean, Cornelia. "Joseph E. Murray, Transplant Doctor and Nobel Prize Winner, Dies at 93." Nov. 27, 2012. *The New York Times.* https://www.nytimes.com/2012/11/28/health/dr-joseph-e-murray-transplant-doctor-and-nobel-winner-dies-at-93.html

Lerner, Barron H. "A Life-Changing Case for Doctors in Training." Mar. 3, 2009. *The New York Times.* https://www.nytimes.com/2009/03/03/health/03zion.html

"Results and Data: 2019 Main Residency Match." *The National Resident Matching Program.* https://mk0nrmp3oyqui6wqfm.kinstacdn.com/wp-content/uploads/2019/04/NRMP-Results-and-Data-2019_04112019_final.pdf

"Active Physicians by Sex and Specialty, 2017." *Association of American Medical Colleges.* https://www.aamc.org/data-reports/workforce/interactive-data/active-physicians-sex-and-specialty-2017

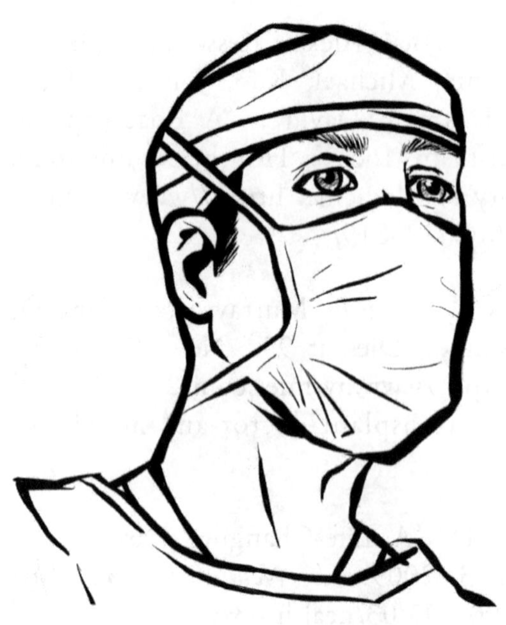

APPENDIX B
HIPPOCRATIC OATH

(1964 Version)

I swear to fulfill, to the best of my ability and judgment, this covenant:

I will respect the hard-won scientific gains of those physicians in whose steps I walk, and gladly share such knowledge as is mine with those who are to follow.

I will apply, for the benefit of the sick, all measures [that] are required, avoiding those twin traps of overtreatment and therapeutic nihilism.

I will remember that there is art to medicine as well as science, and that warmth, sympathy, and understanding may outweigh the surgeon's knife or the chemist's drug.

I will not be ashamed to say, "I know not," nor will I fail to call in my colleagues when the skills of another are needed for a patient's recovery.

I will respect the privacy of my patients, for their problems are not disclosed to me that the world may know. Most especially must I tread with care in matters of life and death. If it is given me to save a life, all thanks. But it may also be within my power to take a life; this awesome responsibility must be faced with great humbleness and awareness of my own frailty. Above all, I must not play at God.

I will remember that I do not treat a fever chart, a cancerous growth, but a sick human being, whose illness may affect the person's family and economic stability. My responsibility includes these related problems if I am to care adequately for the sick.

I will prevent disease whenever I can, for prevention is preferable to cure.

I will protect the environment which sustains us, in the knowledge that the continuing health of ourselves and our societies is dependent on a healthy planet.

I will remember that I remain a member of society, with special obligations to all my fellow human beings, those sound of mind and body as well as the infirm.

If I do not violate this oath, may I enjoy life and art, respected while I live and remembered with affection thereafter. May I always act so as to preserve the finest traditions of my calling and may I long experience the joy of healing those who seek my help.

APPENDIX C
ABOUT THE AUTHOR

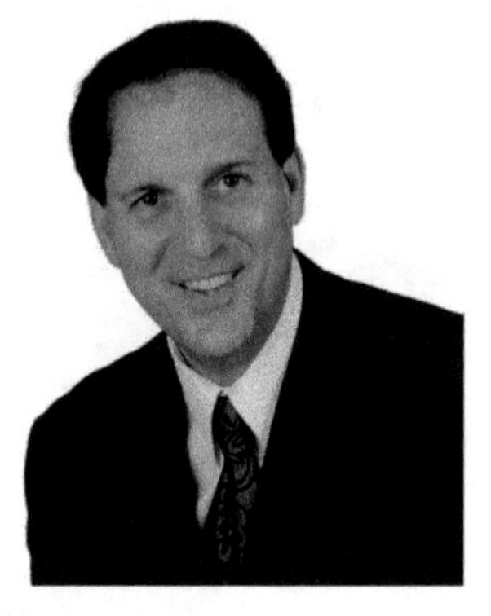

Dr. Joe Garri's long educational path started in Gainesville, Florida. There he attended college and obtained his dental degree at the University of Florida. Upon completion of a general practice residency in dentistry at University Hospital in Jacksonville, Florida, he sought further training and completed a residency in oral and maxillofacial surgery at Harlem Hospital Center in New York City. It was during this residency that Dr. Garri developed an interest in the treatment of children born with cleft lip and palate, and in the care of patients with complex craniofacial issues. To pursue these interests, Dr. Garri decided upon the completion of his oral surgery training, to return to medical school and pursue a career in plastic surgery. He completed medical school at SUNY at Stony Brook, New York, and then a general surgery program at the University of Miami. It was there that he also completed his residency in plastic surgery. Dr. Garri finished his long surgical training at UCLA with a one-year fellowship in craniofacial surgery.

The author of multiple scientific articles and book chapters, Dr. Garri also co-edited a book on craniofacial surgery which was published in 2008. Since the completion of his training, Dr. Garri has remained involved in the education of medical students and young surgeons. He appreciates and enjoys the time he devotes to working with students, surgical residents, and fellows at all levels of training. Dr. Garri lives and practices plastic surgery in Miami Beach, Florida.

Visit his website: www.drgarri.com
www.joegarri.com